"This landmark book establishes positive health science as a new field. The field is concerned with promoting sustainable, positive, healthy lifestyles. This handbook is written by a team of international experts who integrate theory, research, and practices from lifestyle medicine and positive psychology. It will be of interest to students, academics, and practitioners in medicine, nursing, psychology, psychotherapy, coaching, education, and allied healthcare professions."

Alan Carr, *PhD, Professor of Clinical Psychology,*
University College Dublin, IrelandAuthor of "Positive Psychology:
The Science of Wellbeing and Human Strengths."

"This is a truly informative, remarkable book written by experts from throughout the world. It was very heartening to read chapters that reflected and validated my own journey as a clinical psychologist that began with a focus on pathology and "deficits" and moved to a strength-based approach—an approach that highlights each individual's passions, interests, and 'islands of competence,' and prioritizes the nurturing of resilience and healthy lifestyle choices as a major task in our lives.

I was impressed by many, many features of this book, including the clarity with which the concepts of lifestyle medicine, positive psychology, and positive health are described and integrated, the comprehensiveness with which different themes related to these concepts are detailed, and, very importantly, the discussion of a variety of realistic interventions to promote our physical and emotional well-being. There are some books that are written primarily for the professional/scientific community, while others for the lay public. This book will certainly have an enthusiastic audience of professionals from many different disciplines, both clinicians and researchers. Given its subject matter and readability I also believe it will garner a great deal of interest from the lay public. It will become a major resource, to be read and re-read by a diverse audience, all of whom appreciate the importance of understanding and implementing practices related to a positive health model. I recommend this book very highly."

Robert Brooks, *PhD, Faculty, Harvard Medical School (part-time),*
Co-author: The Power of Resilience: Achieving Balance, Confidence,
and Personal Strength in Your Life; Co-author: Reflections on Mortality:
Insights into Meaningful Living

"I love this book so much I want to embrace it and kiss it; I want to send it to everyone I know, as well as everyone I don't know, which means the entire population of our precious planet; I want to shout from the rooftops, 'At last, a book that gets it! Masquerading as a respectable volume of scholarly prose, this book, when unmasked, dances up and down the avenues in delight, its shockingly naked pages thrilling all who read them with an entirely new, breathtakingly spot-on approach to health and life!'

Not only will you love this book and find yourself nodding on every page, you will want your doctor to read it and your best friend; you'll read passages aloud in bed to whomever you sleep with, even your dog; you'll want to jump for joy and share the simultaneously revolutionary and time-honored wisdom displayed, in keeping with good taste, modestly, without the fuss and fanfare it deserves. Instead, the authors let the truth, the unadorned truth, come out of the shadows where Medicine has kept it hidden for centuries, and speak for itself, indeed sing."

Edward Hallowell, *MD, USA, Author of*
"Driven to Distraction" and "ADHD 2.0"

"It is with great enthusiasm that I endorse your newly edited book on Positive Health, which stands as a testament to the collective wisdom and expertise of its distinguished contributors. This remarkable addition to the esteemed 'Routledge International Handbooks' series offers a comprehensive exploration of positive health, empowering readers with invaluable insights and practical guidance to foster well-being and thrive in today's complex world."

Gökmen Arslan, *PhD, Turkey, Associated Professor,*
Mehmet Akif Ersoy University, Burdur, Turkey,
Centre for Wellbeing Science, The University of Melbourne, Australia

"If you are interested in going beyond a reductionist, illness-centered view of health in your personal life, clinical practice, and academic activities, this is the handbook you were waiting for. Combining theoretical and applied knowledge from lifestyle medicine and positive psychology, the panel of eminent authors set the stage for the new science of positive health to the benefit of people and society as a whole."

Prof. Marta Bassi, *PhD, Professor of General Psychology*
at the Medical Faculty, Università degli Studi di Milano, Italy;
Current President of the European Network of Positive Psychology;
Co-author of "Psychological Selection and Optimal Experience
Across Cultures. Social Empowerment through Personal Growth"

"Positive health, thriving in life well beyond the absence of disease. A symbiosis of positive psychology and lifestyle medicine, that offers effective prevention and treatment of chronic disease. This may help to solve many health issues in the world. This book is presented by world experts covering science and theories of positive psychology and lifestyle medicine; applying this evidence to life and clinical practice with wonderful practical how to examples and smart summaries for each section. This is a must read for anyone who wants to be healthy."

Prof. Robert Kelly, *Consultant Cardiology and Lifestyle Medicine,*
University College Dublin Beacon Hospital

"What does it really mean to have health in abundance? And how might we recast our understanding of what health really is? This work answers those questions, among many others and it represents a leap forward in shaping the way we might focus our efforts in healthcare. The international writing team has successfully drawn together systemic principles, a unified concept of mental and physical health, emergent technologies and a deep humanity to uncover what is possible for individual and collective health. Regardless of your role in healthcare, this book will speak to you."

Simon Matthews, *MHlthSc, FASLM, MAPS, DipIBLM, NBC-HWC*
Adjunct Faculty, Avondale University Lifestyle Medicine
and Health Research Centre, Faculty, Wellcoaches School of Coaching,
Producer of Tiny Health Stories: https://www.tinyhealthstories.online

"The field of positive health has been gathering evidence for several decades and is slowly cementing itself in the popular and professional imagination as an essential and effective contribution to global health. This volume, edited and authored by international experts, is a vital, contemporary and comprehensive call to all who wish for and work towards a healthier planet."

Roger Bretherton, *PhD, Associate Professor in Psychology,*
University of Lincoln, United Kingdom

"This text on Positive Health is timely for a topic that is relevant to those interested in and working in the health care sector – those who give of themselves so generously to support other's health and wellbeing. A go-to text for health and wellbeing science students and practitioners who work in this meaningful field."

Suzie Green, *PhD, Honorary Visiting Professor in the School of Psychology,*
University of East London and Founder of The Positivity Institute

"This book is exactly the authentic educational experience that reminds us of the inexplicable foundation of dynamic well-being – positive health."

Joe Raphael, *DrPH, FACLM, MBA, MA, LMFT, CHES,*
HAPM, President, Irvine Christian Counseling and
San Diego Christian Counseling, Board Member,
Global Positive Health Institute

ROUTLEDGE INTERNATIONAL HANDBOOK OF POSITIVE HEALTH SCIENCES

This ground-breaking book combines research and practice in the rapidly growing field of Positive Psychology with the fastest-growing medical speciality of Lifestyle Medicine.

Section 1 maps out the new field of positive health by exploring the scope, content and architecture of this rapidly emerging area of research. It explores research findings and applications derived from Lifestyle Medicine and Positive Psychology that are critical for positive health. Section 2 delves into positive health research, covering topics such as using character strengths to improve health, maximising psychological wellbeing from head to toe, optimising gut health and understanding the relationships between mind and body. Section 3 offers guidance on applying the principles of positive health by describing new Positive Health Interventions (PHIs), introducing innovative positive health coaching models and exploring the contribution of positive psychology to health equity.

The book is ideal for medical doctors, nurses and health professionals interested in helping their patients flourish psychologically and physically. It is an invaluable guide for social workers, positive psychologists, coaches and mental health professionals who want to explore the physiological dimensions of wellbeing.

Jolanta Burke is a Chartered Psychologist and Senior Lecturer (US: Associate Professor) at the Centre for Positive Health, RCSI University of Medicine and Health Sciences, Ireland.

Ilona Boniwell is a Professor of Positive Psychology at the University of East London and the original founder of the UEL's MSc in Applied Positive Psychology.

Beth Frates is a trained physiatrist and a health and wellness coach, with expertise in Lifestyle Medicine and an award-winning teacher at Harvard Medical School.

Liana S. Lianov is President of the Global Positive Health Institute, Assistant Professor, RCSI University of Medicine and Health Sciences, Ireland, and chair of the American College of Lifestyle Medicine Happiness Science and Positive Health Committee.

Ciaran A. O'Boyle is a Professor of Psychology at the RCSI University of Medicine and Health Sciences and the Founding Director of the RCSI Centre for Positive Health Sciences.

THE ROUTLEDGE INTERNATIONAL HANDBOOK SERIES

ROUTLEDGE INTERNATIONAL HANDBOOK OF POSITIVE HEALTH SCIENCES

Positive Psychology and Lifestyle Medicine Research, Theory and Practice

Edited by Jolanta Burke,
Ilona Boniwell, Beth Frates,
Liana S. Lianov and Ciaran A. O'Boyle

Routledge
Taylor & Francis Group

LONDON AND NEW YORK

Cover image: GettyImages/Francesco Vaninetti Photo

First published 2024
by Routledge
4 Park Square, Milton Park, Abingdon, Oxon OX14 4RN

and by Routledge
605 Third Avenue, New York, NY 10158

Routledge is an imprint of the Taylor & Francis Group, an informa business

British Library Cataloguing-in-Publication Data
A catalogue record for this book is available from the British Library

ISBN: 9781032456928 (hbk)
ISBN: 9781032431499 (pbk)
ISBN: 9781003378426 (ebk)

DOI: 10.4324/9781003378426

Typeset in Galliard
by codeMantra

We passionately dedicate this book to the health and wellbeing of our readers, your loved ones and the people you serve. We hope that the knowledge, applications and questions posed will inspire and create ripples of positive influence in our society.

CONTENTS

Contents

FIGURES

TABLES

EDITORS

Dr Jolanta Burke is a Chartered Psychologist and Senior Lecturer (US: Associate Professor) at the RCSI Centre for Positive Health Sciences. She has authored over ten books and researches wellbeing. The Irish Times acknowledged her as one of 30 people who make Ireland a better place. For more info, go to www.jolantaburke.com.

Ilona Boniwell is a Professor of Positive Psychology at the University of East London and the original Founder of the UEL's MSc in Applied Positive Psychology, the first ever degree of this type in Europe. She is one of the world leaders in Positive Psychology, working in the field for over 20 years. Professor Boniwell wrote or edited 12 books, delivered over 200 keynotes and a TEDx, founded the European Network of Positive Psychology, organised the first European Congress of Positive Psychology and was the first Vice-Chair of the International Positive Psychology Association (IPPA). She is also a passionate practitioner of positive psychology. As a CEO of Positran, she consulted the Governments of UAE and Bhutan and many major international companies, including ClubMed, L'Oréal, Unilever, Nestle, EY, Microsoft and BNP Paribas.

Beth Frates, MD, is a trained physiatrist and a health and wellness coach, with expertise in Lifestyle Medicine. Over the years, she has received several teaching accolades from Harvard Extension School and Harvard Medical School. Dr. Frates co-authored The Lifestyle Medicine Handbook: An Introduction to the Power of Healthy Habits, PAVING the Path to Wellness: A Guide to Thriving with a Healthy Body, Peaceful Mind, and Joyful Heart, and The Lifestyle Medicine Pocket Guide.

Liana S. Lianov, MD, MPH, is a leader in lifestyle medicine, having received the 2022 Trailblazer Award from the American College of Lifestyle Medicine. She serves as President and Founder of the Global Positive Health Institute and

Assistant Professor at the Center for Positive Health Sciences, Royal College of Surgeons Ireland.

Dr Ciarán O'Boyle is a Professor of Psychology at the RCSI with over 38 years of experience as an educator, researcher and trainer. He is currently the Director of the RCSI Centre for Positive Health Sciences which he founded in 2019. A psychologist and pharmacologist, he also has postgraduate qualifications in theology and organisational leadership.

CONTRIBUTORS

Qadira M. Ali, MD, MPH, FAAP, DipABLM, Clinical Assistant Professor of Pediatrics, The George Washington School of Medicine and Health Sciences Goldberg Center for Community Pediatric Health, Children's National Hospital Washington, DC, USA.

Gabrielle Bachtel, BA, Lake Erie College of Osteopathic Medicine, Bradenton, FL, USA.

Piotr Bialowolski, PhD, Research Scientist, Human Flourishing Program, Institute for Quantitative Social Science, Harvard University, USA; Associate Professor, Department of Economics, Kozminski University, Poland.

Ilona Boniwell, PhD, Professor of Psychology, School of Psychology, University of East London, London, UK.

David Bowman, M.D., DipABLM, Assistant Professor of Pediatrics; Howard University College of Medicine, Washington, DC (USA); Member, Board of Directors, American College of Lifestyle Medicine (ACLM); Co-Chair, Health Equity Achieved by Lifestyle (HEAL) Initiative, ACLM, USA.

Jolanta Burke, PhD, CPsychol, Senior Lecturer (US: Associate Professor), Centre for Positive Health Sciences, RCSI University of Medicine and Health Sciences, Dublin, Ireland.

Elaine Byrne, PhD, Senior Lecturer (US: Associate Professor), Centre for Positive Health Sciences, RCSI University of Medicine and Health Sciences, Dublin, Ireland.

Tiffani Clingin, BSW, Grad Cert Fam Ther, MAPP, MAASW – Founder, Liberty Health and Happiness, Australia.

Jennifer Donnelly, MSc, PhD Candidate, Centre for Positive Health Sciences, RCSI University of Medicine and Health Sciences, Dublin, Ireland.

Pádraic J. Dunne, PhD, Senior Lecturer (US: Associate Professor), Centre for Positive Health Sciences, RCSI University of Medicine and Health Sciences, Dublin, Ireland.

Beth Frates, MD, President, American College of Lifestyle Medicine; Assistant Clinical Professor, Harvard Medical School, USA.

Anneliese Gill, PhD, Lecturer, Centre for Wellbeing Science, Faculty of Education, University of Melbourne, Melbourne, Australia.

Andrea Giraldez-Hayes, PhD, Senior Lecturer, School of Psychology, University of East London, London, UK.

Dóra Guðrún Guðmundsdóttir, PhD, Director, Public health, Directorate of Health in Iceland, Reykjavík, Director, Graduate Diploma Program on Positive Psychology, University of Iceland, Iceland.

Lucy C. Hone, PhD, Senior Adjunct Fellow at the University of Canterbury, Aotearoa, New Zealand.

Aaron Jarden, PhD, Associate Professor, Centre for Wellbeing Science, Faculty of Education, University of Melbourne, Melbourne, Australia.

Jim Knight, PhD, Senior Partner, Instructional Coaching Group; Centre for Research on Learning, University of Kansas, USA.

Justin Laiti, BSc, PhD Candidate, Centre for Positive Health Sciences, RCSI University of Medicine and Health Sciences, Dublin, Ireland.

Brigitte Lavoie, M.Ps., Psychologist and trainer, Founder of LavoieSolutions, Canada.

Liana S. Lianov, MD, MPH, FACLM, FACPM, DipABLM, President and Founder, Global Positive Health Institute, Sacramento, USA; Assistant Professor, Centre for Positive Health Sciences, RCSI University of Medicine and Health Sciences, Dublin, Ireland.

Croía Loughnane, BA, PGDip, PhD Candidate, Centre for Positive Health Sciences, RCSI University of Medicine and Health Sciences, Dublin, Ireland.

Tadhg Mac Intyre, PhD, Associate Professor, Insight SFI Research Centre for Data Analytics/Department of Psychology, Maynooth University, Ireland; TechPA research Group, Inland Norway University of Applied Sciences: Elverum, Norway.

Charles Martin-Krumm, PhD, IPPA Fellow, Professor of Psychology, VCR, School of Psychologists Practitioners of Paris of the Institut Catholique de Paris, Research Unit "Religion, Culture and Society", France; APEMAC, University of Lorraine Research Unit (UR), France; Armed Forces Biomedical Research Institute (IRBA), Brétigny sur Orge, France.

Trudy Meehan, PhD, DClinPsych, CPsychol, PsSI, Clinical Psychologist Chartered with the Psychological Society of Ireland; a lecturer and researcher at the Centre for Positive Health Sciences, RCSI University of Medicine and Health Sciences, Ireland.

Gia Merlo, MD, MBA, MEd, DipABLM, FACLM, Clinical Professor of Psychiatry, NYU Grossman School of Medicine, New York, USA.

Karen Morgan, PhD, President, RCSI and UCD Malaysia Campus (RUMC), Penang, Malaysia.

Ryan M. Niemiec, PsyD, Chief Science and Education Officer, VIA Institute on Character, USA.

Ciaran A. O'Boyle, PhD, Professor of Psychology, Centre for Positive Health Sciences, RCSI University of Medicine and Health Sciences, Dublin, Ireland.

Róisín O'Donovan, PhD, Postdoctoral Researcher, Centre for Positive Health Sciences, RCSI University of Medicine and Health Sciences, Dublin, Ireland.

Çağla Sanri, MSc, PhD, Lecturer, Centre for Wellbeing Science, Faculty of Education, University of Melbourne, Melbourne, Australia.

Ciara Scott, MDentCh, MSc, PhD Candidate, Centre for Positive Health Sciences, RCSI University of Medicine and Ch Health Sciences, Dublin, Ireland.

Annalisa Setti, PhD, Senior Lecturer, School of Applied Psychology and Environmental Research Institute, University College Cork, Ireland.

Svala Sigurðardóttir, MD, PhD candidate in public Health, Department of health sciences University of Iceland, Iceland and Department of Clinical medicine, Aarhus University, Denmark.

Christian van Nieuwerburgh, PhD, Professor of Coaching and Positive Psychology – Centre for Positive Health Sciences, RCSI University of Medicine and Health Sciences, Dublin, Ireland.

Alyssa M. Vela, PhD, Assistant Professor of Surgery and Psychiatry and Behavioral Sciences, Department of Surgery, Division of Cardiac Surgery, Northwestern University Feinberg School of Medicine, Chicago, IL (USA).

Dianne Vella-Brodrick, PhD – Professor and Gerry Higgins Chair in Positive Psychology, Centre for Wellbeing Science, Faculty of Education, University of Melbourne, Melbourne, Australia.

Dorota Weziak-Bialowolska, PhD, Associate Professor, Centre for Evaluation and Analysis of Public Policies, Faculty of Philosophy, Jagiellonian University, Poland; Faculty Affiliate; Human Flourishing Program, Institute for Quantitative Social Science, Harvard University, USA.

FOREWORD

It is inspiring to review and provide a foreword to this International Handbook. It is a fantastic introduction to Positive Health Sciences. With 20 chapters delivered by 36 authors, representing professional backgrounds as diverse as the geographies they span – Iceland to New Zealand, there is truly something novel and developmental for every reader interested in the future of health sciences.

In a world of 8 billion people – facing the individual health consequences of loneliness and despair, as well as non-communicable diseases, and the threat of whole population health consequences from infectious diseases such as Covid-19 and climate emergencies – a re-imagined approach to health and healthcare is urgently needed.

The chapters in this Handbook bring together the broad areas of thinking and research in Positive Psychology and in Lifestyle Medicine. Many of the concepts discussed have heretofore remained in professional silos, with inadequate opportunities to both engage with and challenge them outside the professional settings within which they have evolved. The chapters thus provide the reader with summaries of areas they already endorse and work within, and also concise introductions to areas that are quite unfamiliar. The chapter on motivation, for instance, gives a condensed tutorial on theoretical developments over three decades in Health Psychology.

The overall sense from the Handbook is one of promise – many differing strands of research and observation support the benefits of a re-directed approach to health – seeing positive health, as the book says, as 'both a destination and a journey', with positive health being 'any movement towards thriving....'. Positive health is thus not a perfection destination but an orientation that supports improved well-being in itself and in the context of the inevitable health challenges we will face in life. The promises evident from research summarised here as aligned with immunology and gut medicine, among other life sciences, signal that there is still much to learn and understand by increased research cooperation across the many boundaries of the sciences informing health and medicine. The chapter on health equity is a timely reminder that the challenges of cross-disciplinary work are not just in aligning positive health sciences with the natural sciences, but also in developing concepts, interventions and policies that enhance fairness and equity.

From my perspective, guiding the aspirations for transformational education of a diverse health sciences faculty in our institutional strategy, the interest in Lifestyle Medicine and Positive Psychology by faculty has been surpassed by the thirst for education and direction in these areas by our medical and other health-care discipline students. Topics that are elective today, yet selected to study by the majority of already busy students, will soon become core in many curricula. This Handbook will accelerate the cross-boundary partnerships that are now needed to advance significant developments such that Positive Health Sciences can become a force for change in how populations can understand and construc-tively engage in advancing their own health and the health of others.

Hannah McGee, PhD, DSc, FEHPS, MRIA
Deputy Vice Chancellor for Academic Affairs,
RCSI University of Medicine and Health Sciences, Dublin,
Ireland. President, European Health Psychology Society, 1998–2000.

PART I

Mapping out the field of Positive Health

Positive Health is an emerging field of science and practice with great potential to save millions of lives yearly, improve people's wellbeing, and reduce their symptoms of illness and disease. To help understand the contribution and potential of Positive Health, in Chapter 1, the book editors, led by Prof. Ciaran O'Boyle from the Centre for Positive Health Sciences, RCSI University of Health Sciences (Ireland), define and conceptualise the new field of Positive Health. This chapter is a "must" read to understand how positive psychology and lifestyle medicine evolve into the science of Positive Health. In Chapter 2, Prof. Gia Merlo from the New York University Grossman School of Medicine (USA) leads a chapter on Lifestyle Medicine breakthroughs and Gabrielle Bachtel from the College of Osteopathic Medicine (USA) present Lifestyle Medicine breakthroughs. In Chapter 3, Prof. Ilona Boniwell from the University of East London (United Kingdom) explores the breakthroughs in Positive Psychology. These chapters will provide us with the necessary foundation to understand how both fields differ and overlap and to what extent they complement each other to improve the health and wellbeing of people worldwide.

1   DOI: 10.4324/9781003378426-1

1

POSITIVE HEALTH

An emerging new construct

*Ciaran A. O'Boyle, Liana Lianov, Jolanta Burke,
Beth Frates and Ilona Boniwell*

How do we define health?

Health, although appearing to be a simple construct, is in fact highly complex, slippery, socially constructed and regularly changing in meaning (Berwick, 2020; Huber et al., 2011; Kelman, 1975; Leonardi, 2018; Turner, 2021; Yull et al., 2010). Many people consider themselves to be healthy if they are not sick and many health professionals still see health and disease as fundamentally binary – a person is either sick or healthy. This conceptualisation of health and disease as opposites reflects, in part, the traditional biomedical model where definitions of health are based on the absence of disease (Thompson et al., 2018). The model is deeply ingrained and, in essence, considers the body as a machine which occasionally malfunctions. The goals of the healthcare system are to fix it, to ensure that the malfunction doesn't get worse or try to maximise the quality of life of the patient who is living with the malfunction (O'Boyle, 2001; Rees et al., 2005; Ring et al., 2005). This approach also reflects Cartesian dualism which conceptually separated mind and body as different entities (Lai & Chang, 2022) and which has had a tenacious hold on models of health and illness.

There is no doubt that the biomedical model has been very successful in relation to communicable diseases and acute conditions and also, to some degree, in relation to some chronic conditions. However, broader conceptualisations of health including the World Health Organization's (WHO) definition of health as "complete physical, mental and social wellbeing and not merely the absence of disease or infirmity", have highlighted the limitations of this traditional biomedical view, and the bio-psycho-social view of health (Engel, 1977, 1980) has increasingly become widely accepted. The WHO definition has itself been criticised on the grounds that: (i) it results in an over-medicalisation of society; (ii) the pattern of diseases has changed from infectious to chronic and many people

DOI: 10.4324/9781003378426-2

cope reasonably well with the challenges of such chronic diseases and (iii) the term "complete" is difficult to define and measure (Huber et al., 2011). Thus, there is a need to develop new models of health and wellbeing.

Positive health

Our interest in this book is in the emerging construct of 'positive health'. This is an approach to health and wellbeing which, while recognising the importance of factors that drive disease and illness, also focuses on the processes that underpin optimal health and well-being (Antonovsky, 1996; Huber et al., 2016, 2022; Labarthe et al., 2016; Lianov, 2019; Ryff & Singer, 1998; Seligman, 2008; Singer & Ryff, 2001). Defining health as the absence of illness or disease does not get to the heart of what it means to be well and thriving (Ickovics & Park, 1998; Ryff & Singer, 1998). Essentially, the positive health model focuses on health as states of well-being rather than states of ill-being and this represents a much broader conceptualisation of health that is relevant for everyone not just those who are ill or suffering from disease or disability (Cloninger et al., 2012; Huber et al., 2011; Ryff & Singer, 1998, 2000; Seligman, 2008). This approach also incorporates a further shift from conceptualisations of mind and body as separate entities to a systems approach that sees these as an integrated "whole" and further considers the setting of this "whole" in the context of the wider social and community environment (Berwick, 2020; Godlee, 2011; Huber et al., 2016).

The development of this approach to positive health is similar to the rationale used by Seligman and Csikszentmihalyi (2000) to articulate the principles of positive psychology. These authors argued that that psychology and psychiatry had done reasonably well to develop an understanding of mental illnesses such as depression, anxiety and substance abuse. But these disciplines had done very poorly in explicating key elements of mental health such as positive emotions, engagement, flow, purpose and meaning, positive relationships and positive accomplishments. In similar vein, Keyes (2007) made the point that eradicating mental illness will not guarantee a mentally healthy population. Proposing that mental health belongs to a separate continuum to mental illness, he argued that the absence of mental health, called languishing, is as bad as major depression. For Keyes, the strategy must be to seek to prevent and treat mental illness AND to promote flourishing in individuals otherwise free of mental illness but not mentally healthy (Keyes, 2007; Ryff & Keyes, 1995). Similarly, modern medicine and healthcare generally have done reasonably well with the treatment of infectious and acute conditions and the management of chronic conditions, but have much less to say about complete physical, mental and social health optimised in terms of flourishing and thriving (Marvasti & Stafford, 2012).

In this chapter, and throughout the book, we describe and draw on a number of emerging approaches that can be incorporated into an overall emerging construction called by us and others 'positive health' where health is seen as the presence of wellbeing and not merely the absence of disease. Currently, our working definition of positive health is as follows:

"Positive health is both a destination and a journey. As a destination it signifies the pinnacle of physical, mental, social, emotional, and meaningful thriving. As a journey, it reflects the fact that any movement towards thriving is a positive health journey."

Drivers for change in formulating health

There are several significant drivers for a broader conceptualisation of health, one that includes its positive dimensions and that focuses to a greater degree than heretofore on lifestyle factors and behaviour. These include:

1 The rapidly increasing incidence and prevalence of non-communicable diseases associated with changes in lifestyle and the ageing of populations, and the ongoing and future challenge that this creates for conventional healthcare systems (Marvasti & Stafford, 2012; WHO, 2018). In this context, the UN sustainable goal (number 3) setting a target of at least a 30% reduction in premature mortality due to non-communicable diseases by 2030 is a challenging one (Roth et al., 2020). However, research shows that 80% of chronic diseases and premature death could be prevented by behavioural changes such as not smoking, being physically active and adhering to a healthy diet (Katz et al., 2018).

2 The global burden of non-communicable diseases will increase as the population ages. According to the World Health Organisation (2023), in 2010 the number of people aged 60 years and older was 1 billion. This number will increase to 1.4 billion by 2030 and 2.1 billion by 2050.

3 The rapidly increasing incidence and prevalence of mental health problems, exacerbated by the COVID pandemic, but already present as an underlying trend, challenges the capacity of conventional approaches to treatment and will require new approaches that can be delivered at scale (WHO, 2021). Among the drivers of "diseases of despair" are substance use disorders, isolation and loneliness.

4 The increasing incidence and prevalence of mental health problems in the young is particularly concerning. Increasing digital use for social connection can lead to inauthentic/poor quality social connections without the benefits of positivity resonance and this can negatively impact mental health (Sohn, 2022; U.S. Surgeon General, 2021).

5 The increasing cost of medical and surgical interventions especially for chronic diseases and the associated rising cost of healthcare (Fazal et al., 2022).

6 The rapidly increasing delineation of new physiological systems and mechanisms such as the microbiome-gut-brain axis, epigenetics, neuroplasticity, metaflammation and psycho-neuro-immunology provide new ways of thinking about mind–body interactions in health and disease and provide new avenues for intervention in both (Davis, 2021).

7 The increasing understanding of the importance of both personal empowerment and systems design. The WHO sees health as influenced by five factors – genetics, social circumstances, environmental exposures, behavioural patterns and healthcare (WHO, 2021). This broader conceptualisation was also reflected in the WHO Ottawa Charter for Health Promotion which made "health for all" its guiding aim and which encouraged "starting from health, to think in systems, to empower people and to address the determinants of health" (WHO, 2012).

8 The burgeoning growth of the "wellness" industry estimated recently as worth $1.5 trillion and growing at 5–10% per year (Callaghan et al., 2021) and the need for an evidence base to protect the public.

9 The intersection of SARS-CoV2 infection and obesity. Current metrics show that people infected with COVID-19 who also have chronic health conditions are at increased risk for severe illness compared with previously healthy individuals. In fact, aside from age, chronic disease was the greatest predictor of poor outcome (Frates & Rifai, 2020; Smirmaul et al., 2020).

10 The emergence of the Wellbeing Economy movement that refers to an economic system that is designed to deliver social justice on a healthy planet. Promoted by the Wellbeing Economy Government Partnerships (Scotland, New Zealand, Iceland, Wales, Finland and Canada), the Wellbeing Economy Alliance, OECD WISE Centre and WHO, it seeks to prioritise wellbeing, health, sustainability and equity over more traditional economic indicators like Gross Domestic Product (GDP). Key scholars within the field already consider the broad scope of health to stretch from intensive care to public wellbeing policies, reflecting the inter-connectedness between health, mental health and wellbeing (Exton, 2023).

All of these factors have become significant drivers for change and have helped stimulate the emergence of positive health sciences.

Disciplinary foundations of positive health

While there are many formulations that are relevant for understanding positive health, our particular interest at this point is in the contributions of disciplines such as positive psychology, health psychology and lifestyle medicine. We are also particularly interested in the ideas and constructs articulated by Aaron Antonovsky in his formulation of salutogenesis (Antonovsky, 1979, 1987, 1996; Mittlemark & Bauer, 2017).

Health psychology is a well-established interdisciplinary field concerned with the application of psychological knowledge, principles and techniques to health, illness and healthcare (Cornish & Gillespie, 2009; Marks et al., 2020; Ogden, 2023). In the present context, the bio-psycho-social model of health (Engel, 1977, 1980), the Whole Person Care model (Thomas et al., 2018) and various theories and models of behavioural change are especially relevant for positive health. The latter include the transtheoretical model (Prochaska et al., 2007), the health belief model (Rosenstock, 1974), the theory of reasoned action and its derivatives (Fishbein & Ajzen, 1975), motivational interviewing (Miller & Rollnick, 2012) and health coaching (Frates et al., 2019, Burke et al., 2023, Van Nieuwerburg & Knight, this volume).

Positive psychology[1] has also added a significant perspective on behavioural change and is highly relevant for the formulation of positive health (Boniwell, 2012; Bonniwell & Tunariu, 2019; Burke et al., 2023). Positive psychology, in its modern formulation, was initiated with the deliberate intention of studying the positive aspects of human experience that are conducive to human flourishing (Seligman & Csikszentmihalyi, 2000). Essentially, positive psychology is the scientific study of human flourishing, and derived from this is an applied approach to optimal functioning (Burke et al., 2023; Ince, 2011). Positive psychology can also be defined as the study of the strengths and virtues that enable individuals, communities and organisations to thrive (Weziak-Bialowolska et al., this volume). Early formulations focused primarily on positive states and experiences of individuals but later formulations integrate negative states and experiences and also focus on systems as well as individuals (Lomas et al., 2020).

Lifestyle medicine is a rapidly developing clinical specialty defined by the American College of Lifestyle Medicine as

> the use of evidence-based lifestyle therapeutic interventions – including a whole food plant-based eating pattern, regular physical activity, restorative sleep, stress management, avoidance of risky substances, and positive social connection – as a primary modality, delivered by clinicians trained and certified in this speciality, to prevent, treat, and often reverse chronic disease.
> *(for good overviews see: Egger et al., 2017; Frates et al., 2019; Kelly & Clayton, 2021; Lianov, 2019; Rippe, 2021)*

The definition of lifestyle medicine places changing people's behaviour at the core of clinical practice and this approach is growing in importance with the increasing prevalence of non-communicable diseases and the associated escalating healthcare costs (Benigas et al., 2022; Bodai et al., 2018). In 2010, a blue ribbon panel lead by one of the authors published a paper describing the competencies necessary for a physician to practice primary care-based lifestyle medicine (Lianov & Johnson, 2010). These consisted of leadership, knowledge, assessment skills, management skills and office and community support. Lifestyle medicine is seen as a distinct field of medicine aimed at "treating the cause" of most modern diseases though lifestyle changes. Lifestyle changes are prescribed as the first line and most important therapy for disease treatment and reversal (Kelly & Clayton, 2021). Other disciplines that have embraced elements of positive health include integrative medicine, behavioural medicine, preventive medicine and public health medicine (Kelly & Clayton, 2021) and there are also some interesting developments in primary care (Huber et al., 2022).

One of the approaches that is increasingly informing thinking and research on positive health (particularly in public health) is that of salutogenesis,[2] an approach first described by the medical anthropologist Aaron Anonovsky (Antonovsky, 1979). Antonovsky's early research focused on the mechanisms of stress and coping in particular diseases. He subsequently became interested in how the experience of stressors, and adaptation to them, could develop an individual's subsequent coping resources. Originally interested in what makes people sick (i.e. the traditional pathogenic approach), he came to see health and illness not as binary phenomena but rather as a continuum ranging from dis-ease to ease (i.e. good health) on which everyone was located. The question for him became what moves people towards the positive end of the dis-ease/ease continuum. The question was not "what makes people sick?" but rather "what makes people healthy?". In order to capture this shift in the paradigm he coined the new term salutogenesis, meaning the origins of health. He urged that "this orientation would prove to be more powerful a guide for research and practice than the pathogenic orientation" (Antonovsky, 1979, 1987, 1996; Mittlemark and Bauer, 2017; Pelikan, 2022). For a thorough, up to date, consideration of the theory and applications of salutogenesis consult the open source "Handbook of Salutogenesis" (Mittelmark et al., 2022).

Salutogenesis refers to the study of the origins of health and assets for health as opposed to the origins of disease and risk factors. A crucial element of the model is the sense of coherence defined as

> … a global orientation that expresses the extent to which one has a pervasive, enduring though dynamic feeling of confidence that one's internal and external environments are predictable and that there is a high probability that things will work out as well as can reasonably be expected.
>
> *(Antonovsky, 1979, 1987)*

One's sense of coherence is a major factor in one's health as it provides one with confidence that stimuli in one's internal and external environment are structured, predictable and explicable, that one has the resources needed to meet the demands one encounters and that these demands are challenges worthy of investment and engagement (Antonovsky, 1987).

There are four main limitations of the current models that inform positive health. First, they are all componential models, and it is widely assumed that higher levels of functioning on all components necessarily result in the highest possible wellbeing. However, the prevalence of flourishing differs significantly across the various models (see Hone et al., 2015 for review), meaning that an optimum level of wellbeing is difficult to define. Moreover, some research suggests that too much of a good thing may cause harm (e.g. Gruber et al., 2011; Nerstad et al., 2019). Therefore, high scores on each one of the components may not necessarily lead to the highest levels of overall wellbeing. Second, Moneta (2013) referred to component models of wellbeing as "bodybuilder" models. In training, bodybuilders prioritise some muscles over others depending on the desired outcome. Applying this principle to health and wellbeing would mean that there are core components and additional optional elements

(Huppert & So, 2013). Currently, most models consider all elements of wellbeing as being of equal importance. However, in reality, some components may be more important than others (Table 1.1).

Table 1.1 Selected conceptualisations of health and wellbeing that are relevant for positive health

Authors	*Key elements relevant for the positive health construct*
Antonovsky (1979, 1987, 1996)	Ease – dis-ease continuum Sense of coherence: Degree to which life is seen as comprehensible, manageable, meaningful
Burke and Dunne (2022)	Positive relationship between the six pillars of lifestyle medicine and psychological flourishing.
Diener et al. (1999)	Subjective Wellbeing: satisfaction with life; high positive affect; low negative affect.
Dodge et al. (2012) Wassell and Dodge (2015)	Wellbeing: Balance point between an individual's resources and challenges, autonomy and intensity, support and demand.
Donaldson et al. (2021)	Developed the PERMA profiler further in the context of work, adding physical health (biological, functional and psychological), growth mindset, prospection, physical environment and economic security (income, medical spending and financial savings)
Foster and Keller (2007) Miller and Foster (2010)	Wellness: Physical, emotional/psychological, social, intellectual, spiritual, occupational, environmental, cultural, economic, climate.
Frates et al. (2019) Lianov (2019) Egger et al. (2017) Rippe (2021)	Lifestyle Medicine: Nutrition; Physical Activity; Sleep; Elimination or Moderation of Risky Substance use; Stress management; Relationships
Gallup Organisation (Rath & Harter, 2010)	Wellbeing: career, social, financial, physical, community wellbeing
Keyes et al. (2002) Ryff and Keyes (1995) Keyes (1998)	Subjective wellbeing: life satisfaction and the balance between positive and negative affect Psychological wellbeing: autonomy, purpose, growth, positive relations, mastery, self-acceptance. Social wellbeing: social contribution, social integrations, social actualisation, social acceptance and social coherence.
Huber et al. (2016) Huber et al. (2022)	Positive Health: bodily functions, mental functions and perception, spiritual/existential, dimension, quality of life, social and societal, participation and daily functioning. Spider diagram representation of positive health
Huppert and So (2013)	Identified core features of flourishing as positive emotions, engagement, interest, meaning, and purpose. Additional features are self-esteem, optimism, resilience, vitality, self-determination and positive relationships.
Labarthe et al. (2016)	Positive cardiovascular health

(Continued)

Table 1.1 (Continued)

Authors	Key elements relevant for the positive health construct
Lianov et al. (2020)	Incorporating positive emotion assessments, positive psychology intervention prescriptions, etc., along with positive psychology for health coaching, into primary and specialty medical care
O'Boyle (1996, 2009) Joyce et al. (1999)	Individual quality of life; Schedule for The Evaluation of Individual Quality of Life
OECD (2023)	Wellbeing Framework: Income and wealth; Work and job quality; Housing, Health, Knowledge and skills, Environment quality, Subjective well-being, Safety, Work–life balance, Social connections, Civil engagement.
OECD (2013)	Subjective Wellbeing: Good mental states, including all of the various evaluations, positive and negative, that people make of their lives and the affective reactions of people to their experiences.
Robinson and Oades (2020)	Mental Fitness at Work: Strength (meaning, purpose, social support, strengths); Flexibility (mindfulness, positive emotions); Endurance (self-efficacy, competence, autonomy, resilience)
Ryan and Deci (2001)	Self-determination theory: meeting key needs of autonomy, competence and relatedness
Ryff and Singer (1998)	Positive Health
Ryff and Singer (1998, 2004); Ryff (2014)	Wellbeing: Eudomonia: autonomy, environmental mastery, personal growth, positive relationships, purpose in life, self-acceptance
Schulte et al. (2015)	Workplace Wellbeing: Subjective well-being, objective wellbeing, composites.
Seligman (2008)	Positive Health
Seligman (2004) Butler and Kern (2016)	Authentic Happiness: PERMA: Positive emotions; Engagement; Relationships; Meaning and purpose; Accomplishment. PERMA-H adds Health
The World Health Organisation (2020)	Health: Complete physical mental and social wellbeing and not merely the absence of disease or infirmity.
The World Health Organisation (2022)	Mental Health: State of wellbeing in which an individual can realise his or her own potential, can cope with the normal stresses of life, can work productively and fruitfully, and can contribute to her or his own community
Vanderweele (2017) Wellbeing Economy Alliance (2023)	Flourishing seen is a state of complete human wellbeing; a broader concept than psychological wellbeing. Elements: close relationships, meaning and purpose, happiness and life satisfaction, physical and mental health, character and virtue; Optional: financial and material stability. Mental Health: People enabled to thrive with their basic human needs (including autonomy and relatedness) met Relationship to nature understood and valued Fundamental needs are met within societ

Third, there is little overall agreement about what precisely constitutes health and wellbeing; hence, the development of a wide variety of models (Ryff et al., 2020; Willen et al., 2022). Furthermore, the emphasis on flourishing *per se* differs across the different models (Hone et al., 2015) and this is a consideration in attempting to formulate a model of positive health. Fourth, none of the models considers the interaction of various components with each other. For example, the PERMA model (Seligman, 2011) does not consider the impact of high levels of one component on others. How are we to interpret an individual scoring high in 'life meaning' but low in 'positive emotions' or vice versa? Could scoring high in one have an impact on the other?

Principles of positive health

The propensity to define health as an absence of illness or disease, while still quite widespread, provides little understanding of what it actually means to be really well, to flourish and to thrive (Huber et al., 2016; Ryff & Singer, 1998). Cloninger et al. (2012) cite extensive epidemiological and clinical evidence that the absence of mental and physical disorders does not assure the presence of indicators of positive health and subjective wellbeing, such as resilience, hardiness, life satisfaction, positive emotional balance or self-realization of one's growth potential. Ickovics and Park (1998) suggested that a paradigm shift from illness to health was necessary, in which thriving represents something more than a return to equilibrium following a challenge. These authors suggested a "value-added" model of health whereby and individual or a community could go beyond survival and recovery from a stressor or illness, to thrive. The rapidly growing body of research relating to post-traumatic growth is just one example of how such a perspective has taken hold over the last thirty or so years (Tedeschi et al., 2018).

In an important early paper setting out the contours of positive health, Ryff and Singer (1998) elucidated three principles underlying their conceptualisation of positive health. First, they considered positive health as being a fundamentally philosophical as opposed to a medical issue and proposed that the philosophical understanding of the goods in life (having a purpose, quality connections with others possessing self-regard and mastery) was the appropriate and necessary starting point. Second, they proposed a comprehensive wholistic approach to positive health which incorporates both physical and mental health and their interconnections. Third, they proposed that positive health be construed as a multidimensional dynamic process rather than a discrete end state. Here, wellbeing was seen as an issue of engagement in living, involving expression of a broad range of human potentialities: intellectual, social, emotional and physical.

In line with the emergence of positive psychology, Seligman (2008) argued for the development of a new construct of positive health as a state that went beyond the mere absence of disease. Positive health is not only desirable in its own right but is also likely to act as a buffer against physical and mental illness.

Huber et al. (2016) proposed the concept of positive health be based on health being defined as the ability to adapt and self-manage in the face of social, physical and emotional challenges. In this model, the six proposed dimensions of positive health are: bodily functions; mental functions and perception; the spiritual/existential dimension; quality of life; social and societal participation; daily functioning. This model has led to the development of a positive health tool that can be used in clinical practice to provide a values-based assessment of patients' health (Bock et al., 2021).

Labarthe et al. (2012, 2016) provide a useful example of a major branch of medicine, cardiology, taking on board some of the ideas associated with positive health. Here, positive cardiovascular health, which aims to improve the cardio-vascular health of all, is seen as a logical outgrowth of preventive cardiology. The American Heart Association adopted the improvement of cardiovascular health of all Americans as one of its strategic impact goals in 2012. The authors see this new focus as a "quiet revolution" in cardiovascular healthcare that has the potential to develop novel approaches at both patients and population levels (see also Boehm et al., 2012).

A working model of positive health

We have set out in Figure 1.1 our current attempt to provide a model of posi-tive health that includes not only considerations of illness and disease, but also attempts to incorporate the positive dimension of wellbeing, represented at its apotheosis as a state of thriving.

We find it useful to think of the continuum in terms of a scale running from –10 at the severe disease end through 0 representing many people's con-ceptualisation of health as "not ill" to +10 representing thriving mentally, physi-cally and socially and in terms of having meaning in one's life.

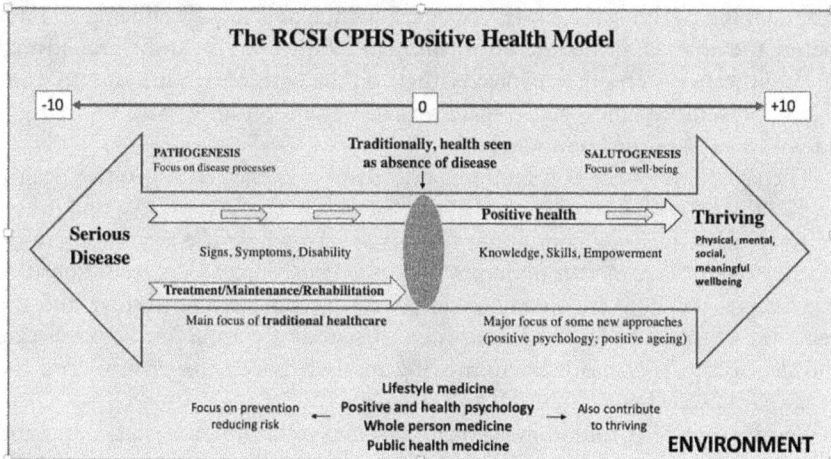

Figure 1.1   A working model of positive health. The model draws on some of the work of: Antonovsky (1979, 1987, 1996); Ryff and Singer (1998); Seligman and Csikszentmihalyi, (2000), Travis and Ryan (2004); WHO (2022).

We conceptualise positive health by representing it as a continuing journey and a direction. We had, at first located it at the end of the continuum on the right but this did not reflect (i) the fact that positive health interventions could also benefit those who are ill and (ii) many people suffering from a disease or disability consider aspects of their overall health to be good. We see positive health in terms of any rightward movement on the continuum from any point. This is similar to Ryff and Singer's (1998) construction of positive health as a multidimensional dynamic process rather than a discrete end state.

We locate the whole continuum, which relates to individual health and disease, in the broader context of the environment which has major implications for both an individual's position on the continuum and their direction of travel along it.

In conceptualising the disease section of the continuum in terms of a 0 to −10 scale, the focus is on the pathological processes that drive disease and illness. Pathogenesis is still the dominant lens in medicine and healthcare generally. The key questions are (i) what are the drivers of illness and disease and (ii) how can we intervene? The goals of healthcare can be seen here as focused on treatment, maintenance and rehabilitation. Most treatment approaches are aimed at: (a) cure: moving the patient to the right from a negative state to the neutral state (from a minus score to 0, or above); (b) maintenance – preventing patients from moving further left on the negative scale; (c) palliative: maximising the quality of life for patients on the negative section of the spectrum.

Prevention, the primary goal of public health and lifestyle medicine, is also largely focused on ensuring that the individual, in particular, does not move from 0 (or from any lower level), in a negative direction (i.e. risk abatement; prevention).

People commonly think of health as the absence of disease or illness, a binary process illustrated here as the ellipse and level 0 on the continuum. The WHO in formulating its constitution was very clear that health meant much more than this, defining health as "complete physical, mental and social wellbeing and not merely the absence of disease or impairment". However, it can be argued that our healthcare systems have evolved largely on the basis of treating and, to some extent, preventing illness and disease with less attention being paid to the right side (0 to +10) of the continuum.

The right side of the continuum is primarily concerned with positive health, i.e. health and wellbeing, over and above the absence of disease. We find it useful to think of this as a continuum from 0 to +10 where the focus is more on the salutogenic factors that underpin thriving. This is more the case for positive psychology which, at least early on, drew a line between the positive and the negative. With salutogenesis health is construed as a continuum between ease and dis-ease, without a distinction being made between the positive and the negative or really between health and disease.

Positive health is multidimensional and involves conceptualising mind and body systems as intimately interlinked in complex multidimensional relationships.

Research aimed at determining the physiological substrates of the positive end of the spectrum is at an early stage of development and the key question is whether such substrates overlap with and/or mirror the pathological processes on the negative end of the spectrum or whether at least some of them might be distinct. Identifying such salutary factors and their biological substrates will be important directions for research. The broaden and build theory in positive psychology may be an example of a distinctly positive neuro-psychological process (Garland et al., 2010).

Positive health interventions are relevant for everyone, both ill and well. The aim is to move people or help them move themselves to the right on the continuum no matter what their starting point (Lianov et al., 2020).

As with positive psychology, the interventions that move someone in a positive direction along the negative side of the spectrum are not necessarily the same interventions that can move someone up the positive side. Positive psychology is more concerned with moving people from 0 to +10 although its interventions are also relevant for those on the negative section of the scale.

A limitation of the model as represented here is that it is possible for someone to be on the negative side of the spectrum in terms of, for example, their physical health but be on the positive side in terms of, for example, their mental or social health and various other combinations are possible. The Huber spider diagram of positive health captures this diversity more effectively (Huber et al., 2022).

It is not only a question of where someone is located on the spectrum but also which direction are they facing and the direction and speed of travel along it.

Physiology of positive health

To date, the focus of much of the research in medicine and the health sciences has understandably been on disease processes. Research on the physiological mechanisms linking mind and body has also focused primarily on the negative consequences of factors such as stress, trauma and ageing. Whereas a large body of research exists detailing the relationship between functioning of the brain and that of systems such as the autonomic, endocrine and immune systems, most of this research has focused on negative outcomes. It is becoming clear that well-being and ill-being may have biological, psychological, social and spiritual causes that are only partially overlapping (Cloninger et al., 2012; Ryff et al., 2006; Seals et al., 2016) and attempting to understand the body during states of wellness rather than under conditions of illness is essentially a paradigm shift in thinking (Ryff et al., 2004). The positive health construct points to the intriguing possibility that the physiological mechanisms underlying thriving may be unique and may not merely mirror those underlying disease and illness (Lee et al., 2019; Lindfors et al., 2005; Ryff et al., 2006; Steptoe, 2019; Steptoe et al., 2015). For example, the impact of wellbeing on secretion patterns of such hormones as cortisol, serotonin and oxytocin is not just the opposite to that of stress and distress (Huppert, 2009).

The emergence of the construct of positive health is occurring at the same time as are exciting discoveries of new biological and psychobiological mechanisms that may help explain the systemic relationships (both positive and negative) between mind, brain and body. In addition to new evidence for the positive impacts on wellbeing of diet, sleep, physical activity, social relationships, stress management and decreased substance use (Frates et al., 2019), we are also starting to understand the complex inter-relatedness of human systems. Relevant research includes inter alia that on the microbiota-gut-brain axis (Cryan et al., 2019; Sherwin et al., 2018), epigenetics (Feinberg, 2008; Hofker et al., 2014), metaflammation (Hotamisligil, 2006; Littrell, 2015), neuroplasticity (Turner, 2022) and psychoneuroimmunology (Kusnecov & Anisman, 2014).

Evidence for the interaction between positive states and physiological function is also to be found in neurobiology. For example, Fredrickson's broaden-and-build theory holds that positive emotions broaden individuals' thought-action repertoires, enabling them to draw flexibly on higher-level connections and wider than usual ranges of percepts, ideas and actions. The resulting broadened cognition in turn creates behavioural flexibility that, over time, builds personal resources, such as mindfulness, resilience, social closeness and even physical health. The theory proposes that the impact of short-term positive emotions on attentional and cognitive processes leads to gradual, long-term growth via changes in brain function that are mediated by neuro-plastic alterations in brain structure (Garland et al., 2010).

At a macro level, evidence exists for a two-way relationship between subjective wellbeing and physical health (Martin-Maria et al., 2017). Poor health usually leads to reduced subjective wellbeing, while high levels of wellbeing can reduce physical health impairments. The likelihood is that wellbeing contributes to the effective functioning of many biological systems. This may help increase resistance to disease and also help promote rapid recovery in the face of illness or adversity (Ryff et al., 2004). Evidence shows that subjective wellbeing is associated with longer survival (Steptoe et al., 2015; Kenny, 2022) and positive states such as optimism have also been shown to be associated with decreased mortality (Lee et al., 2019; Rozanski et al., 2019). The slowing of ageing processes in those who adopt a positive attitude to growing older is thought to be mediated through a number of physiological processes including inflammatory and epigenetic mechanisms (Kenny, 2022; Seals et al., 2016).

Wicked questions

Defining "positive"

The positive health construct is emerging in a manner similar to that which characterised the emergence of positive psychology. In both cases, one of the challenges relates to the definition of "positive" (Worth & Smith, 2018). Human beings by their very nature actively construct their world including their own unique perspectives on such matters as *inter alia* self, others, illness, quality of life, health and wellbeing. Individual factors such as age, gender, personality, experience and culture all have a bearing on such constructions. The phenomenological nature of such perspectives poses a challenge for researchers and health practitioners as to how such unique perspective of the individual can be measured and accommodated. Such challenges are likely to be met, at least in part, through the development of tools that provide the opportunity for the individual to express their own unique perspectives (Bock et al. 2021; Huber et al., 2022; Joyce et al., 1999). In addition to instruments such as these, new models of positive health coaching seek to incorporate the perspectives of individuals and balance these with the complementary inputs of the health professional as expert and partner (Van Nieuwerburgh and Knight, this volume).

Personalising positive health and healthcare

Personalised medicine is a medical model that aims to use molecular profiling, medical imaging and lifestyle data to provide tailor-made prevention and treatment strategies at the right time for defined groups of individuals. The International Consortium for Personalised Medicine predicts that, by 2030, the primary focus of healthcare will have shifted from treatment to risk definition, patient stratification and personalised health promotion and disease prevention strategies of particular value for ageing societies (Vicente et al., 2020). The broader construct of positive health raises many questions about the targets of personalised medicine and healthcare, the interactions between psychological, physical and environmental systems and the extent to which a personalised approach can be applied not only to treat and prevent disease and illness but also to optimise wellbeing.

The person and the system

While the construct of positive health places significant emphasis on the importance of empowering individuals to enhance their own health and wellbeing, there are many factors that influence health that are beyond the individual's control. According to the WHO, the factors that influence health are genetics, social circumstances, environmental exposures, behavioural patterns and healthcare (WHO, 2021). In most countries, main marker of success is GDP and the main goal of economic policy is to drive growth, no matter what the cost. The construct of positive health, incorporating as it does the concept of thriving, raises the question as to whether the major focus of government policies should be the creation of a happy, thriving population in which all individuals can optimise their potential and live a life suffused with meaning. In this, it seems to align with the wellbeing economy that looks at the societal and systemic level, focusing on creating economic systems and policies that promote the wellbeing of all citizens and the planet, providing a framework for policymakers, organizations and institutions to guide economic decision-making and proposing concrete solutions, such as well-being budgeting and judging policies by their cost-effectiveness in terms of WELLBYs, or wellbeing years (Layard & De Neve, 2023). In her book, *Doughout Economics: 7 Ways to Think Like a 21st Century Economist*, the English economist Kate Raworth poses the question of how such a change in focus can be achieved in the context of the numerous challenges humanity will have to face in the coming decades: climate change, resources depletion, increasing inequalities, environmental pollution and biodiversity loss (Raworth, 2017). The emerging construct of positive health can help inform this debate.

Takeaways

- Positive health is an emerging construct which, while not ignoring the factors underlying disease, ageing and illness, focuses on the factors that underpin wellbeing across the lifespan.
- Positive health is relevant for everyone: those who have an illness, disease or disability and those who do not.
- Improving health requires a systems approach that focuses on individual, collective and environmental factors.
- Minds, brains and bodies are closely intertwined and are mutually interdependent. The physiological bases of thriving may be unique and may not simply mirror pathological processes.

Notes

1 Authentic Happiness, University of Pennsylvania: www.authentichappiness.org; Center for Positive Organizations, Ross School of Business, University of Michigan: https://positiveorgs.bus.umich.edu/; Centre for Wellbeing Science, University of Melbourne: https://education.unimelb.edu.au/cpp; Greater Good Science Center, University of Berkeley: http://greatergood.berkeley.edu; International Positive Psychology Association (IPPA): http://www.ippanetwork.org; VIA Institute of Character Strengths: www.viacharacter.org
2 Global Working Group on Salutogenesis (IUPHE): https://www.iuhpe.org/index. php/en/global-working-groups-gwgs/gwg-on-salutogenesis; Society for Theory and Research on Salutogenesis (STARS): https://www.stars-society.org/; The Handbook of Salutogenesis (2022). https://link.springer.com/book/10.1007/978-3-030-79515-3; University of Zurich. Center of Salutogenesis https://www.ebpi.uzh.ch/en/aboutus/departments/publichealth/poh/salutogenesis.html

References

Antonovsky, A. (1979). *Health, stress and coping.* Jossey-Bass.

Antonovsky, A. (1987). *Unravelling the mystery of health - How people manage stress and stay well.* Jossey-Bass.

Antonovsky, A. (1996). The salutogenic model as a theory to guide health promotion. *Health Promotion International, 11,* 11–18.

Benigas, S., Shurney, D., & Stout, R. (2022). Making the case for lifestyle medicine. *The Journal of Family Practice, 71*(Suppl. 1 Lifestyle), S2–S4. https://doi.org/10.12788/jfp.0296

Berwick, D.M. (2020). The moral determinants of health. *JAMA, 324*(3), 225–226.

Bock, L.A., Noben, C.Y.G., Yaron, G., George, E.L.J., Masclee, A.A.M., Essers, B.A.B., & Van Mook, W.N.K.A. (2021). Positive health dialogue tool and value-based healthcare: A qualitative exploratory study during residents' outpatient consultations. *BMJ Open, 11,* e052688. https://doi.org/10.1136/bmjopen-2021-052688

Bodai, B.I., Nakata, T.E., Wong, W.T., Clark, D.R., Lawenda, S., & Tsou, C. et al. (2018). Lifestyle medicine: A brief review of its dramatic impact on health and survival. *Permante Journal, 22,* 17–25.

Boehm, J.K. & Kubzansky, L.D. (2012). The heart's content: The association between positive psychological well-being and cardiovascular health. *Psychological Bulletin, 138,* 655–691.

Boehm, J.K., Vie, L.L., & Kubzansky, L.D. (2012). The promise of well-being interventions for improving health risk behaviors. *Current Cardiovascular Risk Reports, 6,* 511–519.

Boniwell, I. (2012). *Positive psychology in a nutshell.* Open University Press.

Bonniwell, I., & Tunariu, A.D. (2019). *Positive psychology: Theory, research and applications* (2nd ed.). Open University Press.

Burke, J., & Dunne, P.J. (2022). Lifestyle medicine pillars as predictors of psychological flourishing. *Frontiers in Psychology,* 13, https://doi.org/10.3389/fpsyg.2022.963806

Burke, J., Dunne, P.J., Meehan, T., O'Boyle, C.A., & Van Nieuwerburgh, C. (2023). *Positive health: 100+ research-based positive psychology and lifestyle medicine tools to enhance your wellbeing.* Routledge.

Butler, J., & Kern, M.L. (2016). The PERMA-Profiler: A brief multidimensional measure of flourishing. *International Journal of Wellbeing, 6*(3), 1–48.

Callaghan, S., Losch, M., Pione, A., & Teichner, W. (2021). *Feeling good: The future of the $1.5 trillion wellness market.* McKinsey Institute.

Cloninger, C.R., Salloum, I.M., & Mezzich, J.E. (2012). The dynamic origins of health and wellbeing. *International Journal Person Centred Medicine, 2*(2), 179–187. https://doi.org/10.5750/ijpcm.v2i2.213

Cornish, F., & Gillespie, A. (2009). A pragmatist approach to the problem of knowledge in health psychology. *Journal of Health Psychology, 14*(6), 800–809. ISSN 1359-1053. https://doi.org/10.1177/1359105309338974

Cryan, J.F., O'Riordan, K.J., Cowan, C.S.M., Sandhu, K.V., Bastiaanssen, T.F.S., Boehme, M., Codagnone, M.G., Cussotto, & Dinan, T.G. et al. (2019). The microbiota-gut-brain axis. *Physiological Review, 99*(4)1877–2013. https://doi.org/10.1152/physrev.00018.2018. PMID: 31460832.

Davis, D.M. (2021). *The secret body: How the new science of the human body is changing the way we live.* Vintage.

Diener, E., Suh, E.M., Lucas, R.E., & Smith, H.L. (1999). Subjective wellbeing: Three decades of progress. *Psychological Bulletin, 125,* 276–302.

Dodge, R., Daly, A., Huyton, J., & Sanders, L. (2012). The challenge of defining wellbeing. International Journal of Wellbeing, 2(3), 222–235.

Donaldson, S.I., van Zyl, L.E., & Donaldson, S.I. (2022). PERMA+4: A framework for work-related wellbeing, *Frontiers in Psychology,* 12. https://doi.org/10.3389/fpsyg.2021.817244. https://www.frontiersin.org/articles/10.3389/fpsyg.2021.817244.

Egger, G., Binns, A., Rössner, S., & Sagner, M. (2017). *Lifestyle medicine: Lifestyle, the environment, and preventive medicine in health and disease* (3rd ed.). Academic Press.

Engel, G.L. (1977). The need for a new medical model: A challenge for biomedicine. *Science, 196,* 129–135.

Engel, G.L. (1980). The clinical application of the biopsychosocial model, American. *Journal of Psychiatry, 137,* 535–544.

Exton, C. (2023). *Putting well-being metrics into policy action. Where do we stand?* Presented at the Wellbeing Economy Forum, Reykjavik, Iceland. June 14–15

Fazal, F., Saleem, T., Ur Rehman, M.E., Haider, T., Khalid, A.R., Tanveer, U., Mustafa, H., Tanveer, J., & Noor, A. (2022). The rising cost of healthcare and its contribution to the worsening disease burden in developing countries. *Annals of Medicine and Surgery, 82,* 104683. https://doi.org/10.1016/j.amsu.2022.104683

Feinberg, A.P. (2008). Epigenetics at the epicenter of modern medicine. *JAMA, 299*(11):1345–1350. https://doi.org/10.1001/jama.299.11.1345

Fishbein, M., & Ajzen, I. (1975). *Belief, attitude, intention and behaviour: An introduction to theory and research.* Addison-Wesley.

Foster, L.T., & Keller, C.P. (2007). Defining wellness and its determinants. In L.T. Foster & C.P. Keller (Eds.), The British Columbia atlas of wellness (pp. 9–19). Western Geographical Press.

Frates, B., Bonnet, J.P., Joseph, R., & Peterson, J.A. (2019). *The lifestyle medicine handbook: An introduction to the power of healthy habits.* Healthy Learning.

Frates, E.P., & Rifai, T. (2020). Making the case for "COVID-19 Prophylaxis" with lifestyle medicine. *American Journal of Health Promotion: AJHP, 34*(6), 689–691. https://doi.org/10.1177/0890117120930536c

Garland, E.L., Fredrickson, B., Kring, A.M., Johnson, D.P., Meyer, P.S., & Penn, D.L. (2010). Upward spirals of positive emotions counter downward spirals of negativity: Insights from the broaden-and-build theory and affective neuroscience on the treatment of emotion dysfunctions and deficits in psychopathology. *Clinical Psychology Review, 30*(7), 849–864.

Godlee, F. (2011). What is health? *British Medical Journal, 343,* d4817.

Gruber, J., Mauss, I.B., & Tamir, M. (2011). A dark side of happiness? How, when, and why happiness is not always good. *Perspectives on Psychological Science: A Journal of the Association for Psychological Science, 6*(3), 222–233. https://doi.org/10.1177/1745691611406927

Hofker, M.H., Fu, J., & Wijmenga, C. (2014). The genome revolution and its role in understanding complex diseases. *Biochimica et Biophysica Acta, 1842,* 1889–1895.

Hone, L.C., Jarden, A., Duncan, S., & Schofield, G.M. (2015). Flourishing in New Zealand workers: Associations with lifestyle behaviors, physical health, psychosocial, and work-related indicators. *Journal of Occupational and Environmental Medicine, 57*(9), 973–983. https://www.jstor.org/stable/48500540

Hotamisligil, G. (2006). Inflammation and metabolic disorders. *Nature, 444,* 860–867 https://doi.org/10.1038/nature05485

Huber, M., Jung, H.P., & van den Brekel-Dijkstra, K. (2022). *Handbook of positive health in primary care: The Dutch example.* Houten.

Huber, M., Knottnerus, J.A., Green, L., van der Horst, H., Jadad, A.R., & Kromhout, D. et al. (2011). How should we define health? *BMJ, 343,* d4163.

Huber, M., van Vliet, M., Giezenberg, Winkens, B., Heerkens, Y., Dagnelie, P.C., & Knottnerus, K.A. (2016). Towards a 'patient-centred' operationalisation of the new dynamic concept of health: A mixed methods study. *BMJ Open,* e010091. https://doi.org/10.1136/bmjopen-2015-010091

Huppert, F.A. (2009), Psychological well-being: Evidence regarding its causes and consequences. *Applied Psychology: Health and Well-Being, 1,* 137–164. https://doi-org.proxy.library.rcsi.ie/10.1111/j.1758-0854.2009.01008.x

Huppert, F.A., & So, T.T. (2013). Flourishing across Europe: Application of a new conceptual framework for defining well-being. *Social Indicators Research, 110,* 837–861.

Ickovics, J.R., & Park, C.L. (1998). Paradigm shift: Why a focus on health is important. *Journal of Social Issues, 54*(2), 237–244.

Ince, S. (2011). *Positive psychology: Harnessing the power of happiness, mindfulness, and personal growth.* Harvard Medical School Special Health Report, Harvard, MA.

Joseph, S., & Sagy, S. (2022). Positive psychology and its relation to salutogenesis. In M.B. Mittelmark et al. (eds.), *The Handbook of Salutogenesis,* https://doi.org/10.1007/978-3-030-79515-3_23

Joyce, C.R.B., O'Boyle, C.A., & McGee (1999). *Individual quality of life. Approaches to conceptualisation and measurement in health.* Routledge.

Katz, D.L., Frates, E.P., Bonnet, J.P., Gupta, S.K., Vartiainen, E., & Carmona, R.H. (2018). Lifestyle as medicine: The case for a true health initiative. *American Journal of Health Promotion: AJHP, 32*(6), 1452–1458. https://doi.org/10.1177/0890117117705949

Kelly, J., & Clayton, J.S. (2021). *Foundation of lifestyle medicine board review manual.* American College of Lifestyle Medicine.

Kelman, S. (1975). The social nature of the definition problem in health. *International Journal of Health Services, 5*(4), 625–642. https://doi.org/10.2190/X5H6-TC5W-D36T-K7KY

Kenny, R.A. (2022). *Age proof: The new science of living a longer and healthier life.* Lagom.

Keyes, C.L.M. (1998). Social well-being. *Social Psychology Quarterly, 61,* 121–140.

Keyes, C.L.M. (2007). Promoting and protecting mental health as flourishing. *American Psychologist, 62*(2), 95–108.

Keyes, C.L., Shmotkin, D., & Ryff, C.D. (2002). Optimizing well-being: The empirical encounter of two traditions. *Journal of Personality and Social Psychology, 82*(6), 1007–1022.

Kusnecov, A.W., & Anisman, H. (2014). *The Wiley-Blackwell handbook of psychoneuroimmunology.* John Wiley.

Labarthe, D.R. (2012). From cardiovascular disease to cardiovascular health: A quiet revolution?. *Circulation: Cardiovascular Quality and Outcomes, 5*(6), e86–e92. https://doi.org/10.1161/CIRCOUTCOMES.111.964726

Labarthe, D.R., Kubzansky, L.D., Boehm, J.K., Lloyd-Jones, D.M., Berry, J.D., & Seligman, M.E. (2016). Positive cardiovascular health: A timely convergence. *Journal of the American College of Cardiology, 68*(8), 860–867. https://doi.org/10.1016/j.jacc.2016.03.608

Lai, A.G., & Chang, W.H. (2022). There is no health without mental health: Challenges ignored and lessons learned. *Clinical and Translational Medicine, 12*(6), e897. https://doi.org/10.1002/ctm2.897

Layard, R., & De Neve, J.E. (2023). *Wellbeing: Science and policy.* Cambridge University Press.

Lee, L.O., James, P., Zevon, E.S., Kim, E.S., Trudel-Fitzgerald, C., Spiro, A., 3rd, Grodstein, F., & Kubzansky, L.D. (2019). Optimism is associated with exceptional longevity in 2 epidemiologic cohorts of men and women. *Proceedings of the National Academy of Sciences of the United States of America, 116*(37), 18357–18362. https://doi.org/10.1073/pnas.1900712116

Leonardi, F. (2018). The definition of health: Towards new perspectives. *International Journal of Health Services. 48*(4), 735–748. https://doi.org/10.1177/0020731418782653

Lianov, L.S. (2019). *Roots of positive change: Optimizing health care with positive psychology. chesterfield.* American College of Lifestyle Medicine.

Lianov, L.S., Barron, G.C., Fredrickson, B., Hashmi, S., Klemes, A., Krishnaswami, J., & Lee, J. et al. (2020). Positive psychology in health care: Defining key stakeholders and their roles. *TBM, 10,* 637–647. https://doi.org/10.1093/tbm/ibz150

Lianov, L.S., & Johnson, M. (2010). Physician competencies for prescribing lifestyle medicine. *JAMA, 304*(2), 202–203.

Lindfors, P., Lundberg, O., & Lundberg, U. (2005). Sense of coherence and biomarkers of health in 43 year old women. *International Journal of Behavioural Medicine, 12*(2), 98–102.

Littrell, J. (2015). *Neuroscience for psychologists and other mental health professionals: Promoting wellbeing and treating mental illness.* Springer.

Lomas, T., Waters, L., Williams, P., Oades, L., & Kern, M. (2020). Third wave positive psychology: Broadening towards complexity. *Journal of Positive Psychology, 16,* 10.1080/17439760.2020.1805501.

Marks, D.F., Murray, M., & Estacio, E.V. (2020). *Health psychology: Theory, research and practice.* Sage.

Martin-Maria, N., Miret, M., & Caballero, F. et al. (2017). The impact of subjective well-being on mortality: A meta-analysis of longitudinal studies in the general population. *Psychosomatic Medicine, 79,* 565–575.

Marvasti, F.F., & Stafford, R.S. (2012). From sick care to health care — reengineering prevention into the U.S. System. *New England Journal of Medicine, 367*(10), 889–891.

Miller, G., & Foster, L. (2010). *Critical synthesis of wellness literature.* University of Victoria, Faculty of Human and Social Development & Department of Geography.

Available at www.geog.uvic.ca/wellness/Critical_Synthesis%20of%20Wellness%20 Update (accessed January 2018).

Miller, W.R., & Rollnick, S. (2012). *Motivational interviewing: Helping people change* (3rd ed.). The Guilford Press.

Mittlemark, M.B., & Bauer, G.F. (2017). The meanings of salutogenesis. In: M.B. Mittelmark, S. Sagy, M. Eriksson, G.F. Bauer, J.M. Pelikan, B. Lindström, & G.A. Espnes (Eds.), *The Handbook of Salutogenesis.* Springer. https://link.springer.com/book/10.1007/978-3-319-04600-6

Mittelmark, M.B., Bauer, G.F., Vaandrager, L., Pelikan, J.M., Sagy, S., Eriksson, M., Lindström, B., & Meier Magistretti, C. (2022). The Handbook of Salutogenesis (2nd ed.). Springer International Publishing. https://doi.org/10.1007/978-3-030-79515-3

Moneta, G. (2013). *Positive psychology: A critical introduction.* Bloomsbury Publishing.

Nerstad, C.G.L., Wong, S.I., & Richardsen, A.M. (2019). Can engagement go awry and lead to burnout? The moderating role of the perceived motivational climate. *International Journal Environmental Research and Public Health, 16*(11):1979. https://doi.org/10.3390/ijerph16111979

O'Boyle, C.A. (1996). Quality of life in health care. In G. Albrecht & R. Fitzpatrick (Eds.), *Advances in medical sociology* (vol. 5, pp. 159–180). JAI Press.

O'Boyle, C.A. (2009). Quality of life. In: M. Watson, C. Lucas, A. Hoy, & J. Wells (Eds.), *Oxford handbook of palliative care* (2nd ed., pp. 51–59). Oxford University Press.

Ogden, J. (2023). *Health psychology* (7th ed.). McGraw-Hill.

Organisation for Economic Co-operation and Development (OECD) (2023). *Measuring well-being and progress: Well-being research.* Available at https://www.oecd.org/wise/measuring-well-being-and-progress.htm (Accessed January 2023).

Organisation for Economic Co-operation and Development (OECD) (2013). *OECD guidelines on measuring subjective well-being,* OECD Publishing. http://dx.doi.org/10.1787/9789264191655-en

Prochaska, J.O., Norcross, J.C., & DiClemente, C.C. (2007). *Changing for good.* William Morrow.

Rath, T., & Harter, J. (2010). *Wellbeing: The five essential elements.* Gallup Press.

Raworth, K. (2017). *Doughnut economics: 7 ways to think like a 21st century economist.* Chelsea Green Publishing.

Rees, J., Clarke, M.G., Waldron, D., O'Boyle, C., Ewings, P., & MacDonagh, R. (2005). The measurement of response shift in patients with advanced prostate cancer and their partners. *Health and Quality of Life Outcomes, 3*(1), 21–33.

Ring, L., Hoefer, S., Heuston, F., Harris, D., & O'Boyle, C.A. (2005). Response shift masks the treatment impact on patient reported outcomes (PROs): The example of individual quality of life in edentulous patients. *Health & Quality of Life Outcomes 3,* 55: 3:1.

Rippe, J.M. (2021). *Manual of lifestyle medicine.* CRC Press.

Robinson, P., & Oades, L.G. (2020). Mental fitness at work. In L.G. Oades, M.F. Steger, A. Delle Fave, & J. Passmore (Eds.), *The Wiley-Blackwell handbook of the psychology of positivity and strengths-based approaches at work* (pp. 150–170). Wiley.

Rosenstock, I. (1974). Historical origins of the health belief model. *Health Education Monographs, 2*(4), 328–335.

Roth, G.A., Mensah, G.A., Johnson, C.O., Addolorato, G., Ammirati, E., Baddour, L.M., Barengo, N.C., Beaton, A.Z., Benjamin, E.J., Benziger, C.P., Bonny, A., Brauer, M., Brodmann, M., Cahill, T.J., Carapetis, J., Catapano, A.L., Chugh, S.S., Cooper, L.T., Coresh, J., Criqui, M., ... & GBD-NHLBI-JACC Global Burden of Cardiovascular Diseases Writing Group (2020). Global burden of cardiovascular diseases and risk factors, 1990–2019: Update from the GBD 2019 study. *Journal of the American College of Cardiology, 76*(25), 2982–3021. https://doi.org/10.1016/j.jacc.2020.11.010

Rozanski, A., Bavishi, C., Kubansky, L.D., & Cohen, R. (2019). Association of optimism with cardiovascular events and all-cause mortality: A systematic review and meta-analysis. *JAMA Network Open*, 2(9): e1912200. https://doi.org/10.1001/jamanetworkopen.2019.12200

Ryan, R.M., & Deci, E.L. (2001). On happiness and human potentials: A review of research on hedonic and eudaimonic well-being. *Annual Review of Psychology*, 52(1), 141–166.

Ryff, C.D. (2014). Psychological well-being revisited: Advances in the science and practice of eudaimonia. Psychotherapy and Psychosomatics, 83(1), 10–28.

Ryff, C.D., Dienberg Love, G., Urry, H.L., Muller, D., Rosenkranz, M.A., Friedman, E.M., Davidson, R.J., & Singer, B. (2006). Psychological well-being and ill-being: Do they have distinct or mirrored biological correlates? *Psychotherapy and Psychosomatics*, 75(2), 85–95. [PubMed: 16508343]

Ryff, C.D., & Keyes, C.L.M. (1995). The structure of psychological well-being revisited. Journal of Personality and Social Psychology, 69(4), 719–727. https://doi.org/10.1037/0022-3514.69.4.719

Ryff, C.D., Boylan, J.M., Kirsch, J.A. (2020). Disagreement about recommendations for measurement of well-being. *Preventive Medicine, 139, 106049.* https://doi.org/10.1016/j.ypmed.2020.106049

Ryff, C.D., & Singer, B. (1998). The contours of positive human health. *Psychological Inquiry, 9*(1), 1–28.

Ryff, C.D., & Singer, B. (2000). Interpersonal flourishing: A positive health agenda for the new millennium. *Personality & Social Psychology, 4*(1), 30–44.

Ryff, C.D., Singer, B.H., & Dienberg Love, G. (2004). Positive health: Connecting well-being with biology. *Philosophical Transactions of the Royal Society of London. Series B, Biological Sciences, 359*(1449), 1383–1394. https://doi.org/10.1098/rstb.2004.1521

Schulte, P.A., Guerin, R.J., Schill, A.L., Bhattacharya, A., Cunningham, T.R., Pandalai, S.P., Eggerth, D., & Stephenson, C.M. (2015). Considerations for incorporating "Well-Being" in public policy for workers and workplaces. American Journal of Public Health, 105(8), e31–e44.

Seals, D.R., Justice, J.N., & LaRocca, T.J. (2016). Physiological geroscience: Targeting function to increase healthspan and achieve optimal longevity. *The Journal of Physiology, 594*(8), 2001–2024. https://doi.org/10.1113/jphysiol.2014.282665

Seligman, M.E.P. (2004). *Authentic happiness: Using the new positive psychology to realize your potential for lasting fulfillment.* Free Press.

Seligman, M.E.P. (2008). Positive health. *Applied Psychology: An International Review, 57*, 3–18; 10.1111/j.1464-0597.2008.00351.x

Seligman, M.E.P. (2011). Flourish: A visionary new understanding of happiness and well-being. Free Press.

Seligman, M.E.P., & Csikszentmihalyi, M. (2000). Positive psychology: An introduction. *American Psychologist, 55*(1) 5–14

Sherwin, E., Dinan, T.G., & Cryan, J.F. (2018). Recent developments in understanding the role of the gut microbiota in brain health and disease. *Annals of the New York Academic Science, 1420*, 5–25.

Singer, B.H., & Ryff, C.D. (2001). *New horizons in health: An integrative approach.* National Research Council (US) Committee on Future Directions for Behavioural and Social Sciences Research at the National Institutes of Health. Washington (DC): National Academies Press (US). PMID: 20669490.

Smirmaul, B.P.C., Chamon, R.M., de Moraes, F.M., Rozin, G., Moreira, M.A.S.B., de Almeida, R.G., & Guimarães, S.T. (2020). Lifestyle medicine during (and after) the COVID-19 pandemic. *American Journal of Lifestyle Medicine.* https://doi.org/10.1177/1559827620950276

Sohn, E. (2022). Depression in the young. *Nature, 608*, S39–S41.

Steptoe, A. (2019). Happiness and health. Steptoe A. Happiness and health. *Annual Review of Public Health, 40*, 339–359. https://doi.org/10.1146/annurev-publ-health-040218-044150. Epub 2019 Jan 2.PMID: 30601719.

Steptoe, A., Deaton, A., & Stone, A.A. (2015). Subjective wellbeing, health and ageing. *Lancet, 85*, 640–648

Tedeschi, R.G., Shakespeare-Finch, J., Taku, K., & Calhoun, L.G. (2018). *Post traumatic growth: Theory, research and applications.* Taylor and Francis Ltd.

Thomas, H., Mitchell, G., Rich, J., & Best, M. (2018). Definition of whole person care in general practice in the English language literature: A systematic review. *BMJ Open 8*, e023758. 10.1136/bmjopen-2018-023758

Thompson, S. (2018). Positive psychology, mental health and the false promise of the medical model. In: N.J.L. Brown, T. Lomas, & F.T. Eiroa-Orosa (Eds.), *The routledge international handbook of critical positive psychology* (pp. 70–83). Routledge.

Travis, J.W., & Ryan, R.S. (2004). *The wellness workbook, 3rd ed: How to achieve enduring health and vitality.* Celestial Arts.

Turner, B.S. (2021). The history of the changing concepts of health and illness: Outline of a general model of illness categories. In: S.C. Scrimshaw, S.D. Lane, R.A. Rubinstein, & J. Fisher (Eds.), *The sage handbook of social studies in health and medicine*, (pp. 81–102). Sage.

Turner, R. (2022). *Cognitive and brain plasticity: Current research.* Murphy and Moore.

U.S. Surgeon General, (2021). *Youth mental health. U.S. surgeon general advisory*, https://www.hhs.gov/surgeongeneral/priorities/youth-mental-health/index.html

VanderWeele, T.J. (2017). On the promotion of human flourishing. *Proceedings of the National Academy of Sciences, 114*(31), 8148–8156.

van Dierendonck, D., & Lam, H. (2022). Interventions to enhance eudaemonic psychological well-being: A meta-analytic review with Ryff's Scales of Psychological Well-being. *Applied Psychology: Health and Well-Being*, 1–17. https://doi-org.proxy.library.rcsi.ie/10.1111/aphw.12398

Van Nieuwerburg, C., & Knight, J. (this volume).

Vicente, A.M., Ballensiefen, W., & Jönsson, J.I. (2020). How personalised medicine will transform healthcare by 2030: The ICPerMed vision. *Journal of Translational Medicine, 18*(1), 180. https://doi.org/10.1186/s12967-020-02316-w

Wassell, E.D., & Dodge, R. (2015). A multidisciplinary framework for measuring and improving wellbeing. *International Journal of Sciences: Basic and Applied Research (IJSBAR), 21*(2), 97–107. Retrieved from https://www.gssrr.org/index.php/JournalOfBasicAndApplied/article/view/3760

Wellbeing Economy Alliance. (2023). *What is well-being economy?* Retrieved from https://weall.org/what-is-wellbeing-economy

Willen, S.S., Williamson, A.F., Walsh, C.C., Hyman, M., & Tootle, W. (2022). Rethinking flourishing: Critical insights and qualitative perspectives from the U.S. Midwest. *SSM - Mental Health, 2*, https://doi.org/10.1016/j.ssmmh.2021.100057

World Health Organisation (2012). *The Ottawa charter for health promotion.* https://www.who.int/publications/i/item/ottawa-charter-for-health-promotion

World Health Organisation (2018). *Noncommunicable Diseases.* https://www.who.int/news-room/fact- sheets/detail/noncommunicable-diseases

World Health Organisation (2021). *Social determinants of health.* https://www.who.int/health-topics/social-determinants-of-health#tab=tab_1)

World Health Organisation (2022). *Basic documents 49th edition.Constitution.* Available at https://apps.who.int/gb/bd/pdf_files/BD_49th-en.pdf#page=6

World Health Organisation (2022). *World mental health report: Transforming mental health for all.* https://www.who.int/teams/mental-health-and-substance-use/world-mental-health-report

World Health Organisation (2023). *Ageing.* https://www.who.int/health-topics/ageing#tab=tab_1

Worth, P., & Smith, M. (2018). Critical positive psychology: A creative convergence of two disciplines. In: N.J.L. Brown, T. Lomas, & F.J. Eiroa-Orosa (Eds.), *The Routledge international handbook of critical positive psychology.* Routledge, 3–11.

Yull, C., Crinson, I., & Duncan, E. (2010). *Key concepts in health studies.* Sage.

2

LIFESTYLE MEDICINE BREAKTHROUGHS

Gia Merlo and Gabrielle Bachtel

As a powerful driver of health behavior change, positive emotions need to be leveraged in clinical practice coaching, lifestyle medicine (LM), and health care broadly by each health care team member. Evidence is mounting that positive emotions can promote healthy behaviors and, in turn, health behaviors, the pillars of LM – a predominantly plant-based eating pattern, physical activity, adequate and high-quality sleep, avoiding substance use, managing stress, and social connection – can increase positive emotions (Lianov, 2023). Moreover, positive activities offer direct physiologic benefits, serving as additional, independent health protective factors. Therefore positive psychology (PP) interventions that lead to subjective and psychological wellbeing should be considered for both self-care and health care. These combined healthy lifestyle and PP habits have the potential to achieve positive health, a state of total wellbeing that includes physical, mental, emotional, social, and spiritual health for greater longevity, quality of life, and capacity to bounce back and grow from inevitable adverse life experiences (Lianov et al., 2019, 2022). We can transform health care and self-care to facilitate positive health beyond that achieved by traditional health practices.

This chapter reviews the most recent data in LM that have major implications in PP, describes how advances in LM have furthered our understanding of evidence-based literature in PP, reports new breakthroughs in LM, and identifies how this data can be connected and applied to PP in patient care.

The American College of Lifestyle Medicine (ACLM) describes LM as follows:

Lifestyle medicine is a medical specialty that uses therapeutic lifestyle interventions as a primary modality to treat chronic conditions including, but not limited to, cardiovascular diseases, type 2 diabetes, and obesity. Lifestyle medicine-certified clinicians are trained to apply

DOI: 10.4324/9781003378426-3   24

evidence-based, whole-person, prescriptive lifestyle change to treat and, when used intensively, often reverse such conditions. Applying the six pillars of lifestyle medicine...also provides effective prevention for these conditions.

(ACLM, 2022)

LM incorporates and emphasizes patients' psychosocial wellbeing, wellness and life goals, sense of purpose, motivation and readiness to initiate change, and therapeutic alliance with their healthcare providers. Increasing evidence suggests that lifestyle-based strategies can effectively improve brain health, emotional wellbeing, and overall health and wellbeing (Morton, 2018; Rippe, 2018). Positive lifestyle changes under the framework of the six pillars of LM can facilitate human flourishing (optimal functioning and wellbeing) (Burke & Dunne, 2022). LM concepts can be practiced by healthcare providers; utilized by individuals outside of clinical settings; and applied to groups, institutions, and communities. To achieve these aims, the disciples of LM have organized key lifestyle interventions into six pillars that include: (1) nutrition emphasizing whole food, plant-predominant eating pattern, (2) physical activity, (3) adequate sleep, (4) stress management, (5) harm reduction of risky substances, and (6) positive social connections (ACLM, 2022).

Nutrition

Multiple studies have pointed to the relationship between plant-predominant eating patterns and decreased risk of chronic diseases, longevity, mindful dietary choices, happiness, wellbeing, life satisfaction, positive affect, psychological resilience, self-regulation, improved mental health outcomes, mood, and cognitive function. The ACLM and many leading health organizations recommend a plant-predominant eating pattern that involves the daily consumption of more fruits, vegetables, nuts, seeds, and whole grains and less red meat and sugar to improve human and environmental health on a global scale (Willett et al., 2019). Diet improvements could prevent one in every five deaths worldwide (Afshin et al., 2019). Notably, suboptimal consumption of healthy foods (e.g., fruits, vegetables, nuts, seeds, whole grains) is the leading global cause of preventable deaths. Diets with insufficient nutrient-dense plant foods, fiber, and prebiotics may induce chronic, systemic, low-grade inflammation that can increase risk of chronic diseases, morbidity, and mortality (Furman et al., 2019). Higher levels of fruit and vegetable intake are correlated to decreased risk of chronic diseases and greater longevity (Conner et al., 2014). This association remains significant across all demographic and health circumstances.

Making mindful dietary choices is a health investment in future happiness and wellbeing (Mujcic & Oswald, 2016). There is a positive association between wellbeing, life satisfaction, happiness, positive affect, physical health, and consumption of fruits and vegetables (Blanchflower et al., 2012). Of note, consumption of increased varieties and amounts of fruit and vegetables results in significant, dose-dependent increases in life-satisfaction points and happiness; fruit and vegetable intake may predict improvements in wellbeing.

Consumption of fruits and vegetables is linked to key indicators of flourishing and psychological resilience, such as greater eudemonic wellbeing (the combination of experience and feelings – or lack thereof – associated with a life of purpose, meaning, and engagement) and eudemonic behaviors (e.g., creativity, curiosity) (Conner et al., 2014). Individuals eating more fruits and vegetables report higher average eudemonic wellbeing, eudemonic behaviors, and positive affect than those who consume fewer fruits and vegetables. The American Psychological Association (APA) defines psychological resilience as follows: "Resilience is the process and outcome of successfully adapting to difficult or challenging life experiences, especially through mental, emotional, and behavioral flexibility and adjustment to external and internal demands" (APA, 2022). Common mental disorders, such as depression, anxiety, stress, and insomnia, in conjunction with comorbidities (i.e., chronic conditions), can have significant negative effects on psychological resilience (Lam et al., 2021). Research has revealed increased incidence and intensity of depressive symptoms with lower vegetable intake (Agarwal et al., 2015). Daily fruit consumption has been found to reduce self-reported anxiety (Conner et al., 2014). Notably, those who adhere to a plant-based diet typically report improved mental health, vitality, work productivity, and dietary satisfaction in comparison to control groups.

Cumulatively, current literature suggests that there may be negative consequences in short-term mood and mental states in the setting of diets high in animal products. An important concept in the formation and adherence to a plant-based diet is an emphasis on plant foods and relative restriction or complete elimination of animal products and fats. Long-chain omega-3 fatty acid intake has been linked to mood (Lange, 2020). Of note, omega-3 fatty acids are precursors to anti-inflammatory signaling molecules with regulatory functions on neurochemicals in the brain. Plant-predominant eating patterns that restrict animal sources of proteins incorporate lower quantities of long-chain omega-3 and omega-6 fatty acids in comparison to omnivorous diets are associated with better self-reported mood than omnivores (Beezhold & Johnston, 2012). Data also suggests that dietary elimination of meat, fish, and poultry, in comparison to an omnivorous diet, may increase individuals' capacity to cope with mental stress.

The gut microbiome has also been implicated in the management of chronic conditions and the promotion of emotional resilience. Consumption of highly processed foods can induce increased intestinal permeability, which can facilitate toxin distribution throughout the entire body. By nature of the brain–gut connection, the nervous system can be affected significantly by poor diet and thus, create an environment in which emotional resilience, mood, cognitive functioning, and positive health assets may be negatively impacted (Bodai et al., 2018).

Physical activity

Exercise is an effective, evidence-based therapeutic lifestyle intervention to extend longevity, promote mental/brain health, protect brain plasticity, and prevent, manage, and treat chronic conditions; it has been referred to as a "miracle drug that can benefit every part of the body and substantially expand lifespan" in literature (Wen & Wu, 2012). Mental health factors play a crucial role in the reduction of risks and health consequences of lifestyle-related diseases and influence the promotion and success of exercise interventions (Merlo & Vela, 2021).

Across the lifespan, mental/brain health and psychosocial function regulate health-promoting behaviors and exercise habits. A sedentary lifestyle has a direct negative effect on mortality, mental/brain health, and health-promoting dietary choices (Leibow et al., 2020). The authors suggest that lack of exercise is a worldwide predictor of poor health outcomes, such as early morbidity and mortality. The current Federal guidelines released by the Office of Disease Prevention and Health Promotion, *Physical Activity Guidelines for Americans,* advocate for 150 minutes of moderate-intensity physical activity with two days of muscle-strengthening activity per week (ODPHP, 2021). A recent National Health Interview Survey conducted by the Centers for Disease Control (CDC) in 2020 revealed that, of all adults aged 18 and over, nearly half did not meet the guidelines for aerobic activity or muscle-strengthening activity (Elgaddal et al., 2022).

Research has largely suggested a bidirectional relationship between physical activity and brain/mental health (Zhao et al., 2020). Notably, exercise can have a positive influence on mental health conditions, such as anxiety and depression, and mental health outcomes. Increased levels/volume of exercise have been associated with higher levels of happiness, positive mood, positive affect, and mental wellbeing (Richards et al., 2015). Improvements in physical activity and health-promoting behaviors can be predicted by positive affect. For this paper, positive affect will be defined according to the APA: "the internal feeling state (affect) that occurs when a goal has been attained, a source of threat has been avoided, or the individual is satisfied with the present state of affairs"; inversely, negative affect will be defined as: "the internal feeling state (affect) that occurs when one has failed to achieve a goal or to avoid a threat or when one is not satisfied with the current state of affairs" (APA, 2022). Positive affect increases health-promoting and goal-directed behaviors through the cultivation of a future-oriented mindset and self-efficacy (Peifer et al., 2020). In this chapter, self-efficacy will describe "an individual's belief in his or her capacity to execute behaviors necessary to produce specific performance attainments" (APA, 2022).

The mediation between physical activity, quality of life, and life satisfaction is likely driven by self-regulated positive subjective experiences, positive affect, self-efficacy, and overall health status. Studies have shown that the positive correlation of physical activity with quality of life is applicable to all populations, exercise modalities, and settings (McAuley & Morris, 2007). Negative affect and symptoms of depression and anxiety have been correlated with low exercise

27

volume (Leibow et al., 2020). Chronic noncommunicable diseases (NCDs) and poor physical and mental health outcomes have been linked to negative affect. The exercise-induced increased ratio of positive affect to negative affect determines overall psychosocial functioning through positive feedback on emotional and behavioral regulation (Leibow et al., 2020). Positive emotions and self-regulation are significant contributors to psychological resilience that can modulate thought processes, emotions, and behaviors to align with future-oriented goals (Weidner et al., 2015). Thus, exercise can increase one's capacity to flourish.

Increased susceptibility to NCD onset and functional decline due to advanced age and unhealthy lifestyle behaviors can result in reduced mental/brain health and quality of life as the aging process progresses. Physical activity can maintain and enhance physical and psychological functioning across the lifespan. Higher levels of fitness, in comparison to lower levels of fitness, may prevent declines in age-related mental/brain health (McAuley & Morris, 2007; Zhao et al., 2020). Notably, high-fit individuals have less gray and white matter tissue loss and quicker and more accurate performance of various cognitive, motor, and perceptual activities than their low-fit counterparts. Exercise stimulates angiogenesis (growth of new blood vessels) and increases blood flow and supply to the brain, which improves cognition (Kwak et al., 2018). Physically active individuals also display less Alzheimer's disease biomarkers, enhanced brain glucose metabolism and hippocampal volume, attenuated beta-amyloid burden, and better immediate memory, visuospatial ability, speed, and flexibility than sedentary individuals (Okonkwo et al., 2014).

Social connection

How we think and feel about ourselves – the cognitive and affective domains, respectively, of self-interpretation – are significant determinants of overall wellbeing (Kansky & Diener, 2017). There is a strong link between wellbeing and positive adaptations in key areas of functioning, such as social relationships. Social relationships can significantly influence positive health outcomes through their impacts on health behaviors, brain/mental health, physical health, and mortality risk (Umberson & Karas Montez, 2010). Healthy social relationships have been directly correlated with individual capacity to flourish, whereas the lack or deficiency of human connections has been linked to poorer physical and psychosocial outcomes (Borelli et al., 2020).

The link between flourishing and positive connection is thought to be modulated through psychophysiologic mechanisms of positive emotions (Kok et al., 2013). Positive emotions are an innate set of tools that can be accessed through behavior changes. Positive emotions (e.g., happiness, life satisfaction), as delineated by the broaden-and-build theory, are experiential parameters that impact our behaviors by motivating us to broaden and build the resources that stimulate these rewarding psychophysiologic responses; this positive reinforcement cycle supports a future-oriented mindset that is more likely to coordinate health-promoting behaviors (Fredrickson, 2004). Positive psychological resilience, the execution of protective thoughts, behaviors, and actions that contribute to adaptability and recovery in the setting of stress- or trauma-inducing events, has been linked to positive emotions (Xu & Roberts, 2010). Positive emotions can reverse the physiological consequences of negative emotions. Healthy social connection is not only associated with positive psychological resilience, but also cognitive resilience. Cognitive resilience is the capacity of one's cognitive functions to maintain structural durability and volume of the brain in the face of aging and disease processes.

There are protective neurocognitive benefits to the reception or perception of social support (Bennett et al., 2006). A specific form of social support called *supportive listening* has been associated with increased cognitive resilience. Those with a high level of listener availability, compared to those with a low listener availability, have increased protection against Alzheimer's disease, stroke, and dementia. Methods of social support that cultivate true connection may work through pathways related to neuroplasticity, neurogenesis, social behavior, executive functioning, and/or brain-derived neurotrophic factor-dependent neurogenesis (Salinas et al., 2017). In general, higher quality and quantity of social interactions can lead to higher cognitive reserve and enhanced brain networks with the capacity to compensate for and protect against neurological diseases (Sundström et al., 2019).

Loneliness can increase amyloid cortical burden and is a neuropsychiatric indicator of risk for progression to Alzheimer's disease and related disorders (Donovan et al., 2016; Biddle et al., 2019). Negative emotions and behavioral symptoms may precede the onset of cognitive impairment and progression of neuropathologies. The limbic, cortical, and subcortical areas of the brain that support social cognition are involved in processes such as semantic and episodic memory and formulate thoughts and feelings of self, non-self, and social environments (Bennett et al., 2006). The nature and strength of one's subjective perceptions of social belonging are linked to psychosocial functioning, overall wellbeing, and the volumes and structures of these specific brain regions involved in emotion, memory, and perception. Loneliness is based on individual cognitive processes and perception and is independent of actual social network size (Düzel et al., 2019). Although high-quality relationships have additional health benefits, even brief social interactions or contact with others who are not family or close friends have been associated with higher levels of happiness, emotional wellbeing, sense of social embeddedness, and thus, positive health outcomes (Sandstrom & Dunn, 2014).

Restorative sleep

The relationship between sleep and wellbeing is bidirectional. Inadequate sleep interferes with cognitive and emotional functioning. Importantly, insufficient quantity or quality of sleep diminishes one's ability to make healthful dietary choices, manage stress through health-promoting coping mechanisms, engage in positive social interactions, maintain healthy interpersonal relationships, and have enough energy and motivation to exercise (Merlo & Vela, 2021). According to a review on the primary health consequences of insufficient sleep, sleep deprivation causes reduced happiness, savoring of positive experiences, sociability, cognitive and prefrontal cortex function, and immunity, as well as increased negative mood, memory dysfunction, appetite, risk of weight gain and cardiometabolic disorders, and insulin resistance (Chattu et al., 2018). Of note, insufficient sleep has been associated with 7 of the 15 leading causes of mortality. On average, one-third of the human lifespan is spent sleeping. The National Sleep Foundation recommends that adults sleep for a minimum of 7 hours on a nightly basis (Hirshkowitz et al., 2015). However, over one-third of all adults in the U.S. report sleeping less than 7 hours per night (CDC, 2022).

Sleep has a causative relationship with mental health problems (Freeman et al., 2020). Sleep loss or lack of quality sleep can alter one's reactions and psychological resiliency to daily stressors and positive events (Sin et al., 2020). Those who sleep well are more satisfied with life and exhibit increased likelihood and capacity to maintain more positive mindsets (Shin & Kim, 2018). Inversely, life satisfaction may increase sleep quality. Poor sleep has been correlated with depression and low mood, as it may reduce positive affect experienced due to positive events and increase negative affect caused by stressors (Morton, 2018). New synaptic connections are created during the restorative processes of sleep to facilitate the consolidation of new information and memories attained during the day; of note, sleep-deprived individuals are more likely to retain memories with negative connotations. Therefore, sleep deprivation may induce a negative mindset. There is a dose-dependent decline in tasks requiring attention as awake-time accumulates (Krause et al., 2017). Cognitive functions, such as attention, a goal-oriented behavior, can be significantly impacted by sleep loss.

Lifestyle habits, health status, and inflammatory markers associated with insufficient sleep have deleterious impacts on mental and physical health and mediate mortality related to sleep (Hall et al., 2015). Adults who lack consistent sleep patterns and have later sleep timing have poorer health outcomes than those with earlier sleep timing, consistent sleep patterns, and catch-up sleep on the weekends (Chaput et al., 2020).

Stress management

Both real and perceived distress, over time, deteriorate mental and physiological homeostatic processes and lead to greater susceptibility to chronic disease and negative health consequences (Segrin & Passalacqua, 2010). Persistent exposure to excessive stress has negative impacts on all components of individual wellbeing (Guidi et al., 2020). While some stress motivates goal-oriented behaviors to accomplish life tasks, high levels of psychological stress are associated with innumerable comorbidities. Greater than three-quarters of all healthcare visits are related to chronic levels of excessive stress (Avey et al., 2003).

Exposure to excessive levels of stress or trauma can eventually lead to burnout; according to the APA, burnout is the

> physical, emotional, or mental exhaustion accompanied by decreased motivation, lowered performance, and negative attitudes toward oneself and others. It results from performing at a high level until stress and tension, especially from extreme and prolonged physical or mental exertion or an overburdening workload, take their toll.
>
> *(APA, 2022)*

Stress and burnout have a reciprocal and reinforcing relationship that can compound negative physical, mental, and emotional health impacts.

Exposure to chronic stress reduces psychological resiliency and overall wellbeing by inciting long-term changes in the physiological crosstalk pathways involved in the mind-body connection (Bottaccioli et al., 2018). A field of study known as psychoneuroendocrineimmunology has recently emerged to research the links between psychological, nervous, immune, endocrine, and metabolic systems. The physiological impact of excessive levels of chronic stress on neurological, immune, cardiovascular, digestive, and reproductive systems may correspondingly worsen mental health; the relationship between stress and physical and mental health is significant across the lifespan (Merlo & Vela, 2021). Acute stress can produce transient inflammatory responses throughout the entire body, including the brain (Merlo & Vela, 2021). Those with depressive symptoms have been found to exhibit increased rates of stress-induced inflammation, suggesting a link between emotional dysregulation and mental wellbeing and psychological resiliency and inflammation (Fagundes et al., 2013). Stress management techniques, early interventions, and healthy lifestyle behaviors may protect against the deleterious pro-inflammatory effects of stress that may otherwise alter clinical outcomes, overall wellbeing, quality of life, and brain neurocircuitry, function, and structure.

Stress management can improve one's ability to cope and strengthen resilience in the face of life stressors that could otherwise lead to unhealthy lifestyle habits or poor health outcomes. Those who experience stress management interventions (i.e., positive psychology interventions [PPIs]) report less stress, physical and mental complaints, and increased ability to relax after work (Bono et al., 2013). Those who utilize their personal strengths, which can lead to more positive experiences and better overall wellbeing, exhibit increased wellbeing over time, as well as lower levels of perceived stress and enhanced positive affect, vitality, and self-esteem (Wood et al., 2011). The use of unhealthy lifestyle behaviors, including misusing risky substances and overeating processed foods, as coping strategies can further exacerbate stress levels and stress-induced negative health outcomes (Bremner et al., 2020). Therefore, lifestyle interventions and healthy methods of stress management and coping may prove an effective modality in the development of long-term resilience and flourishing in patients.

Mindfulness practices can increase positive perception and positive affect related to life stressors by attenuating distress through the upward spiral of positive psychological processes and facilitating awareness of the present moment (Garland et al., 2011). Gratitude, reappraisal, and mindfulness activities may increase individual resilience by allowing patients to view stressful life events or circumstances as opportunities for personal growth and, thus, have increased capacity to flourish in the setting of unpredictable life events. For example, patients with breast cancer exhibited increased capacity for improvements in quality of life, hope, optimism, life satisfaction, wellbeing, and life meaning in patients with breast cancer (Casellas-Grau et al., 2013).

Harm reduction of risky substances

LM approaches can facilitate recovery from, avoidance of, and addiction to risky substances by emphasizing healthy social connections, the savoring of positive experiences, and patient-centered decisions that align with patients' life meaning, personal strengths, and health goals. Healthy lifestyle behaviors and positive psychological interventions can reduce risk of substance use harm by increasing psychological resiliency, enhancing mental health, and improving overall wellbeing (Horigian et al., 2020). Though ACLM currently uses the term Avoiding Risky Substances for this pillar, we believe that it is more accurately denoted as Substance Use Harm Reduction.

Use of risky substances (e.g., alcohol, drugs) has various adverse effects on overall wellbeing. Risky substance and prescription medication misuse have a bidirectional association with mental health (Merlo & Vela, 2021). Negative affect is associated with symptoms of mental health conditions, such as depression and anxiety, and can alter individuals' self-regulatory and motivational behaviors; substance use is often used to cope with negative affect related to mental illness (Treeby & Bruno, 2012). Those with poor mental health, high levels of loneliness, and/or chronic conditions are more likely to use risky substances (Esmaeelzadeh et al., 2018; Wu et al., 2018). In turn, substance use can cause further harm to mental and physical health.

Strengthening positive health assets (i.e., self-efficacy), assessing personal strengths, and practicing motivational interviewing may offer distinct benefits to patients who struggle with risky substance use, as they provide additional positive health benefits and an immediate non-substance-related reward. Self-efficacy, one's perception or belief of his or her ability to execute certain goal-oriented behaviors can predict health/treatment outcomes related to the use of risky substances (Kadden & Litt, 2011). A study investigating factors related to smoking cessation in patients with various mental health conditions noted that self-efficacy and motivation are significantly influenced by risk-benefit perception; participants reported expectations of worsened mental health and anxiety symptoms and loss of a coping strategy and pleasure caused by smoking cessation (Kerr et al., 2013).

Healthy lifestyle interventions and positive psychological approaches may decrease the likelihood of desiring and using risky substances among patients

(Krentzman, 2013; Stone, 2022). Mindfulness-based practices, paired with reappraisal and savoring strategies, may disrupt the onset and progression of addictive behaviors by enhancing attention (a goal-oriented behavior); positive affect; decision-making abilities; control of cognitive functioning; working memory; and self-awareness of natural-reward processing (Field et al., 2020; Garland, 2016). For instance, mindfulness and experience-savoring practices have been found to attenuate risks of opioid misuse in chronic pain patients treated with opioids through enhanced mental health and decreased pain severity (Garland et al., 2019). In a study consisting of happiness, personal strengths, optimism, and gratitude interventions in alcohol-misusing adolescents, participants exhibited significant improvements in positive emotions, optimism, future goal orientation, levels of happiness, and overall wellbeing, as well as reduced alcohol dependence and drug use (Akhtar & Boniwell, 2010). Moreover, a vast body of evidence supports the association between smoking cessation and enhanced quality of life; positive mood; and attenuated stress, anxiety, and depression. The benefits obtained from avoidance of substance use are not dependent of having a mental health disorder. (Taylor et al., 2014).

Especially in recent years, the advances in LM have furthered our understanding of the evidence-based literature in PP. PPIs are evidence-based approaches and activities designed to increase positive emotions, positive cognitive processes and perceptions, and positive behaviors. LM and PP reinforce each other due to the bidirectional relationship between health-promoting behaviors and overall wellbeing; positive emotions can foster health-promoting behaviors, while health-promoting behaviors can amplify positive emotions. The nexuses between LM and PP include nutrition, physical activity, sleep health, social connections and PP activities, stress reduction, and the avoidance of risky substances, as illustrated by PERMA, a model for flourishing. PERMA describes positive emotion (P), engagement (E), relationships (R), meaning (M), and accomplishment (A) as the elements of wellbeing (Seligman, 2018).

Those who adhere to three to six pillars of LM are more likely to flourish (Burke & Dunne, 2022). Participants of a ten-week multimodal lifestyle intervention project that combined PP strategies with LM approaches (e.g., positive speech practices, dynamic movement, social engagement, sleep, nutritious diet, service) exhibited moderate improvements in levels of vitality and stress reduction and significant improvements in life satisfaction, mental health, depression, and anxiety from baseline to postintervention (Morton et al., 2017). A narrative review on PP and hope as LM modalities in therapeutic encounters suggested their practical application in patient healthcare due to the importance of hope for improvement, the patient's active role in health promotion, and significance of behavior changes in patients' journeys to overall wellbeing (Duncan et al., 2020). Personal lifestyle behavior changes have been demonstrated to enhance primary health outcomes and, in turn, positively impact psychological outcomes (Borelli et al., 2020).

Applications

LM approaches can facilitate the achievement of numerous healthcare goals, such as enhancing physical benefits; improving quality of life; promoting mental/brain health and treating mental illness; maintaining positive, satisfying, and effective interactions between patients and providers; encouraging unconscious motivation for health-promoting changes in behavior; and enriching overall patient wellbeing. The clinical applications of LM have the potential to align with existing frameworks for flourishing (i.e., PERMA). PP, the study of flourishing, plays an essential role in improving quality of life; increasing healthy behaviors; enhancing physical, mental/brain, spiritual, and social health; successfully managing stress; and fostering productive, satisfying, and supportive interactions between healthcare providers and their patients (Lianov, 2019, 2023).

Conclusion

Patient-centered LM is a method of individualized health promotion and treatment that integrates the biopsychosocial model of health, and personal strengths, weaknesses, and life goals of patients to create respectful, empowering, and effective patient-provider collaborations (Roy et al., 2014). Practicing healthy lifestyle behaviors (such as adopting a plant-predominant eating pattern; engaging in physical activity; attaining adequate sleep; reducing substance use harm; managing stress; and sustaining healthy social connections that increase positive emotions, engagement, relationships, meaning, and accomplishment) is key to increasing individual, institutional, and societal wellbeing.

A health-promoting healthcare system must identify mechanisms that allow individuals and populations to support and enhance their health in ways that maintain the integrity of personal belief systems but also facilitate structured, meaningful, achievable, and sustainable healthcare. Health is a lifelong, multi-faceted, ever-changing product of the entanglement of biological, psychological, social, environmental, and spiritual systems. Global models and approaches to population health have, historically, been designed on the basis of societal deficits, such as health-damaging behaviors, disease, and deprivation (Morgan & Ziglio, 2007). Disregard for LM approaches to healthcare negates the concept that health and wellness cannot be fully understood through the study of pathogenesis and inherently supports the perspective that health is generated through the elimination of risk factors for disease. Half of all premature deaths in the U.S. are due to behavioral and other preventable factors (National Academy of Sciences, 2015). The provision of healthcare services with the aim of treating sickness no longer has the capacity to quell the public health crises of chronic disease, many of which are lifestyle-related.

Increasing evidence shows that a life of happiness, fulfillment, purpose, engagement, and balanced psychological and social components are both a consequence and cause of good health and a long and healthy life. Since the inception of PP, leaders in the field have propounded that healthcare providers must implement clinical applications that integrate their knowledge of medicine and PP to empower patients with tools, techniques, and strategies that effectively cultivate healing, overall wellbeing, and flourishing (Van Cappellen et al., 2017). Recent breakthroughs in LM elucidate the role of the six pillars of LM in the achievement of overall health and wellbeing, as well as the promotion of human flourishing.

In this chapter, we've also laid out the empirical evidence for the link of PP to each of the six pillars of LM, as well as health behavior changes and we made recommendations for application in self-care and health care. Chapter 20 provides delves further into the role of PP in LM. Future research will advance the evidence base and best practices for PP in medicine.

The overarching conclusion is that the application of PP to physical health and in LM and health care is promising. A short-term goal can be to harness the field's research-informed approaches, activities, and interventions based on the individual's interests, while the work to build the evidence base for health care continues (Millstein & Lianov, 2019; Park et al., 2014; Pressman et al., 2019). Medical practitioners and positive psychologists can advance the integration of PP into medicine and health care by collaborating on translational research, disseminating research-informed educational and training programs and developing practical clinical applications (Lianov et al, 2019).

Takeaways

General

- This chapter which describes lifestyle medicine breakthroughs, including the application of positive psychology approaches, reinforces several key take aways on the role of positive psychology in lifestyle medicine in Chapter 20.
- LM can achieve healthcare system goals by improving overall wellbeing among patients, institutions, and society as a whole.
- LM approaches and PP concepts have a reciprocal and reinforcing relationship in the adherence to and promotion and sustainability of healthy lifestyle behaviors that promote flourishing.
- Providers who incorporate LM approaches to patient treatment plans can facilitate patients' adoption and maintenance of health-promoting behaviors, as well as equip patients with lifestyle tools that have the potential to increase flourishing and quality of life across the lifespan.

Practical

- Recent breakthroughs in LM elucidate existing literature of PP related to overall wellbeing, quality of life, and flourishing.
- The biopsychosocial model of health has a bidirectional relationship to lifestyle behaviors and habits.

- Application of the six pillars of LM aligns with PERMA, a positive psychological framework of human flourishing, and can facilitate health-promoting behavior changes that further enhance patients' overall wellbeing.

Wicked questions

1 How does clinical application of the six pillars of LM relate to the biopsychosocial model of health?
2 How can LM applications improve patient quality of life across the lifespan?
3 How can research breakthroughs in LM be integrated into clinical care to best support human flourishing and lifelong patient benefits from the healthcare system? (similar to LL1)

References

Afshin, A., Sur, P. J., Fay, K. A., Cornaby, L., Ferrara, G., Salama, J. S., Mullany, E. C., Abate, K. H., Abbafati, C., Abebe, Z., Afarideh, M., Aggarwal, A., Agrawal, S., Akinyemiju, T., Alahdab, F., Bacha, U., Bachman, V. F., Badali, H., Badawi, A., ... & Murray, C. J. (2019). Health effects of dietary risks in 195 countries, 1990–2017: A systematic analysis for the global burden of disease study 2017. *The Lancet, 393*(10184), 1958–1972. https://doi.org/10.1016/s0140-6736(19)30041-8

Agarwal, U., Mishra, S., Xu, J., Levin, S., Gonzales, J., & Barnard, N. D. (2015). A multicenter randomized controlled trial of a nutrition intervention program in a multiethnic adult population in the corporate setting reduces depression and anxiety and improves quality of life: The GEICO study. *American Journal of Health Promotion, 29*(4), 245–254. https://doi.org/10.4278/ajhp.130218-quan-72

Akhtar, M., & Boniwell, I. (2010). Applying positive psychology to alcohol-misusing adolescents. *Groupwork, 20*(3), 6–31. https://doi.org/10.1921/095182410x576831

American Psychological Association. (2022). *APA Dictionary of Psychology*. American Psychological Association. Retrieved December 22, 2022, from https://dictionary.apa.org/burnout

American Psychological Association. (2022). *APA Dictionary of Psychology*. American Psychological Association. Retrieved December 22, 2022, from https://dictionary.apa.org/negative-affect

American Psychological Association. (2022). *APA Dictionary of Psychology*. American Psychological Association. Retrieved December 20, 2022, from https://dictionary.apa.org/positive-affect

American Psychological Association. (2022). *Resilience - American Psychological Association*. Resilience. Retrieved December 22, 2022, from https://www.apa.org/topics/resilience/

American Psychological Association. (2022). *Self-efficacy teaching tip sheet*. American Psychological Association. Retrieved December 22, 2022, from https://www.apa.org/pi/aids/resources/education/self-efficacy

Avey, H., Matheny, K. B., Robbins, A., & Jacobson, T. A. (2003). Health care providers' training, perceptions, and practices regarding stress and health outcomes. *The Journal of the National Medical Association, 95*(9), 833, 836–845

Beezhold, B. L., & Johnston, C. S. (2012). Restriction of meat, fish, and poultry in omnivores improves mood: A pilot randomized controlled trial. *Nutrition Journal, 11*(1). https://doi.org/10.1186/1475-2891-11-9

Bennett, D. A., Schneider, J. A., Tang, Y., Arnold, S. E., & Wilson, R. S. (2006). The effect of social networks on the relation between alzheimer's disease pathology and level of cognitive function in old people: A longitudinal cohort study. *The Lancet Neurology*, 5(5), 406–412. https://doi.org/10.1016/s1474-4422(06)70417-3

Biddle, K. D., d'Oleire Uquillas, F., Jacobs, H. I. L., Zide, B., Kirn, D. R., Rentz, D. M., Johnson, K. A., Sperling, R. A., & Donovan, N. J. (2019). Social engagement and amyloid-β-related cognitive decline in cognitively normal older adults. *The American Journal of Geriatric Psychiatry*, 27(11), 1247–1256. https://doi.org/10.1016/j.jagp.2019.05.005

Blanchflower, D. G., Oswald, A. J., & Stewart-Brown, S. (2012). Is psychological well-being linked to the consumption of fruit and vegetables? *Social Indicators Research*, 114(3), 785–801. https://doi.org/10.1007/s11205-012-0173-y

Bodai, B. I., Nakata, T. E., Wong, W. T., Clark, D. R., Lawenda, S., Tsou, C., Liu, R., Shiue, L., Cooper, N., Rehbein, M., Ha, B. P., McKeirnan, A., Misquitta, R., Vij, P., Klonecke, A., Mejia, C. S., Dionysian, E., Hashmi, S., Greger, M., ... & Campbell, T. M. (2018). Lifestyle medicine: A brief review of its dramatic impact on health and survival. *The Permanente Journal*, 22(1). https://doi.org/10.7812/tpp/17-025

Bono, J. E., Glomb, T. M., Shen, W., Kim, E., & Koch, A. J. (2013). Building positive resources: Effects of positive events and positive reflection on work stress and health. *Academy of Management Journal*, 56(6), 1601–1627. https://doi.org/10.5465/amj.2011.0272

Borelli, J. L., Smiley, P. A., Kerr, M. L., Hong, K., Hecht, H. K., Blackard, M. B., Falasiri, E., Cervantes, B. R., & Bond, D. K. (2020). Relational savoring: An attachment-based approach to promoting interpersonal flourishing. *Psychotherapy*, 57(3), 340–351. https://doi.org/10.1037/pst0000284

Bottaccioli, A. G., Bottaccioli, F., & Minelli, A. (2018). Stress and the psyche-brain-immune network in psychiatric diseases based on psychoneuroendocrineimmunology: A concise review. *Annals of the New York Academy of Sciences*, 1437(1), 31–42. https://doi.org/10.1111/nyas.13728

Bremner, J., Moazzami, K., Wittbrodt, M., Nye, J., Lima, B., Gillespie, C., Rapaport, M., Pearce, B., Shah, A., & Vaccarino, V. (2020). Diet, stress and mental health. *Nutrients*, 12(8), 2428. https://doi.org/10.3390/nu12082428

Burke, J., & Dunne, P. J. (2022). Lifestyle medicine pillars as predictors of psychological flourishing. *Frontiers in Psychology*, 13. https://doi.org/10.3389/fpsyg.2022.963806

Casellas-Grau, A., Font, A., & Vives, J. (2013). Positive psychology interventions in breast cancer. A systematic review. *Psycho-Oncology*, 23(1), 9–19. https://doi.org/10.1002/pon.3353

Centers for Disease Control and Prevention. (2022, September 12). *Sleep and sleep disorders data and statistics.* Centers for Disease Control and Prevention. Retrieved December 13, 2022, from https://www.cdc.gov/sleep/data_statistics.html

Chaput, J.-P., Dutil, C., Featherstone, R., Ross, R., Giangregorio, L., Saunders, T. J., Janssen, I., Poitras, V. J., Kho, M. E., Ross-White, A., Zankar, S., & Carrier, J. (2020). Sleep timing, sleep consistency, and health in adults: A systematic review. *Applied Physiology, Nutrition, and Metabolism*, 45(10(Suppl. 2)). https://doi.org/10.1139/apnm-2020-0032

Chattu, V. K., Sakhamuri, S. M., Kumar, R., Spence, D. W., BaHammam, A. S., & Pandi-Perumal, S. R. (2018). Insufficient sleep syndrome: Is it time to classify it as a major noncommunicable disease? *Sleep Science*, 11(2). https://doi.org/10.5935/1984-0063.20180013

Conner, T. S., Brookie, K. L., Richardson, A. C., & Polak, M. A. (2014). On carrots and curiosity: Eating fruit and vegetables is associated with greater flourishing in daily life. *British Journal of Health Psychology*, 20(2), 413–427. https://doi.org/10.1111/bjhp.12113

Donovan, N. J., Okereke, O. I., Vannini, P., Amariglio, R. E., Rentz, D. M., Marshall, G. A., Johnson, K. A., & Sperling, R. A. (2016). Association of higher cortical amyloid burden with loneliness in cognitively normal older adults. *JAMA Psychiatry*, *73*(12), 1230. https://doi.org/10.1001/jamapsychiatry.2016.2657

Duncan, A. R., Jaini, P. A., & Hellman, C. M. (2020). Positive psychology and hope as lifestyle medicine modalities in the therapeutic encounter: A narrative review. *American Journal of Lifestyle Medicine*, *15*(1), 6–13. https://doi.org/10.1177/1559827620908255

Düzel, S., Drewelies, J., Gerstorf, D., Demuth, I., Steinhagen-Thiessen, E., Lindenberger, U., & Kühn, S. (2019). Structural brain correlates of loneliness among older adults. *Scientific Reports*, *9*(1). https://doi.org/10.1038/s41598-019-49888-2

Elgaddal, N., Kramarow, E. A., & Reuben, C. (2022, August 30). *Physical activity among adults aged 18 and over: United States, 2020.* Centers for Disease Control and Prevention. Retrieved December 13, 2022, from https://www.cdc.gov/nchs/products/databriefs/db443.htm

Esmaeelzadeh, S., Moraros, J., Thorpe, L., & Bird, Y. (2018). Examining the association and directionality between mental health disorders and substance use among adolescents and young adults in the U.S. and Canada—a systematic review and meta-analysis. *Journal of Clinical Medicine*, *7*(12), 543. https://doi.org/10.3390/jcm7120543

Fagundes, C. P., Glaser, R., Hwang, B. S., Malarkey, W. B., & Kiecolt-Glaser, J. K. (2013). Depressive symptoms enhance stress-induced inflammatory responses. *Brain, Behavior, and Immunity*, *31*, 172–176. https://doi.org/10.1016/j.bbi.2012.05.006

Field, M., Heather, N., Murphy, J. G., Stafford, T., Tucker, J. A., & Witkiewitz, K. (2020). Recovery from addiction: Behavioral economics and value-based decision making. *Psychology of Addictive Behaviors*, *34*(1), 182–193. https://doi.org/10.1037/adb0000518

Fredrickson, B. L. (2004). The broaden–and–build theory of positive emotions. *Philosophical Transactions of the Royal Society of London. Series B: Biological Sciences*, *359*(1449), 1367–1377. https://doi.org/10.1098/rstb.2004.1512

Freeman, D., Sheaves, B., Waite, F., Harvey, A. G., & Harrison, P. J. (2020). Sleep disturbance and psychiatric disorders. *The Lancet Psychiatry*, *7*(7), 628–637. https://doi.org/10.1016/s2215-0366(20)30136-x

Furman, D., Campisi, J., Verdin, E., Carrera-Bastos, P., Targ, S., Franceschi, C., Ferrucci, L., Gilroy, D. W., Fasano, A., Miller, G. W., Miller, A. H., Mantovani, A., Weyand, C. M., Barzilai, N., Goronzy, J. J., Rando, T. A., Effros, R. B., Lucia, A., Kleinstreuer, N., & Slavich, G. M. (2019). Chronic inflammation in the etiology of disease across the life span. *Nature Medicine*, *25*(12), 1822–1832. https://doi.org/10.1038/s41591-019-0675-0

Garland, E. L. (2016). Restructuring reward processing with mindfulness-oriented recovery enhancement: Novel therapeutic mechanisms to remediate hedonic dysregulation in addiction, stress, and pain. *Annals of the New York Academy of Sciences*, *1373*(1), 25–37. https://doi.org/10.1111/nyas.13034

Garland, E. L., Gaylord, S. A., & Fredrickson, B. L. (2011). Positive reappraisal mediates the stress-reductive effects of mindfulness: An upward spiral process. *Mindfulness*, *2*(1), 59–67. https://doi.org/10.1007/s12671-011-0043-8

Garland, E. L., Hanley, A. W., Riquino, M. R., Reese, S. E., Baker, A. K., Salas, K., Yack, B. P., Bedford, C. E., Bryan, M. A., Atchley, R., Nakamura, Y., Froeliger, B., & Howard, M. O. (2019). Mindfulness-oriented recovery enhancement reduces opioid misuse risk via analgesic and positive psychological mechanisms: A randomized controlled trial. *Journal of Consulting and Clinical Psychology*, *87*(10), 927–940. https://doi.org/10.1037/ccp0000390

Guidi, J., Lucente, M., Sonino, N., & Fava, G. A. (2020). Allostatic load and its impact on health: A systematic review. *Psychotherapy and Psychosomatics*, *90*(1), 11–27. https://doi.org/10.1159/000510696

Hall, M. H., Smagula, S. F., Boudreau, R. M., Ayonayon, H. N., Goldman, S. E., Harris, T. B., Naydeck, B. L., Rubin, S. M., Samuelsson, L., Satterfield, S., Stone, K. L., Visser, M., & Newman, A. B. (2015). Association between sleep duration and mortality is mediated by markers of inflammation and health in older adults: The health, aging and body composition study. *Sleep, 38*(2), 189–195. https://doi.org/10.5665/sleep.4394

Hirshkowitz, M., Whiton, K., Albert, S. M., Alessi, C., Bruni, O., DonCarlos, L., Hazen, N., Herman, J., Katz, E. S., Kheirandish-Gozal, L., Neubauer, D. N., O'Donnell, A. E., Ohayon, M., Peever, J., Rawding, R., Sachdeva, R. C., Setters, B., Vitiello, M. V., Ware, J. C., & Adams Hillard, P. J. (2015). National Sleep Foundation's sleep time duration recommendations: Methodology and results summary. *Sleep Health, 1*(1), 40–43. https://doi.org/10.1016/j.sleh.2014.12.010

Horigian, V. E., Schmidt, R. D., & Feaster, D. J. (2020). Loneliness, mental health, and substance use among us young adults during COVID-19. *Journal of Psychoactive Drugs, 53*(1), 1–9. https://doi.org/10.1080/02791072.2020.1836435

Kadden, R. M., & Litt, M. D. (2011). The role of self-efficacy in the treatment of substance use disorders. *Addictive Behaviors, 36*(12), 1120–1126. https://doi.org/10.1016/j.addbeh.2011.07.032

Kansky, J., & Diener, E. (2017). Benefits of well-being: Health, social relationships, work, and resilience. *Journal of Positive Psychology and Wellbeing, 1*(2), 129–169.

Kerr, S., Woods, C., Knussen, C., Watson, H., & Hunter, R. (2013). Breaking the habit: A qualitative exploration of barriers and facilitators to smoking cessation in people with enduring mental health problems. *BMC Public Health, 13*(1). https://doi.org/10.1186/1471-2458-13-221

Kok, B. E., Coffey, K. A., Cohn, M. A., Catalino, L. I., Vacharkulksemsuk, T., Algoe, S. B., Brantley, M., & Fredrickson, B. L. (2013). How positive emotions build physical health. *Psychological Science, 24*(7), 1123–1132. https://doi.org/10.1177/0956797612470827

Krause, A. J., Simon, E. B., Mander, B. A., Greer, S. M., Saletin, J. M., Goldstein-Piekarski, A. N., & Walker, M. P. (2017). The sleep-deprived human brain. *Nature Reviews Neuroscience, 18*(7), 404–418. https://doi.org/10.1038/nrn.2017.55

Krentzman, A. R. (2013). Review of the application of positive psychology to substance use, addiction, and recovery research. *Psychology of Addictive Behaviors, 27*(1), 151–165. https://doi.org/10.1037/a0029897

Kwak, S.-E., Lee, J.-H., Zhang, D., & Song, W. (2018). Angiogenesis: Focusing on the effects of exercise in aging and cancer. *Journal of Exercise Nutrition & Biochemistry, 22*(3), 21–26. https://doi.org/10.20463/jenb.2018.0020

Lianov L. (2023). The role of positive psychology in lifestyle medicine. *American Journal of Lifestyle Medicine.* 0(0). https://doi.org/10.1177/15598276231184157 (*AJLM OnLineFirst*).

Lianov L (2022). Positive health practice for clinical practitioners: Workshop series. [PowePoint Slides]. Global Positive Health Institute. https://positivehealth.world.

Lianov, L.S., Fredrickson, B.,Barron, C., Krishnaswami, J., Wallace, A. (2019) Positive psychology in lifestyle medicine and health care: Strategies for Implementation. *AJLM, 13*(5), 480–486.

Lam, J. A., Murray, E. R., Yu, K. E., Ramsey, M., Nguyen, T. T., Mishra, J., Martis, B., Thomas, M. L., & Lee, E. E. (2021). Neurobiology of loneliness: A Systematic Review. *Neuropsychopharmacology, 46*(11), 1873–1887. https://doi.org/10.1038/s41386-021-01058-7

Lange, K. W. (2020). Omega-3 fatty acids and mental health. *Global Health Journal, 4*(1), 18–30. https://doi.org/10.1016/j.glohj.2020.01.004

Leibow, M. S., Lee, J. W., & Morton, K. R. (2020). Exercise, flourishing, and the positivity ratio in seventh-day adventists: A prospective study. *American Journal of Health Promotion, 35*(1), 48–56. https://doi.org/10.1177/0890117120930392

McAuley, E., & Morris, K. S. (2007). State of the art review: Advances in physical activity and mental health: Quality of life. *American Journal of Lifestyle Medicine, 1*(5), 389–396. https://doi.org/10.1177/1559827607303243

Measuring the risks and causes of premature death. (2015). *National Academies Press (US)*. https://doi.org/10.17226/21656

Merlo, G., & Vela, A. (2021). Mental health in lifestyle medicine: A call to action. *American Journal of Lifestyle Medicine, 16*(1), 7–20. https://doi.org/10.1177/15598276211013313

Millstein, R.A. & Lianov, L. (2019). Positive Psychology Research in Health Care Settings. In Lianov, L. (Ed.). *Roots of Positive Change, Optimizing Healthcare with Positive Psychology*. Chesterfield, MO: American College of Lifestyle Medicine.

Morgan, A., & Ziglio, E. (2007). Revitalising the evidence base for public health: An assets model. *Promotion & Education, 14*(Suppl. 2), 17–22. https://doi.org/10.1177/10253823070140020701x

Morton, D. P. (2018). Combining lifestyle medicine and positive psychology to improve mental health and emotional well-being. *American Journal of Lifestyle Medicine, 12*(5), 370–374. https://doi.org/10.1177/1559827618766482

Morton, D. P., Hinze, J., Craig, B., Herman, W., Kent, L., Beamish, P., Renfrew, M., & Przybylko, G. (2017). A multimodal intervention for improving the mental health and emotional well-being of college students. *American Journal of Lifestyle Medicine, 14*(2), 216–224. https://doi.org/10.1177/1559827617733941

Mujcic, R. & Oswald, A. J. (2016). Evolution of well-being and happiness after increases in consumption of fruit and vegetables. *American Journal of Public Health, 106*(8), 1504–1510. https://doi.org/10.2105/ajph.2016.303260

Office of Disease Prevention and Health Promotion. (2021, August 24). *Physical Activity Guidelines for Americans*. Current guidelines. Retrieved December 13, 2022, from https://health.gov/our-work/nutrition-physical-activity/physical-activity-guidelines/current-guidelines

Okonkwo, O. C., Schultz, S. A., Oh, J. M., Larson, J., Edwards, D., Cook, D., Koscik, R., Gallagher, C. L., Dowling, N. M., Carlsson, C. M., Bendlin, B. B., LaRue, A., Rowley, H. A., Christian, B. T., Asthana, S., Hermann, B. P., Johnson, S. C., & Sager, M. A. (2014). Physical activity attenuates age-related biomarker alterations in preclinical AD. *Neurology, 83*(19), 1753–1760. https://doi.org/10.1212/wnl.0000000000000964

Park, N., Peterson, C., Szvarca, D., Vander Molen, R. J., Kim, E. S., & Collon, K. (2014). Positive psychology and physical health. *American Journal of Lifestyle Medicine, 10*(3), 200–206. https://doi.org/10.1177/1559827614550277

Peifer, C., Schönfeld, P., Wolters, G., Aust, F., & Margraf, J. (2020). Well done! effects of positive feedback on perceived self-efficacy, flow and performance in a mental arithmetic task. *Frontiers in Psychology, 11*. https://doi.org/10.3389/fpsyg.2020.01008

Pressman, S., Jenkins, B.N., & Moskowitz, S.D. (2019). Positive affect and health: What do we know and where next should we go? *Annual Review of Psychology, 70*, 627–650.

Richards, J., Jiang, X., Kelly, P., Chau, J., Bauman, A., & Ding, D. (2015). Don't worry, be happy: Cross-sectional associations between physical activity and happiness in 15 European countries. *BMC Public Health, 15*(1). https://doi.org/10.1186/s12889-015-1391-4

Rippe, J. M. (2018). Lifestyle medicine: The health promoting power of daily habits and practices. *American Journal of Lifestyle Medicine, 12*(6), 499–512. https://doi.org/10.1177/1559827618785554

Roy, M., Levasseur, M., Couturier, Y., Lindström, B., & Généreux, M. (2014). The relevance of positive approaches to health for patient-centered care medicine. *Preventive Medicine Reports, 2*, 10–12. https://doi.org/10.1016/j.pmedr.2014.11.005

Salinas, J., Beiser, A., Himali, J. J., Satizabal, C. L., Aparicio, H. J., Weinstein, G., Mateen, F. J., Berkman, L. F., Rosand, J., & Seshadri, S. (2017). Associations between social relationship measures, serum brain-derived neurotrophic factor, and risk of stroke and dementia. *Alzheimer's & Dementia: Translational Research & Clinical Interventions, 3*(2), 229–237. https://doi.org/10.1016/j.trci.2017.03.001

Sandstrom, G. M., & Dunn, E. W. (2014). Social Interactions and well-being. *Personality and Social Psychology Bulletin, 40*(7), 910–922. https://doi.org/10.1177/0146167214529799

Segrin, C., & Passalacqua, S. A. (2010). Functions of loneliness, social support, health behaviors, and stress in association with poor health. *Health Communication, 25*(4), 312–322. https://doi.org/10.1080/10410231003773334

Seligman, M. (2018). PERMA and the building blocks of well-being. *The Journal of Positive Psychology, 13*(4), 333–335. https://doi.org/10.1080/17439760.2018.1437466

Shin, J.-eun, & Kim, J. K. (2018). How a good sleep predicts life satisfaction: The role of zero-sum beliefs about happiness. *Frontiers in Psychology, 9.* https://doi.org/10.3389/fpsyg.2018.01589

Sin, N. L., Wen, J. H., Klaiber, P., Buxton, O. M., & Almeida, D. M. (2020). Sleep duration and affective reactivity to stressors and positive events in daily life. *Health Psychology, 39*(12), 1078–1088. https://doi.org/10.1037/hea0001033

Stone, B. M. (2022). Positive psychology for substance use disorders: A rationale and call to action. *Journal of Studies on Alcohol and Drugs, 83*(6), 959–961. https://doi.org/10.15288/jsad.22-00259

Sundström, A., Adolfsson, A. N., Nordin, M., & Adolfsson, R. (2019). Loneliness increases the risk of all-cause dementia and alzheimer's disease. *The Journals of Gerontology: Series B, 75*(5), 919–926. https://doi.org/10.1093/geronb/gbz139

Taylor, G., McNeill, A., Girling, A., Farley, A., Lindson-Hawley, N., & Aveyard, P. (2014, February 13). Change in mental health after smoking cessation: Systematic review and meta-analysis. *BMJ, 348*(1). https://doi.org/10.1136/bmj.g1151

Treeby, M., & Bruno, R. (2012). Shame and guilt-proneness: Divergent implications for problematic alcohol use and drinking to cope with anxiety and depression symptomatology. *Personality and Individual Differences, 53*(5), 613–617. https://doi.org/10.1016/j.paid.2012.05.011

Umberson, D., & Karas Montez, J. (2010). Social relationships and health: A flashpoint for health policy. *Journal of Health and Social Behavior, 51*(1). https://doi.org/10.1177/0022146510383501

Van Cappellen, P., Rice, E. L., Catalino, L. I., & Fredrickson, B. L. (2017). Positive affective processes underlie positive health behaviour change. *Psychology & Health, 33*(1), 77–97. https://doi.org/10.1080/08870446.2017.1320798

Weidner, G., Sieverding, M., & Chesney, M. A. (2015). The role of self-regulation in health and illness. *Psychology, Health & Medicine, 21*(2), 135–137. https://doi.org/10.1080/13548506.2015.1115528

Wen, C. P. & Wu, X. (2012). Stressing harms of physical inactivity to promote exercise. *The Lancet, 380*(9838), 192–193. https://doi.org/10.1016/s0140-6736(12)60954-4

What is lifestyle medicine? American College of Lifestyle Medicine. (2022, December 10). Retrieved December 13, 2022, from https://lifestylemedicine.org/

Willett, W., Rockström, J., Loken, B., Springmann, M., Lang, T., Vermeulen, S., Garnett, T., Tilman, D., DeClerck, F., Wood, A., Jonell, M., Clark, M., Gordon, L. J., Fanzo, J., Hawkes, C., Zurayk, R., Rivera, J. A., De Vries, W., Majele Sibanda, L., ... & Murray, C. J. (2019). Food in the anthropocene: The eat–lancet commission on healthy diets from sustainable food systems. *The Lancet, 393*(10170), 447–492. https://doi.org/10.1016/s0140-6736(18)31788-4

Wood, A. M., Linley, P. A., Maltby, J., Kashdan, T. B., & Hurling, R. (2011). Using personal and psychological strengths leads to increases in well-being over time: A longitudinal study and the development of the strengths use questionnaire. *Personality and Individual Differences, 50*(1), 15–19. https://doi.org/10.1016/j.paid.2010.08.004

Wu, L.-T., Zhu, H., & Ghitza, U. E. (2018). Multicomorbidity of chronic diseases and substance use disorders and their association with hospitalization: Results from Electronic Health Records Data. *Drug and Alcohol Dependence, 192*, 316–323. https://doi.org/10.1016/j.drugalcdep.2018.08.013

Xu, J. & Roberts, R. E. (2010). The power of positive emotions: It's a matter of life or death—subjective well-being and longevity over 28 years in a general population. *Health Psychology, 29*(1), 9–19. https://doi.org/10.1037/a0016767

Zhao, J. L., Jiang, W. T., Wang, X., Cai, Z. D., Liu, Z. H., & Liu, G. R. (2020). Exercise, brain plasticity, and depression. *CNS Neuroscience & Therapeutics, 26*(9), 885–895. https://doi.org/10.1111/cns.13385

3

POSITIVE PSYCHOLOGY BREAKTHROUGHS

Ilona Boniwell

The emerging collaboration between positive psychology and lifestyle medicine suggests an innovative path towards holistic health management. This chapter will explore some ground-breaking discoveries in positive psychology that can be of interest and practical use for practitioners from the field of lifestyle and general medicine. It aims to provide a broad overview of the field of positive psychology, focusing on ten prominent areas of research and privileging meta-review and meta-analytic evidence, whenever available.

Positive psychology has often been delineated into three broad levels of analysis: the subjective level, which pertains to positive subjective experiences; the individual level, which involves the study of positive individual traits; and the group level, which is concerned with positive institutions and communities that contribute to better citizenship and overall well-being. These three levels collectively contribute to our understanding of the pathways to human flourishing (Seligman & Csikszentmihalyi, 2000).

As the most commonly accepted framework, the three levels of positive psychology will be used to guide the chapter structure, with full acknowledgement of the limitations of this original framework. According to Diener (2012), the exploration of 'positive subjective experiences' and 'positive individual traits' has dominated the field, while the investigation into positive institutions has been somewhat overlooked. He comments that positive psychology 'focuses too exclusively on the individual person, rather than considering the impact of neighborhoods, social groups, organizations, and governments in shaping positive behavior' (p. 9).

Positive subjective experience

This level pertains to positive subjective experiences in the past, present, and future, including research areas such as happiness and subjective well-being (SWB),

 DOI: 10.4324/9781003378426-4

which encompasses how people experience the quality of their lives (Seligman & Csikszentmihalyi, 2000), but can also be seen to include eudaimonic well-being, meaning, purpose and positive psychology interventions (PPIs) that aim to enhance positive subjective experience in individuals. Some of these areas are explored below with reference to health outcomes.

Subjective well-being: tangible benefits of life satisfaction and positive emotions

One of the major breakthroughs of positive psychology is the explicit focus on, understanding of and the study of happiness and well-being. So, what is happiness? How do we define it and what is known about the relationship between happiness and health?

Despite Martin Seligman's PERMA model – representing Engagement, positive Relationships, Meaning, and Accomplishments – being seen as positive psychology's predominant happiness framework in collective imagination, it had attracted considerable critique from scholars (Donaldson et al., 2022; Goodman et al., 2018; Wong & Roy, 2018). Scholars have contended that rather than presenting a comprehensive theory of well-being, PERMA merely assembles components already associated with well-being (Wong & Roy, 2018). Furthermore, they argue that the model lacks theoretical grounding for the selection of these components (Donaldson et al., 2022). Critics also suggest that PERMA does not add any unique variance to wider frameworks of well-being, hence rendering it redundant (Goodman et al., 2018).

Instead, the predominant scientific understanding of happiness is best captured by the construct of SWB. SWB is a broad concept that includes evaluations of both positive and negative emotions, as well as cognitive assessments of life satisfaction. Research has linked increased happiness with improved health outcomes, including lower mortality and decreased risk of cardiovascular disease (Chida & Steptoe, 2008). A significant body of research has demonstrated a link between high SWB and better mental health outcomes, including lower levels of depression, anxiety, and stress. For instance, a study by Keyes (2005) found that individuals who report higher levels of SWB are less likely to suffer from mental illnesses. Ngamaba, Panagioti, and Armitage's 2017 meta-analysis examined the relationship between SWB and health status, establishing a moderate-to-strong association between these variables. This indicates that individuals with better health status generally report higher levels of SWB, and vice versa. Associations between health status and SWB remained largely consistent regardless of whether health status was measured objectively or subjectively, and across samples from both the general population and those with chronic medical conditions. However, this association was notably stronger when SWB was defined in terms of life satisfaction rather than happiness. It was also more pronounced in studies conducted in developing countries compared to those in developed nations.

Positive emotions, another important component of SWB, can help individuals build personal resources and resilience, contributing to better mental health

(Cohn et al., 2009; Fredrickson et al., 2008). Research has indicated that individuals with positive affect often adopt healthier behaviors and have better adherence to medical recommendations (Pressman & Cohen, 2005). Possible mechanisms for the beneficial effects of positive emotions on health outcomes include better immune function, lower inflammation, better sleep, and improved stress response (Steptoe, Dockray, & Wardle, 2009). Interventions focused on promoting positive emotions have been found to increase psychological well-being and reduce depression (Fredrickson, 2001). These strategies have been employed in lifestyle medicine to alleviate chronic disease-related stress, improve patient engagement, and increase overall patient satisfaction (Cohn et al., 2009).

When happiness is not enough: eudaimonic well-being, meaning and purpose

The concept of happiness is multifaceted and complex. Traditional measures of happiness represented by SWB are largely considered to be hedonic, emphasizing pleasure attainment and pain avoidance (Boniwell & Henry, 2007). Yet, many argue that it does not capture the entirety of what it means to be "happy" (Huta & Waterman, 2014).

Eudaimonic well-being, which focuses on the concept of self-realization and living according to one's true self, has been widely studied for its influence on health outcomes. Unlike hedonic well-being, eudaimonic well-being encompasses deeper life satisfaction derived from leading a purposeful and meaningful life. Research, such as that by Ryff et al. (2004), shows a positive correlation between eudaimonic well-being and mental health. Individuals with a higher sense of purpose, personal growth, and self-acceptance report lower levels of depression, anxiety, and psychological distress. People with higher eudaimonic well-being are reported to be more proactive about their health. They tend to engage in healthy behaviors like regular exercise, balanced diet, and routine check-ups, leading to better health outcomes (Henderson et al., 2013).

Despite a large multiplicity of constructs within the notion of eudaimonic well-being (Huta & Waterman, 2014), most researchers agree on meaning and purpose as defining constructs. Research by Steger et al. (2006) found that individuals who perceive their lives as having more purpose report better mental health outcomes, including lower levels of depression and anxiety. A meta-analysis by Hooker et al. (2018) concluded that higher levels of purpose in life are linked to lower levels of psychological distress, including depression and anxiety. Other research has extended this to include physical health outcomes. For instance, a study by Kim et al. (2013) found that older adults who reported having a sense of purpose in life showed a reduced risk of suffering from strokes. Their subsequent research (Kim et al., 2020) also found that having a higher sense of purpose in life is associated with a lower risk of physical health conditions like stroke and heart disease. Czekierda et al. (2017) meta-analysis found significant small to moderate-size associations between the presence of meaning in life and physical health, with stronger associations for subjective health indicators.

A meta-analysis by Cohen et al. (2016) demonstrated that a sense of purpose was associated with both preventive health care behaviors and use of preventive health care services, implying that individuals who perceive their lives as meaningful might be more proactive about maintaining their health. Individuals with a higher sense of purpose have been found to engage in healthier behaviors, such as exercise, good sleep hygiene, and not smoking. This could potentially explain the protective effects on physical health (Czekierda et al., 2017).

Positive psychological interventions and health outcomes

Positive psychology interventions (PPIs) are scientifically supported approaches designed to cultivate positive emotions, behaviors, and cognitions. These interventions are characterized by their focus on positive methodologies and/or the evaluation of positive outcomes. PPIs offer practical and easily implementable methods that can be incorporated into daily routines, allowing individuals to intentionally engage in activities that promote well-being and enhance positive psychological states (Sin & Lyubomirsky, 2009, p. 467). It is difficult to decide whether to position PPIs as part of positive experience, given that they lead to positive subjective outcomes, or at the individual level, given that these are activities that individuals undertake intentionally. PPIs range from simple activities like gratitude expression to complex programmes, and have been found to promote positive feelings and reduce depressive symptoms and stress (Sin & Lyubomirsky, 2009), which is the finding that is nowadays confirmed by nearly 200 meta-analyses and even one mega-analysis (Carr et al., 2023). To aid comprehension and remembering of PPIs Boniwell and Tunariu (2019) has suggested a comprehensive ACTIONS framework that stands for Active, Calming, Thinking, Identity, Optimizing, Nourishing and Social interventions. Carr et al.'s (2023) mega-analysis has also identified four major PPI categories, including mindfulness, mind-body, physical exercise-based interventions and other PPIs, with mind-body PPIs such as yoga judged as particularly effective. Although all of the above categories would have a merit to be considered separately in this chapter, a brief overview of mindfulness and nature-based interventions can serve as illustration of beneficial health outcomes.

Mindfulness meditation

The concept of mindfulness, defined as active, present-focused attention, has been a significant contribution from positive psychology (Kabat-Zinn, 2003). Mindfulness-based interventions like Mindfulness-Based Stress Reduction (MBSR) are demonstrated to be effective in stress and mental health management (Kabat-Zinn, 2003), both in healthy individuals (e.g., Khoury et al., 2015) and individuals with chronic illnesses and even cancer (Gotink et al., 2015; Zhang et al., 2015). Not only multi-component mindfulness interventions have demonstrable impact, stand-alone mindfulness exercises have also been found effective in reducing anxiety and depression (Blanck et al., 2018). Furthermore, mindfulness has been found to be effective in chronic pain management (Cherkin et al., 2016), improved blood pressure and other cardiovascular health indicators (Loucks et al., 2015), improved immune response (Davidson et al., 2003) and better self-care behaviors in chronic conditions such as hypertension and diabetes (Hughes et al., 2013).

Experience of nature

The beneficial effects of nature on human well-being are another breakthrough in positive psychology (Kaplan, 1995). Regular exposure to natural environments can have direct physical and mental health benefits. This includes improved cardiovascular health, lower blood pressure, and increased longevity, reduced rumination and alleviation of symptoms of depression and anxiety (Bratman et al., 2012; Maas et al., 2009). Recognizing these effects, 'green prescriptions' in healthcare have gained popularity, showing a decrease in symptoms of depression and anxiety (Barton & Pretty, 2010).

Using PPIs with patients

Given the evidence behind overall PPIs effectiveness, lifestyle medicine has incorporated PPIs to motivate healthier behaviors, enhance coping skills, and increase medical advice adherence, thereby influencing health outcomes (Proyer et al., 2014). Other health professionals may consider integrating PPIs in their treatment plan. However, in doing so, it is important to consider the specific evidence related to the use of PPIs with patients struggling with acute and chronic health conditions. A review of eight studies by Iddon, Dickson and Unwin (2016) tested the impact of PPIs on individuals with non-malignant chronic pain, indicating improvements in psychological well-being, hope, pain self-efficacy, happiness, and life satisfaction. Additionally, Müller et al. (2016) demonstrated the efficacy of a personalized computer-based PPI in enhancing well-being and reducing pain for individuals dealing with physical disabilities, including spinal cord injury, multiple sclerosis, neuromuscular disease, or post-polio syndrome. A study by Peters et al. (2017) analyzed an internet-based multi-component PPI program, "Happy Despite Pain", and compared it with a CBT intervention in fibromyalgia patients, using a waitlist control group. They observed comparable effects on happiness and depression from both treatments, although neither had an effect on physical disability. A recent study by Kalisch et al. (2022) has looked into the use of PPIs with Ehlers-Danlos Syndromes (EDS) patients. EDS are hereditary conditions that can be chronic and debilitating. EDS patients were divided into three groups: assigned PPI (a five-week on-line program), self-chosen PPI (choosing one's own PPIs to construct a five-week on-line program), and a waitlist control group. Results showed that participants in the self-chosen PPI group reported less fatigue and increased life satisfaction and positive affect compared to the control group after six weeks. This research demonstrated the efficacy of PPI for EDS patients, however only for those individuals who selected their own program contents.

Summary

In summary, positive subjective experience encompasses many areas of research, including happiness, SWB, and eudaimonic well-being. SWB is associated with better mental and physical health outcomes, while eudaimonic well-being, which focuses on meaning and purpose, also seems to contribute to improved health. Positive psychological interventions, such as mindfulness and nature-based experiences, have been found to enhance well-being and have positive effects on mental and physical outcomes. These interventions can be beneficial when integrated into healthcare and treatment plans for individuals with acute and chronic health conditions.

Positive individual traits and characteristics

This level pertains to positive individual traits, such as the capacity for love and work, courage, compassion, resilience, creativity, curiosity, integrity, self-knowledge, moderation, and wisdom. It includes research on character strengths and virtues, but can also be extended to other personality variables deemed "positive". Some of these positive characteristics, such as character strengths, resilience, post-traumatic growth (PTG), positive self-evaluation and balanced time perspective (BTP) will be explored below. Other research areas falling under this level, such as motivational processes, including locus of control, self-regulation and goal setting are considered in Chapter 17 of this volume.

Character strengths and personality

Character strengths and personality traits have been identified as key factors that could potentially influence health outcomes. Broadly speaking, character strengths are positive traits reflected in thoughts, feelings, and behaviors, whereas personality traits are enduring patterns of thoughts, feelings, and behaviors. The "strengths-based approach" in lifestyle medicine allows individuals to leverage their inherent strengths to better manage their health (Proctor et al., 2011). Several studies have linked certain character strengths, such as hope/optimism, and gratitude with better physical and mental health outcomes.

For example, gratitude, or the ability to recognize and appreciate the positive aspects of life, has been associated with lower rates of depression and higher levels of well-being and life satisfaction (Wood, Froh, & Geraghty, 2010). Character strengths of hope, explanatory style and optimism have been extensively examined in the present volume by Martin-Krumm (Chapter 8). Positive psychology's investigation into optimism, characterized by expecting favorable outcomes, reveals that optimists enjoy better health, stronger immune responses, lower risk of cardiovascular disease and longer life spans than pessimists (Boehm & Kubzansky, 2012; Rasmussen et al., 2009; Segerstrom, 2007). Lifestyle medicine has integrated these findings into patient care by offering optimism training to encourage positive visualization and reinforce positive experiences.

It should be noted that character strengths are integral components of individual's personality, although character strengths carry moral connotations, whereas personality traits are seen in a more neutral light. Both character strengths and positive personality traits, however, are connected to the expression of emotions and thoughts and are considered to contribute to an individual's authenticity and moral action (Dametto & Noronha, 2021).

Personality traits, particularly those within the Five Factor Model (extraversion, agreeableness, conscientiousness, neuroticism, and openness), have been examined for their association with health outcomes. Research has consistently found that higher levels of conscientiousness and lower levels of neuroticism are associated with better mental and physical health outcomes, as well as longevity (Kern & Friedman, 2008). For example, conscientious individuals tend to adopt healthier habits, such as regular exercise and balanced diet, and are more likely to follow medical recommendations (Bogg & Roberts, 2004).

Resilience and post-traumatic growth

The study of resilience, a process of effective adaptation to stress or adversity, has been a game-changer in positive psychology. Resilience, or the ability to bounce back from adversity, is one of the most studied character strengths in relation to mental health. Evidence associates resilience with improved health and lower chronic disease risk (Rutter, 2012). Resilience has been associated with a lower risk of depression and anxiety, as well as better recovery from physical illness (Southwick et al., 2014). High resilience levels are associated with lower rates of mental health disorders, including depression and anxiety. It's also linked to faster recovery after experiencing a traumatic event. Emphasizing resilience training has become an integral part of lifestyle medicine, particularly for chronic disease patients, as it boosts their coping skills and life quality (Waugh & Koster, 2015).

The concept of PTG, referring to positive psychological changes that individuals may experience as a result of struggling with highly challenging life circumstances, significantly changed our understanding of trauma nowadays (Tedeschi & Calhoun, 2004). It does not imply that trauma is necessary or beneficial for growth but recognizes that profound personal growth may sometimes occur as a by-product of coping with traumatic experiences. PTG has been found to positively correlate with improved immune system functioning (Bower et al., 2003) and better mental health, specifically lower depression (Helgeson et al., 2006). A recent review by Kunz et al. (2017) found a positive relationship between PTG and lower symptoms of depression in patients with spinal cord injury. These findings have profound implications for lifestyle medicine, particularly in managing patients with traumatic injuries or illnesses, encouraging a focus on growth and transformation alongside recovery (Joseph & Linley, 2010).

Self-evaluation: self-esteem and self-efficacy

Contrary to popular perspectives, the notion of self-esteem has a mixed reputation within the field of contemporary positive psychology. Baumeister et al. (2003) critiqued the popular perspective on self-esteem, arguing that its benefits are often overstated and its negative impacts overlooked and suggesting the lack of strong evidence for a direct causal relationship between high self-esteem and performance outcomes. Furthermore, they questioned the thin line separating healthy self-esteem and harmful narcissism, and proposed that self-esteem is often the result of achievement, not its cause. Baumeister also warned of potential adverse effects from an overemphasis on and over-investment into self-esteem, such as fostering unrealistic expectations, downplaying personal weaknesses, and promoting a tendency to externalize blame. This work implies that self-esteem is an important but complex facet of mental health and personal achievement, requiring careful and nuanced understanding.

Despite these important precautions, a substantial body of research indicates a clear link between self-esteem and health outcomes, with numerous studies suggesting that higher levels of self-esteem are associated with better mental and, in part, physical health outcomes. Low self-esteem appears as a risk factor for mental disorders such as depression and anxiety (Sowislo & Orth, 2013). High self-esteem is also associated with better resilience and coping skills, helping individuals navigate stressful situations more effectively, thereby mitigating the negative impacts of stress on mental health. The relationship between self-esteem and physical health is less direct. High self-esteem appears to be linked to positive health behaviors, such as good sleep hygiene, balanced nutrition, and regular exercise, which, in turn may contribute to better physical health outcomes (Mann et al., 2004).

Let's now turn to another self-evaluation construct. Self-efficacy, as defined by psychologist Albert Bandura (e.g., Bandura et al., 2003), refers to an individual's belief in their capacity to execute the behaviors necessary to achieve specific performance outcomes. It's a crucial component of Bandura's social cognitive theory and is considered a significant determinant of health behavior, health choices, and overall well-being.

Recent research, including meta-analyses, has continued to support the association between high self-efficacy and positive health outcomes. For instance, a meta-analysis by Jiang et al. (2019) found that self-efficacy focused education significantly improves blood sugar level and effective self-management behaviors in diabetic patients. A meta-analysis by Jackson et al. (2014) concluded that pain self-efficacy is associated with lower levels of disability, depression, and pain intensity in chronic pain populations. Self-efficacy has been shown to be a reliable predictor of physical activity, a key aspect of physical health. Significant associations between self-efficacy and physical activity across a range of populations have been demonstrated (Ashford, Edmunds, & French, 2010).

How to increase self-efficacy? Drawing on the established sources of self-efficacy, enhancing self-efficacy involves strategies that bolster the belief in one's capabilities. Crucial approaches include mastery experiences, positive feedback, observing others' successful tasks (vicarious experiences), and social persuasion like verbal encouragement (i.e. encouragement and reassurance). Additionally, managing psychological responses such as stress and mood can contribute to stronger self-efficacy (Maddux, 2002). Focusing on the promotion of recreational physical activity, a meta-analysis by Ashford, Edmunds, and French (2010) concluded that interventions incorporating feedback related to prior individual or others' performance resulted in the most significant levels of self-efficacy, as were vicarious experiences. Conversely, interventions involving persuasion, graduated mastery, and identification of obstacles were associated with lower self-efficacy levels.

Importantly, research seems to suggest that enhanced self-efficacy can lead to increased self-esteem. As people experience success and demonstrate competence – central components of self-efficacy – they are likely to develop a higher self-esteem (Maddux, 2002).

Time perspective

Positive psychology of time is a relatively new but rapidly growing field within positive psychology that focuses on our perspectives towards the past, present, and future and how these perspectives influence our well-being. Time perspective, referring to how individuals mentally categorize experiences into past, present, and future, is a cognitive-motivational construct rather than a conventional personality variable. It is stable yet malleable, influencing decisions and behaviors much like personality traits. However, it can be altered more easily than typical personality traits, positioning it somewhere between stable traits and transient states in terms of its influence on behavior (Zimbardo & Boyd, 1999). An individual's time perspective – that is, their attitudes and beliefs about the past, present, and future – can significantly influence their health-related behaviors and, by extension, their health outcomes. For example, research has shown that individuals with a future-oriented time perspective are more likely to engage in preventative health behaviors such as regular exercise, a balanced diet, and routine medical check-ups, since they are motivated by the future benefits of these actions (Adams & Nettle, 2009; Guthrie et al., 2013). On the other hand, people with a present-oriented time perspective might be more inclined to engage in risky health behaviors, such as smoking, excessive drinking, or unprotected sex, as they place higher value on immediate gratification over future health benefits (Keough, Zimbardo, & Boyd, 1999).

Further, a past-negative time perspective, characterized by a focus on negative or regretful past experiences, has been associated with poorer mental health outcomes, including depression and anxiety (Stolarski, Bitner, & Zimbardo, 2011). Micillo et al. (2022) have carried out a cross-cultural study during the COVID-19 pandemics demonstrating that past negative and present fatalistic perspectives were consistently predictive of anxiety and depression levels in the majority of the nations under study. Also, in many countries, depression was negatively predicted by a positive past orientation.

A BTP has been suggested as an optimal way of thinking about time, where one can flexibly shift among past, present, and future perspectives based on the demands of the present context. BTP is characterized by a moderately high, positive past and future orientation, and a present orientation that is not excessively hedonistic or fatalistic (Boniwell & Zimbardo, 2015). Although relatively little research links BTP with health outcomes, one study found that BTP was associated with more physical activity, possibly because these individuals were more successful in balancing the immediate rewards of relaxation with the future benefits of exercise (Daugherty & Brase, 2010)

Summary

Positive individual traits and characteristics, including character strengths, resilience, and self-evaluation (such as self-esteem and self-efficacy), have been extensively studied in relation to mental and physical health outcomes. These factors have been found to contribute to improved well-being, better coping skills, and positive health behaviors. Understanding and promoting these positive traits can have significant implications for enhancing overall health and promoting a higher quality of life, however, a nuanced understanding of research findings may be important for optimal implementation.

Positive social connections, groups and institutions

The final level concerns the community and includes the study of civic virtues and the institutions that move individuals toward better citizenship: responsibility, nurturance, altruism, civility, moderation, tolerance, and work ethic. It investigates how groups, communities, and societies can support the psychological well-being of their members. In addition to the criticisms addressed in the introduction, the group level can also be seen as potentially too broad in that it is currently unites relational, team, group, organizational, societal and culture-related areas of research.

Positive relationships and love

The role of social connections is thoroughly examined in Chapter 6 of this volume with the focus on child attachment, adult attachment and social support. Available data on the impact of social relationships on health and longevity outcomes suggests their protective role against physical and mental health issues (Santini et al., 2020). For example, it was found that individuals who perceived higher social support had lower inflammation levels, which could reduce the risk of various health conditions. Women generally tend to have larger social networks and engage more in social interactions than men, deriving higher well-being benefits, which could provide them with greater social support in managing stress and adversity (Antonucci & Akiyama, 1987).

Of particular interest to the reader might be a novel conception of love advocated by a prominent positive psychologist Barbara Fredrickson (2013), who views love not as a long-lasting state but rather as micro-moments of positive connection between people. This conceptualization of love extends beyond romantic relationships to include connections with friends, family, and even strangers. Fredrickson and her colleagues have found empirical support for the impact of these micro-moments of love on both psychological and physiological health. For example, experiencing love or positive connection stimulates the release of oxytocin and vagal tone, both of which have wide-ranging impacts on health and well-being (Kok et al., 2013). Oxytocin, known as the "love hormone", is associated with trust and bonding, while vagal tone is linked to the body's capacity to regulate physiological responses, with higher vagal tone linked to better health outcomes. For example, Kok et al. (2013) found that individuals who have positive social connections have better cardiovascular health (as indicated by a healthier profile of heart rate variability).

However, there is a flipside to relationships, with loneliness being strongly associated with heart disease, accelerated ageing, depression, anxiety, and suicidality (Pantell et al., 2013; Valtorta et al., 2016; Xia & Li, 2018).

Positive organizations and workplaces

Positive psychology applications to the workplace include studying how to create positive organizational cultures that promote employee well-being, engagement, and satisfaction. This could involve research into leadership styles, team dynamics, work–life balance, workplace policies, and the physical working environment. Positive psychology breakthroughs in this area include the operationalization of job satisfaction, work engagement, and understanding of their predictor variables or drivers.

Job satisfaction significantly impacts individuals' health outcomes, both mentally and physically. We can go as far as to say that it is crucial for mental health, with consistent findings across various sectors and occupations showing that satisfaction at work correlates with reduced stress, anxiety, and depression levels (Faragher, Cass, & Cooper, 2005). Additionally, physical health is also positively influenced by job satisfaction. Employees expressing greater satisfaction at work report fewer physical issues such as migraines, back pain, and cardiovascular problems. This also extends to improved immune function and generally fewer illnesses (Faragher, Cass, & Cooper, 2005; Gubler, Larkin, & Pierce, 2018). On the other hand, job dissatisfaction is a predictor of earlier retirement and increased health service utilization, indicating an indirect impact on health outcomes (Bültmann et al., 2006).

Work engagement is another significant factor that influences both mental and physical health outcomes. The concept of work engagement refers to a positive, fulfilling work-related state of mind characterized by vigor, dedication, and absorption. Higher levels of work engagement are associated with better mental health outcomes. Engaged workers typically report lower stress levels, less burnout, and fewer symptoms of anxiety and depression (Hakanen, Schaufeli, & Ahola, 2008; Innstrand, Langballe, & Falkum, 2012). Engaged employees report better self-rated health, fewer chronic diseases, and a lower prevalence of sickness absence (Hakanen, & Schaufeli, 2012; Kivimäki et al., 2002; Mazzetti et al, 2023).

However, it's essential to consider that while these correlations exist, the relationship between both job satisfaction and engagement on the one hand and health/mental health outcomes is multifaceted and influenced by multiple factors. This includes work–life balance, leadership style, team dynamics, physical work environment, social support, and individual personality traits (Haar et al., 2014).

Positive education: building well-being and resilience skills as a response to mental health crisis

The mental well-being of children and adolescents has been a crucial concern in recent times. Notably, even prior to the pandemic, research by McCarthy (2019) and Ravens-Sieberer et al. (2020) highlighted the poor mental health status of teenagers globally, with nearly one in three adolescents experiencing anxiety - a condition that worsened in the first year of the pandemic. With the onslaught of COVID-19, reports pointed towards a surge in various psychological issues including depression, anxiety, loneliness, stress, insomnia, and feelings of irritability among this population (Del Ciampo & Del Ciampo, 2021; Jones et al., 2021). A recent longitudinal study by Gotlib et al. (2022) on the neuroanatomical effects of the pandemic on teenagers provides additional cause for concern. Findings suggest that pandemic conditions may be contributing to the premature aging of adolescent brains and triggering changes more typically associated with individuals who are older or have experienced significant adversity during childhood.

Positive education, an educational approach that incorporates well-being and traditional academic learning, focuses on the development of well-being and resilience skills via explicit programmes, a whole-school approach and development of tools that teachers can use sporadically to address emerging classroom needs (Boniwell & Lucciarini, in press). A substantial body of research suggests that positive education and corresponding programs can be beneficial for health outcomes, pointing towards beneficial impact on positive well-being and psychological distress indicators (Boniwell, Osin, & Martinez, 2016; Boniwell et al, 2023; Pluess et al., 2017; Tejada-Gallardo et al., 2020).

Summary

The final level of positive psychology focuses on positive social connections, groups, and institutions. This includes the study of civic virtues, social relationships, love, positive organizations and workplaces, and positive education. Research has shown that social connections and supportive relationships have a protective role in physical and mental health outcomes. Job satisfaction and work engagement are associated with improved mental and physical health in employees, and positive education programs can enhance student well-being and resilience.

Many more areas of positive psychology research and discoveries fall under the third level of inquiry, including positive communities (i.e., community engagement, volunteering, community resilience, and neighborhood characteristics), cultural factors in well-being, cross-cultural positive psychology research, well-being focused public policy and intersection of positive psychology and environmental stewardship that is sometimes referred to as "positive environmental psychology" (pro-environmental attitudes, behaviors, and institutions, as these factors contribute to human well-being and a sustainable planet). While it would have been valuable to scrutinize these research areas through the perspective of health outcomes, space constraints preclude such an examination.

Implications for practice

It's important to note that given its scope, this chapter doesn't provide an exhaustive overview of the broad field of positive psychology, focusing, instead, on brief overviews of a number of selected areas of research. Nevertheless, the areas explored here can serve as a starting point for contemplating potential practical applications.

Based on the ten topic areas examined in this chapter, it's apparent that nearly all studied constructs exhibit a relationship with health outcomes. Crucially, these connections tend to be more pronounced for mental health outcomes and are typically stronger when health status is self-reported rather than objectively measured. This underscores the vital role of individual perceptions in gauging health and well-being. Furthermore, given the largely positive relationships established by research, a special attention needs to be paid to contradictory versus confirmatory information, wherever available.

Despite a large availability of easily accessible models and frameworks, we would urge the practitioners to pay attention to scientifically validated information. For example, the PERMA model unites the definitions and selected predictors of happiness. Conversely, the concept of SWB allows us to differentiate happiness as an outcome from pathways to happiness, typically captured by predictors and correlates of happiness, along with actionable steps that can be embodied by PPIs.

The expanding field of PPIs might seemingly advocate for widespread PPI prescription, considering their potential mental and health benefits. However, a recent study by Kalisch et al. (2022) is intriguing, not only due to its emphasis on allowing patients to choose their interventions autonomously but also because it presents an unexpected lack of significance when comparing "standard" PPI prescription with a control group.

A detailed interpretation of research outcomes is equally vital, as illustrated in the section on self-evaluation. Given the confirmed role of low self-esteem as a risk factor for depression, one might argue that strategies to boost self-esteem could help mitigate the risk of depression onset. However, considering the challenges associated with unstable or inflated self-esteem, research appears to propose that the path to healthy self-esteem is through cultivating self-efficacy.

Finally, positive psychology is designed as an evidence-based science with a strong dependence on measurement and assessment. However, in practice, psychological evaluations often remain inaccessible to many medical and lifestyle medicine practitioners, leading them to depend on intuitive interpretations. To optimize the utility of positive psychological predictors of health outcomes, it's crucial to explore methods that allow practitioners to swiftly and reliably employ a wide range of non-clinical measures associated with positive psychology constructs.

Conclusion

The intersection between positive psychology and lifestyle medicine is constantly evolving, offering an enriched understanding of health and well-being. By integrating these findings, healthcare providers can offer a more comprehensive, evidence-based and patient-centered approach. As research progresses, we anticipate more such enlightening convergences to further enrich lifestyle and general medicine practices.

Takeaways

- Positive psychology is categorized into three primary levels of analysis – subjective, individual, and group – which collectively study positive experiences, traits, and institutions, respectively, to enhance our understanding of human flourishing.
- Nearly all constructs within positive psychology, ranging from SWB to positive relationships, demonstrate a significant correlation with mental and/ or physical health outcomes. Importantly though, a careful examination of available research is essential to derive tangible recommendations for practice.
- In the realm of positive psychology, it's crucial to interpret research outcomes with depth and subtlety, as interventions that prove beneficial in some contexts may not have the same efficacy universally.
- To maximize the benefits of positive psychology in health outcomes, efforts should be made to make psychological assessments more accessible to practitioners. This includes developing methods that allow for swift and reliable application of a wide range of non-clinical measures associated with positive psychology constructs.

Wicked questions

1 How would you integrate the dimension of choice in proposing a PPI or a PPI program to your patients?
2 Prior to reading this chapter, what importance did you attach to the role of self-esteem?

3 Which of your beliefs, if any, were challenged by this chapter?
4 Given the limitations of the three-level framework in positive psychology, what would you suggest instead?

References

Adams, J., & Nettle, D. (2009). Time perspective, personality and smoking, body mass, and physical activity: An empirical study. *British Journal of Health Psychology, 14*(1), 83–105.

Antonucci, T. C., & Akiyama, H. (1987). An examination of sex differences in social support among older men and women. *Sex Roles, 17*(11–12), 737–749.

Ashford, S., Edmunds, J., & French, D. P. (2010). What is the best way to change self-efficacy to promote lifestyle and recreational physical activity? A systematic review with meta-analysis. *British journal of health psychology, 15*(2), 265–288.

Bandura, A., Caprara, G. V., Barbaranelli, C., Gerbino, M., & Pastorelli, C. (2003). Role of affective self-regulatory efficacy in diverse spheres of psychosocial functioning. *Child Development, 74*(3), 769–782.

Barton, J., & Pretty, J. (2010). What is the best dose of nature and green exercise for improving mental health? A multi-study analysis. *Environmental Science & Technology, 44*(10), 3947–3955.

Baumeister, R. F., Campbell, J. D., Krueger, J. I., & Vohs, K. D. (2003). Does high self-esteem cause better performance, interpersonal success, happiness, or healthier lifestyles?. *Psychological Science in the Public Interest, 4*(1), 1–44.

Blanck, P., Perleth, S., Heidenreich, T., Kröger, P., Ditzen, B., Bents, H., & Mander, J. (2018). Effects of mindfulness exercises as stand-alone intervention on symptoms of anxiety and depression: Systematic review and meta-analysis. *Behaviour Research and Therapy, 102,* 25–35.

Boehm, J. K., & Kubzansky, L. D. (2012). The heart's content: the association between positive psychological well-being and cardiovascular health. *Psychological bulletin, 138*(4), 655.

Bogg, T., & Roberts, B. W. (2004). Conscientiousness and health-related behaviors: A meta-analysis of the leading behavioral contributors to mortality. *Psychological Bulletin, 130*(6), 887.

Boniwell, I., & Henry, J. (2007). Developing conceptions of well-being: Advancing subjective, hedonic and eudaimonic theories. *Social Psychology Review, 9*(1), 3–18.

Lucciarini, E., & Boniwell. I. (in press). The Toolbox Approach: towards a novel flexible way of implementing and testing Positive Education. In M. White, F. McCallum & C. Boyle (Eds.) *New Research and Possibilities in Wellbeing Education.* Springer.

Boniwell, I., Osin, E., Kalisch, L., Chabanne, J., & Abou Zaki, L. (2023). SPARK resilience in the workplace: Effectiveness of a brief online resilience intervention during the COVID-19 lockdown. *PloS one, 18*(3), e0271753.

Boniwell, I., Osin, E. N., & Martinez, C. (2016). Teaching happiness at school: Non-randomised controlled mixed-methods feasibility study on the effectiveness of personal well-being lessons. *The Journal of Positive Psychology, 11*(1), 85–98.

Boniwell, I., & Tunariu, A. D. (2019). *Positive psychology: Theory, research and applications.* McGraw-Hill Education (UK).

Boniwell, I., & Zimbardo, P. G. (2015). Balancing time perspective in pursuit of optimal functioning. In S. Joseph (Ed.), *Positive psychology in practice: Promoting human flourishing in work, health, education, and everyday life* (2nd ed., pp. 223–236). Wiley.

Bower, J. E., Kemeny, M. E., Taylor, S. E., & Fahey, J. L. (2003). Finding positive meaning and its association with natural killer cell cytotoxicity among participants in a bereavement-related disclosure intervention. *Annals of Behavioral Medicine, 25*(2), 146–155.

Bratman, G. N., Hamilton, J. P., & Daily, G. C. (2012). The impacts of nature experience on human cognitive function and mental health. *Annals of the New York Academy of Sciences, 1249*(1), 118–136.

Bültmann, U., Rugulies, R., Lund, T., Christensen, K. B., Labriola, M., & Burr, H. (2006). Depressive symptoms and the risk of long-term sickness absence: A prospective study among 4747 employees in Denmark. *Social Psychiatry and Psychiatric Epidemiology, 41*(11), 875–880.

Carr, A., Finneran, L., Boyd, C., Shirey, C., Canning, C., Stafford, O.,... & Burke, T. (2023). The evidence-base for positive psychology interventions: A mega-analysis of meta-analyses. *The Journal of Positive Psychology*, 1–15. DOI: 10.1080/17439760.2023.2168564

Cherkin, D. C., Sherman, K. J., Balderson, B. H., Cook, A. J., Anderson, M. L., Hawkes, R. J., ... & Turner, J. A. (2016). Effect of mindfulness-based stress reduction vs cognitive behavioral therapy or usual care on back pain and functional limitations in adults with chronic low back pain: a randomized clinical trial. *Jama, 315*(12), 1240–1249.

Chida, Y., & Steptoe, A. (2008). Positive psychological well-being and mortality: A quantitative review of prospective observational studies. *Psychosomatic Medicine, 70*(7), 741–756.

Cohen, R., Bavishi, C., & Rozanski, A. (2016). Purpose in life and its relationship to all-cause mortality and cardiovascular events: A meta-analysis. *Psychosomatic Medicine, 78*(2), 122–133.

Cohn, M. A., Fredrickson, B. L., Brown, S. L., Mikels, J. A., & Conway, A. M. (2009). Happiness unpacked: Positive emotions increase life satisfaction by building resilience. *Emotion, 9*(3), 361–368.

Czekierda, K., Banik, A., Park, C. L., & Luszczynska, A. (2017). Meaning in life and physical health: Systematic review and meta-analysis. *Health Psychology Review, 11*(4), 387–418.

Dametto, D. M., & Noronha, A. P. P. (2021). Study between personality traits and character strengths in adolescents. *Current Psychology, 40*, 2067–2072.

Daugherty, J. R., & Brase, G. L. (2010). Taking time to be healthy: Predicting health behaviors with delay discounting and time perspective. *Personality and Individual Differences, 48*(2), 202–207.

Davidson, R. J., Kabat-Zinn, J., Schumacher, J., Rosenkranz, M., Muller, D., Santorelli, S. F., ... & Sheridan, J. F. (2003). Alterations in brain and immune function produced by mindfulness meditation. *Psychosomatic medicine, 65*(4), 564–570.

Del Ciampo, L. A., & Del Ciampo, I. R. (2021). COVID-19 impacts on children's health. *The Einstein Journal of Biology and Medicine, 30*, 20–26.

Diener, E. (2012). Positive psychology: Past, present, and future. In S. J. Lopez & C. R. Snyder (Eds.), *The Oxford handbook of positive psychology* (pp. 6–12). Oxford University Press.

Donaldson, S. I., Van Zyl, L. E., & Donaldson, S. I. (2022). PERMA+4: A framework for work-related wellbeing, performance and positive organizational psychology 2.0. *Frontiers in Psychology, 12*, Article 817244.

Faragher, E. B., Cass, M., & Cooper, C. L. (2005). The relationship between job satisfaction and health: A meta-analysis. *From Stress and Health, 20*(5), 263–278.

Fredrickson, B. L. (2001). The role of positive emotions in positive psychology: The broaden-and-build theory of positive emotions. *American Psychologist, 56*(3), 218–226.

Fredrickson, B. L. (2013). *Love 2.0: How our supreme emotion affects everything we feel, think, do, and become.* Penguin.

Fredrickson, B. L., Cohn, M. A., Coffey, K. A., Pek, J., & Finkel, S. M. (2008). Open hearts build lives: Positive emotions, induced through loving-kindness meditation, build consequential personal resources. *Journal of Personality and Social Psychology, 95*(5), 1045–1062.

Goodman, F. R., Disabato, D. J., Kashdan, T. B., & Kauffman, S. B. (2018). Measuring wellbeing: A comparison of subjective wellbeing and PERMA. *The Journal of Positive Psychology, 13*(4), 321–332.

Gotink, R. A., Chu, P., Busschbach, J. J., Benson, H., Fricchione, G. L., & Hunink, M. M. (2015). Standardised mindfulness-based interventions in healthcare: An overview of systematic reviews and meta-analyses of RCTs. *PloS one, 10*(4), e0124344.

Gotlib, I. H., Miller, J. G., Borchers, L. R., Coury, S. M., Costello, L. A., Garcia, J. M., & Ho, T. C. (2022). Effects of the COVID-19 pandemic on mental health and brain maturation in adolescents: Implications for analyzing longitudinal data. *Biological Psychiatry Global Open Science.* https://www.sciencedirect.com/science/article/pii/S2667174322001422?via%3Dihub

Gubler, T., Larkin, I., & Pierce, L. (2018). Doing well by making well: The impact of corporate wellness programs on employee productivity. *Management Science, 64*(11), 4967–4987.

Guthrie, L. C., Lessl, K., Ochi, O., & Ward, M. M. (2013). Time perspective and smoking, obesity, and exercise in a community sample. *American Journal of Health Behavior, 37*(2), 171–180.

Haar, J. M., Russo, M., Suñe, A., & Ollier-Malaterre, A. (2014). Outcomes of work–life balance on job satisfaction, life satisfaction and mental health: A study across seven cultures. *Journal of Vocational Behavior, 85*(3), 361–373.

Hakanen, J. J., & Schaufeli, W. B. (2012). Do burnout and work engagement predict depressive symptoms and life satisfaction? A three-wave seven-year prospective study. *Journal of Affective Disorders, 141*(2–3), 415–424.

Hakanen, J. J., Schaufeli, W. B., & Ahola, K. (2008). The job demands-resources model: A three-year cross-lagged study of burnout, depression, commitment, and work engagement. *Work & Stress, 22*(3), 224–241.

Helgeson, V. S., Reynolds, K. A., & Tomich, P. L. (2006). A meta-analytic review of benefit finding and growth. *Journal of Consulting and Clinical Psychology, 74*(5), 797–816.

Henderson, L. W., Knight, T., & Richardson, B. (2013). An exploration of the well-being benefits of hedonic and eudaimonic behaviour. *The Journal of Positive Psychology, 8*(4), 322–336.

Hooker, S. A., Masters, K. S., & Park, C. L. (2018). A meaningful life is a healthy life: A conceptual model linking meaning and meaning salience to health. *Review of General Psychology, 22*(1), 11–24.

Hughes, J. W., Fresco, D. M., Myerscough, R., van Dulmen, M. H., Carlson, L. E., & Josephson, R. (2013). Randomized controlled trial of mindfulness-based stress reduction for prehypertension. *Psychosomatic Medicine, 75*(8), 721–728.

Huta, V., & Waterman, A. S. (2014). Eudaimonia and its distinction from hedonia: Developing a classification and terminology for understanding conceptual and operational definitions. *Journal of Happiness Studies, 15*, 1425–1456.

Iddon, J. E., Dickson, J. M., & Unwin, J. (2016). Positive psychological interventions and chronic non-cancer pain: A systematic review of the literature. *International Journal of Applied Positive Psychology, 1*, 133–157.

Innstrand, S. T., Langballe, E. M., & Falkum, E. (2012). Exploring occupational differences in work engagement: A longitudinal study. *Work, 41*(Suppl. 1), 1023–1030.

Jackson, T., Wang, Y., Wang, Y., & Fan, H. (2014). Self-efficacy and chronic pain outcomes: A meta-analytic review. *The Journal of Pain, 15*(8), 800–814.

Jiang, X., Wang, J., Lu, Y., Jiang, H., & Li, M. (2019). Self-efficacy-focused education in persons with diabetes: A systematic review and meta-analysis. *Psychology Research and Behavior Management, 12*, 67–79.

Jones, E. A., Mitra, A. K., & Bhuiyan, A. R. (2021). Impact of COVID-19 on mental health in adolescents: A systematic review. *International Journal of Environmental Research and Public Health, 18*(5), 2470.

Joseph, S., & Linley, P. A. (2010). Positive psychological perspectives on posttraumatic stress: An integrative psychosocial framework. In T. Weiss & R. Berger (Eds.), *Post-traumatic growth and culturally competent practice: Lessons learned from around the globe* (pp. 37–48). Wiley.

Kabat-Zinn, J. (2003). Mindfulness-based interventions in context: Past, present, and future. *Clinical Psychology: Science and Practice, 10*(2), 144–156.

Kalisch, L., Boniwell, I., Osin, E., & Baeza-Velasco, C. (2022). Feeling good despite EDS: The effects of a 5-week online positive psychology programme for Ehlers–Danlos-syndromes patients. *Journal of Contemporary Psychotherapy, 52*(1), 79–87.

Kaplan, S. (1995). The restorative benefits of nature: Toward an integrative framework. *Journal of Environmental Psychology, 15*(3), 169–182.

Keough, K. A., Zimbardo, P. G., & Boyd, J. N. (1999). Who's smoking, drinking, and using drugs? Time perspective as a predictor of substance use. *Basic and Applied Social Psychology, 21*(2), 149–164.

Kern, M. L., & Friedman, H. S. (2008). Do conscientious individuals live longer? A quantitative review. *Health Psychology, 27*(5), 505–512.

Keyes, C. L. (2005). Mental illness and/or mental health? Investigating axioms of the complete state model of health. *Journal of Consulting and Clinical Psychology, 73*(3), 539.

Khoury, B., Sharma, M., Rush, S. E., & Fournier, C. (2015). Mindfulness-based stress reduction for healthy individuals: A meta-analysis. *Journal of Psychosomatic Research, 78*(6), 519–528.

Kim, E. S., Sun, J. K., Park, N., & Peterson, C. (2013). Purpose in life and reduced incidence of stroke in older adults: 'The health and retirement study'. *Journal of Psychosomatic Research, 74*(5), 427–432.

Kim, E. S., Shiba, K., Boehm, J. K., & Kubzansky, L. D. (2020). Sense of purpose in life and five health behaviors in older adults. *Preventive Medicine, 139*, 106172.

Kivimäki, M., Leino-Arjas, P., Luukkonen, R., Riihimäki, H., Vahtera, J., & Kirjonen, J. (2002). Work stress and risk of cardiovascular mortality: Prospective cohort study of industrial employees. *BMJ, 325*(7369), 857.

Kok, B. E., Coffey, K. A., Cohn, M. A., Catalino, L. I., Vacharkulksemsuk, T., Algoe, S. B., Brantley, M., & Fredrickson, B. L. (2013). How positive social connections sustain positive emotions in the face of death. *Psychological Science, 24*(7), 1203–1210.

Kunz, S., Joseph, S., Geyh, S., & Peter, C. (2017). Posttraumatic growth and adjustment to spinal cord injury: Moderated by posttraumatic depreciation? *Psychological Trauma: Theory, Research, Practice, and Policy, 9*(4), 434–444.

Loucks, E. B., Schuman-Olivier, Z., Britton, W. B., Fresco, D. M., Desbordes, G., Brewer, J. A., & Fulwiler, C. (2015). Mindfulness and cardiovascular disease risk: state of the evidence, plausible mechanisms, and theoretical framework. *Current Cardiology Reports, 17*, 1–11.

Maas, J., Verheij, R. A., Groenewegen, P. P., de Vries, S., & Spreeuwenberg, P. (2009). Green space, urbanity, and health: How strong is the relation? *Journal of Epidemiology & Community Health, 60*(7), 587–592.

Maddux, J. E. (2002). Self-efficacy: The power of believing you can. In C. R. Snyder & S. J. Lopez (Eds.), *Handbook of positive psychology* (pp. 277–287). Oxford University Press.

Mann, M., Hosman, C. M., Schaalma, H. P., & De Vries, N. K. (2004). Self-esteem in a broad-spectrum approach for mental health promotion. *Health Education Research, 19*(4), 357–372.

Mazzetti, G., Robledo, E., Vignoli, M., Topa, G., Guglielmi, D., & Schaufeli, W. B. (2023). Work engagement: A meta-analysis using the job demands-resources model. *Psychological Reports, 126*(3), 1069–1107.

McCarthy, P. J. (2019). Positive emotion in sport performance: Current status and future directions. *International Review of Sport and Exercise Psychology, 12*(1), 57–79.

Micillo, L., Rioux, P. A., Mendoza, E., Kübel, S. L., Cellini, N., Van Wassenhove, V., ... & Mioni, G. (2022). Time perspective predicts levels of anxiety and depression during the COVID-19 outbreak: A cross-cultural study. *PLoS One, 17*(9), e0269396.

Müller, R., Gertz, K. J., Molton, I. R., Terrill, A. L., Bombardier, C. H., Ehde, D. M., & Jensen, M. P. (2016). Effects of a tailored positive psychology intervention on well-being and pain in individuals with chronic pain and a physical disability: A feasibility trial. *Clinical Journal of Pain, 32*(1), 32–44.

Ngamaba, K. H., Panagioti, M., & Armitage, C. J. (2017). How strongly related are health status and subjective well-being? Systematic review and meta-analysis. *The European Journal of Public Health, 27*(5), 879–885.

Pantell, M., Rehkopf, D., Jutte, D., Syme, S. L., Balmes, J., & Adler, N. (2013). Social isolation: A predictor of mortality comparable to traditional clinical risk factors. *American Journal of Public Health, 103*(11), 2056–2062

Peters, M. L., Smeets, E., Feijge, M., van Breukelen, G., Andersson, G., Buhrman, M., & Linton, S. J. (2017). Happy despite pain: A randomized controlled trial of an 8-week internet-delivered positive psychology intervention for enhancing well-being in patients with chronic pain. *Clinical Journal of Pain, 33*(11), 962–975.

Pluess, M., Boniwell, I., Hefferon, K., & Tunariu, A. (2017). Preliminary evaluation of a school-based resilience-promoting intervention in a high-risk population: Application of an exploratory two-cohort treatment/control design. *PloS one, 12*(5), e0177191.

Pressman, S. D., & Cohen, S. (2005). Does positive affect influence health?. *Psychological Bulletin, 131*(6), 925.

Proctor, C., Maltby, J., & Linley, P. A. (2011). Strengths use as a predictor of well-being and health-related quality of life. *Journal of Happiness Studies, 12*(1), 153–169.

Proyer, R. T., Gander, F., Wellenzohn, S., & Ruch, W. (2014). Positive psychology interventions in people aged 50–79 years: Long-term effects of placebo-controlled online interventions on well-being and depression. *Aging & Mental Health, 18*(8), 997–1005.

Rasmussen, H. N., Scheier, M. F., & Greenhouse, J. B. (2009). Optimism and physical health: A meta-analytic review. *Annals of Behavioral Medicine, 37*(3), 239–256.

Ravens-Sieberer, U., Kaman, A., Erhart, M., Devine, J., Schlack, R., & Otto, C. (2022). Impact of the COVID-19 pandemic on quality of life and mental health in children and adolescents in Germany. *European Child & Adolescent Psychiatry, 31*(6), 879–889.

Rutter, M. (2012). Resilience as a dynamic concept. *Development and Psychopathology, 24*(2), 335–344.

Ryff, C. D., Singer, B. H., & Dienberg Love, G. (2004). Positive health: connecting well-being with biology. *Philosophical Transactions of the Royal Society of London. Series B: Biological Sciences, 359*(1449), 1383–1394.

Santini, Z. I., Koyanagi, A., Tyrovolas, S., Mason, C., & Haro, J. M. (2020). The association between social relationships and depression: A systematic review. *Journal of Affective Disorders, 260*, 21–33.

Segerstrom, S. C. (2007). Optimism and resources: Effects on each other and on health over 10 years. *Journal of Research in Personality, 41*(4), 772–786.

Seligman, M. E., & Csikszentmihalyi, M. (2000). Positive psychology: An introduction. *American Psychologist, 55*(1), 5–14.

Sin, N. L., & Lyubomirsky, S. (2009). Enhancing well-being and alleviating depressive symptoms with positive psychology interventions: A practice-friendly meta-analysis. *Journal of Clinical Psychology, 65*(5), 467–487.

Southwick, S. M., Bonanno, G. A., Masten, A. S., Panter-Brick, C., & Yehuda, R. (2014). Resilience definitions, theory, and challenges: Interdisciplinary perspectives. *European Journal of Psychotraumatology, 5*(1), 25338.

Sowislo, J. F., & Orth, U. (2013). Does low self-esteem predict depression and anxiety? A meta-analysis of longitudinal studies. *Psychological Bulletin, 139*(1), 213–240.

Steger, M. F., Frazier, P., Oishi, S., & Kaler, M. (2006). The meaning in life question-naire: Assessing the presence of and search for meaning in life. *Journal of Counseling Psychology, 53*(1), 80–93.

Steptoe, A., Dockray, S., & Wardle, J. (2009). Positive affect and psychobiological pro-cesses relevant to health. *Journal of Personality, 77*(6), 1747–1776.

Stolarski, M., Bitner, J., & Zimbardo, P. G. (2011). Time perspective, emotional intel-ligence and discounting of delayed awards. *Time & Society, 20*(3), 346–363.

Tedeschi, R. G., & Calhoun, L. G. (2004). Posttraumatic growth: Conceptual founda-tions and empirical evidence. *Psychological Inquiry, 15*(1), 1–18.

Tejada-Gallardo, C., Blasco-Belled, A., Torrelles-Nadal, C., & Alsinet, C. (2020). Effects of school-based multicomponent positive psychology interventions on well-being and distress in adolescents: A systematic review and meta-analysis. *Journal of Youth and Adolescence, 49*(10), 1943–1960.

Valtorta, N. K., Kanaan, M., Gilbody, S., & Hanratty, B. (2016). Loneliness, social iso-lation and risk of cardiovascular disease in the English longitudinal study of ageing. *European Journal of Preventive Cardiology, 23*(16), 1767–177.

Waugh, C. E., & Koster, E. H. W. (2015). A resilience framework for promoting stable remission from depression. *Clinical Psychology Review, 41*, 49–60.

Wong, P. T. P., & Roy, S. (2018). Critique of positive psychology and positive interven-tions. In N. J. Brown, T. Lomas, & F. J. Eiroa-Orosa (Eds.), *The Routledge interna-tional handbook of critical positive psychology* (1st ed., pp. 142–160). Routledge.

Wood, A. M., Froh, J. J., & Geraghty, A. W. (2010). Gratitude and well-being: A review and theoretical integration. *Clinical Psychology Review, 30*(7), 890–905.

Xia, N., & Li, H. (2018). Loneliness, social isolation, and cardiovascular health. *Antioxi-dants & Redox Signalling, 28*(9), 837–851.

Zhang, M. F., Wen, Y. S., Liu, W. Y., Peng, L. F., Wu, X. D., & Liu, Q. W. (2015). Effectiveness of mindfulness-based therapy for reducing anxiety and depression in patients with cancer: A meta-analysis. *Medicine, 94*(45). https://www.ncbi.nlm.nih.gov/pmc/articles/PMC4912240/

Zimbardo, P. G., & Boyd, J. N. (1999). Putting time in perspective: A valid, reliable individual-differences metric. *Journal of Personality and Social Psychology, 77*(6), 1271.

PART II

Positive health research

It is essential to explore the research, theories and some practice existing in the nexus between positive psychology and lifestyle medicine to understand the rationale underpinning Positive Health practice. With this in mind, in Chapter 4, Prof. Dianne Vella-Brodrick and Dr Annelise Gill from the Centre of Wellbeing Sciences at the University of Melbourne (Australia) delve into the positive psychological concept of wellbeing in the context of physical health. Chapter 5, written by Dorota Weziak-Bialowolska from Jagellonian University (Poland) and the Harvard Institute for Quantitative Social Science (USA), Piotr Bialowolski from Kazminski University (Poland) and the Harvard Institute for Quantitative Social Science and Ryan M. Niemiec from VIA Character Institute (USA), explored the impact of Character Strengths on the body and how they can be applied in the context of lifestyle medicine.

In Chapter 6, we explore the research on relationships, an integral part of positive psychology and one of the pillars of lifestyle medicine. Written by Dr Çağla Sanri and Dr Aaron Jarden from the Centre of Wellbeing Sciences, University of Melbourne (Australia), the chapter delves into positive psychological concepts that can be applied in the Lifestyle Medicine context to improve health, not only psychological wellbeing. In Chapter 7, Dr Trudy Meehan from the Centre for Positive Health Sciences, RCSI University of Medicine and Health Sciences (Ireland) explores the psychological and physiological impact of positive emotions. Chapter 8, authored by Dr Lucy C. Hone from the University of Canterbury (New Zealand), Tiffani Clingin from Liberty Health and Happiness (Australia) and Brigitte Lavoie Founder of LavoieSolutions (Canada) examines the body and mind link in the context of resilience. In Chapter 9, Prof. Charles Martin-Krumm from the University of Lorraine Research Unit

 DOI: 10.4324/9781003378426-5

(France) explores direct and indirect approaches to optimism and their psychological and physiological markers. Finally, in Chapter 10, Dr Pádraic J Dunne from the Centre for Positive Health Sciences, RCSI University of Medicine and Health Sciences (Ireland), examines positive psychology's role in psychobiotics and gut health.

4

FLOURISHING FROM HEAD TO TOE

An interdisciplinary approach

Dianne Vella-Brodrick and Anneliese Gill

In the quest to understand how humans can feel well and function optimally many theories, approaches and models have been presented from scholars and practitioners specialising in a range of disciplines. Naturally, proponents from each discipline have tended to focus primarily on their area of specialisation. For example, those from medicine have focused on the physical state of the body and those from psychology have focused on how our brain and state of mind can function for optimal wellbeing. Although, these specialised perspectives have contributed many valuable insights, they have also led to highly siloed and fragmented approaches to understanding and promoting human health and wellbeing.

Mind-body connection

There are instances where there is a greater acknowledgement that the body can influence the mind (somatopsychic) and the mind can influence the body (psychosomatic); in other words, that the mind and body are inter-connected. This is evident from fields of inquiry such as psychosomatic medicine which emphasises the interplay between psychological and physiological factors in the onset, progression, and treatment of physical illness. Psychosomatic medicine can involve a range of interventions such a medication, psychotherapy, stress management techniques and lifestyle changes.

There are many specific examples of the mind-body connection. One of the most basic examples is the placebo effect. More specifically, peoples' belief in a treatment can lead to real physiological changes, despite them not receiving the actual treatment. Psychological states such as depression, anxiety and anger can also amplify the perceptions of pain while other psychological states can

 DOI: 10.4324/9781003378426-6

decrease pain experiences (Peters, 2015). In other words, pain is not only a consequence of the nociceptive input but it can also be shaped by psychological factors.

Psychoneuroimmunology research examines the ways in which psychosocial factors are related to or can influence the immune system, inflammation, and overall physical health. For example, a review by Pressman and Cohen (2005) found that positive affect is associated with improved immune function, including antibody production and natural killer cell activity. Cohen et al. (2006) found that individuals reporting a positive emotional style were less likely to develop a cold or flu after being exposed to the virus in a laboratory setting. Fancourt and Steptoe et al. (2020) found that individuals who experienced higher levels of eudaimonic wellbeing had lower levels of inflammatory cytokines, which are markers of inflammation that have been linked to a range of chronic diseases. In addition, positive psychological wellbeing, especially optimism, has been linked with higher cardiovascular health as well as restorative health behaviours (Boehm & Kubzansky, 2012).

The gut-brain axis is a well-established connection between the digestive system and the brain. The brain and gut communicate through the vagus nerve, and imbalances in the gut microbiome have been linked to a variety of psychiatric and neurological conditions, such as depression and Parkinson's disease (Foster & McVey Neufeld, 2013; Liang et al., 2018). Psychological stress and emotions can also affect the functioning of the digestive system and contribute to conditions such as irritable bowel syndrome (IBS) and inflammatory bowel disease (IBD).

Various mind–body practices, such as meditation, yoga, and tai chi, have been shown to have physical health benefits. For example, a study by Witek-Janusek et al. (2008) examined the effects of a mindfulness-based stress reduction program on stress and immune function in patients with breast cancer. Results showed that the women who completed the mindfulness program re-established their NK cell activity and cytokine production, and displayed improved coping, quality of life and cortisol levels relative to a control group who demonstrated ongoing reductions in immune function, quality of life and coping. A study by Petrie et al. (2004) found that HIV-infected patients who wrote about positive experiences for 20 minutes a day had higher levels of CD4+ T cells, which help to fight infections, than those who wrote about neutral topics.

Disciplinary silos

Despite such compelling evidence in support of mind body connections, there are still respected disciplines that continue to focus predominantly on the physical and objective aspects of humans or the psychosocial dimensions. Two fields of inquiry – lifestyle medicine and positive psychology – will be examined in this chapter to seek to understand both the strengths and limits of their primary mind or body focus.

Lifestyle medicine

Lifestyle medicine is a medical approach that focuses on preventing, managing and treating chronic diseases by making healthy lifestyle choices. This approach recognises that many of the most common chronic diseases, such as heart disease, type 2 diabetes, obesity, and some forms of cancer, are largely preventable through the adoption of healthy behaviours. Examples of these lifestyle behaviours include; following a healthy diet, engaging in regular physical activity, managing stress, getting enough sleep and avoiding tobacco and excess alcohol consumption. Lifestyle medicine also emphasises the importance of personalised care and a patient-centred approach. Instead of treating only the symptoms of a disease, lifestyle medicine aims to identify the root causes of health problems in order to help patients make sustainable lifestyle changes that will improve their overall health and wellbeing. Lifestyle medicine has been found to be more effective and cost efficient in preventing and reversing a wide range of chronic diseases than traditional medicine alone (McDonald, 2022).

There is a move towards lifestyle medicine practitioners working in interdisciplinary teams to provide more holistic care to patients and include stress management and relationships as key lifestyle areas that warrant attention. In support of this approach physician competencies for prescribing lifestyle medicine have expanded to include positive health components that go beyond traditional risk factors and incorporate activities that promote physical, mental and emotional flourishing. The role of connectedness and positive psychology has recently been recognised as a core competency for lifestyle medicine practitioners and will be used by American Board of Lifestyle Medicine as part of the certification process in this field (Lianov et al, 2022). Within this competency area, lifestyle medicine practitioners are encouraged to explain how lifestyle, positive emotions and flourishing are inter-related. They are expected to integrate positive psychology activities, including social connectedness, in their health behaviour change counselling to promote emotional wellbeing and flourishing.

This is a good sign that future lifestyle medicine practitioners will have a more holistic approach to their practice. However, much of the focus to date, has been on improving health behaviours, such as increasing physical activity, eating nutritious food or reducing alcohol intake. What is often missing is an understanding of the psychological factors such as depression, life satisfaction and optimism, that can play a key role in influencing physical health. For example, depression can negatively affect sleep, which in turn can reduce energy levels and physical activity.

Positive psychology

Positive psychology is a scientific field that studies the positive aspects of human behaviour, such as happiness, wellbeing, positive emotions, and flourishing. It focuses on the strengths and virtues that enable individuals and communities to thrive, rather than solely on pathology and dysfunction. Positive psychology was developed as a response to the traditional focus of psychology on mental illness and disorder. Instead of solely treating mental health problems, positive psychology seeks to understand and promote positive emotions, character strengths and virtues that can enhance people's lives.

Positive Psychology approaches have traditionally overlooked the role of the body in optimal psychological functioning. For example, PERMA (Seligman, 2011) is one of the most influential wellbeing models. It underscores the importance of Positive Emotion, Engagement, Relationships, Meaning, and Accomplishment for human flourishing but it does not include the influence of physical health on wellbeing. However, some proponents of positive psychology, such as Friedman and Kern (2014) and Norrish (2015), have argued that physical health is a significant correlate of psychosocial functioning and should therefore be a core component of flourishing. This has led to the development of models and tools that include a physical component. For example, Geelong Grammar School have added a Positive Health dimension to the PERMA model, which refers to optimal physical and psychological health (Norrish et al., 2013). Similarly, the PERMA Profiler developed by Butler and Kern (2016) includes a Physical Health subscale.

There seems to be growing recognition that more holistic and interdisciplinary approaches to health and wellbeing may lead to more favourable and sustained health and wellbeing outcomes.

Holistic approaches to health and wellbeing

Why is it important to focus on holistic health and wellbeing? There are clear associations between levels of physical activity, physical health, and psychological wellbeing. Positive psychology, for example, is linked to physical health through a range of pathways, including reduced stress, improved immune function, health-promoting behaviours, and increased longevity. By promoting positive emotions and wellbeing, positive psychology can help individuals develop 'mental fitness', physical fitness and embodiment, enabling then to lead healthier and more fulfilling lives.

Mental fitness

The concept of "Mental Fitness" has been used by multiple authors in psychology. For example, Robinson et al. (2015) conducted a Delphi study with a panel of 25 experts to define mental fitness. They defined mental fitness as "the modifiable capacity to utilise resources and skills to flexibly adapt to challenges or advantages, enabling thriving" (p. 53). Four guiding principles were also developed; mental fitness is a positive concept, it is easily understood by the layperson, it is measurable and it can be enhanced through various interventions, similarly to physical fitness. One of the key recommendations was that the development of mental fitness activities could be designed with the intention to simultaneously build mental and physical fitness.

Physical activity

Similarly, being physically fit and active reduces the risk of cardiovascular disease, cancer, obesity, sleep disorders, and depression, and protects against age-related cognitive decline and dementia (Aked et al., 2008; Australian Institute of Health and Welfare, 2018). In addition, participating in physical activity is associated with reduced negative psychological states such as anxiety and enhanced positive emotions, coping mechanisms and self-concept (Aked et al., 2008; Dishman, 1997; Fox, 2000; Hoffmann, 1997).

It is therefore not surprising that being physically active has also been identified as one of the core components of the 'five ways to wellbeing'. This health literacy campaign emerged from the 2008 Mental Capital and Wellbeing project conducted by the UK government as part of its *Foresight* program (Aked et al., 2008). Synthesising research from around the world, the goal was to identify simple everyday actions or behaviours that people of all ages could implement to enhance personal well-being. Five key actions were proposed relating to social relationships (Connect), physical activity (Be Active), awareness (Be Aware), learning (Keep Learning) and giving (Help Others). The messaging around the 'Be Active' theme emphasises the importance of engaging in personally enjoyable physical activities that 'feel good' even if they are slower paced (such as walking or stretching) as opposed to high intensity workouts (Aked et al., 2008). The beauty of this approach is in its simplicity. Individuals can self-determine and activate their own way to wellbeing without having to undertake or engage in any specialised interventions.

Positive psychology and embodiment

From a Positive Psychology perspective, the body could be viewed as fundamental to experiencing and promoting subjective and psychological wellbeing as there are numerous physical mechanisms in addition to physical activity "which assist momentary experiences of pleasure or longer lasting feelings of meaning and self-development" (Hefferon & Boniwell, 2011, p. 176). Encouragingly the field of Positive Psychology is beginning to recognise the importance of addressing the physical and somatic mechanisms of wellbeing in conjunction with the cognitive and emotional dimensions (Hefferon, 2013, 2015). This somatopsychic approach includes a focus on physical health and activity but also encompasses embodiment, that is, understanding how individuals subjectively use, perceive, connect with and relate to their bodies in response to the world around them.

Kate Hefferon is a researcher and psychologist who has conducted extensive research on embodiment. Her work has explored how engaging in physical activity can enhance wellbeing by improving body image, reducing stress, and increasing self-esteem. She has also examined how mindfulness practices, such as meditation, can improve body awareness and decrease negative thoughts and emotions related to body image. A key aspect of her work is understanding how

69

embodiment can be incorporated into psychotherapy and counselling and she has developed an approach called "embodied self-awareness," which involves using physical sensations and movements to help clients connect with their emotions and gain insight into their psychological experiences.

The concept of embodiment is integral to optimal functioning and refers to the subjective felt experience of our own body (Brani et al., 2014). Broadly speaking, thoughts, feelings and behaviour will be mediated by the subjective awareness of and response to changing bodily sensations and states in relation to the environment (Hefferon, 2015; Meier, Schnall, Schwarz, & Bargh, 2012). For example, physiological sensations such as temperature and heart rate, posture, and body language can influence thoughts, emotions, and behaviour, including social interactions (Briñol, Petty, & Wagner, 2009; Vacharkulksemsuk & Fredrickson, 2012). Thus, embodiment theory does not distinguish the mind as being separate to the body, rather, it views all psychological processes as being intricately intertwined with and influenced by the body (Vilvoskaya, 2021). This has important implications for Positive Psychology as it offers a wider perspective from which to promote wellbeing and importantly, one that moves away from a purely cognitive and emotional focus.

Practice

How we understand, care for, position, move, nourish and connect with our body can have a large impact on subjective and psychological wellbeing (Hefferon, 2015). Hefferon's work underscores the importance of incorporating physical experiences and practices into interventions aimed at improving mental health and wellbeing. There are numerous ways in which embodiment principles can be integrated into Positive Psychology and lifestyle medicine practices to promote wellbeing. These include:

Enhancing Body Awareness: Body awareness refers to the ability to notice, acknowledge, and correctly identify body sensations and connect them with appropriate emotions. Although heightened body awareness can be associated with maladaptive functioning, helping individuals to have a better understanding of their bodies' signals and sensations rather than misinterpreting, overlooking or suppressing them is associated with improved subjective and psychological wellbeing (Hefferon, 2013).

Biofeedback: This is a method used to help individuals become aware of their physiological responses so they can learn to control these for improved physical and mental wellbeing. Biofeedback typically involves the use of sensors and instruments that measure physiological responses such as heart rate, muscle tension, skin temperature, and brain waves. The results of these measurements are then used to help individuals develop greater self-awareness and control over their physical and mental responses. Biofeedback has be shown to improve health (e.g., reducing the frequency and intensity of headaches and migraines, insomnia, chronic pain) and psychological wellbeing (e.g., managing stress and anxiety). Given that an individual's level of wellbeing can be made visible through the body's physiological processes, providing individuals with biodata could serve as a powerful wellbeing training tool (Austad & Gendron, 2018).

Human Touch: Increasing interpersonal touch through massage therapy, hugging and reflexology can reduce anxiety and depression, improve physical functioning, enhance feelings of joy, contentment and serenity (subjective wellbeing) and strengthen connections and bonds with significant others (psychological wellbeing: Hefferon & Boniwell, 2011).

Nutrition: Maintaining a healthy diet and body weight can prevent disease and cognitive decline (Hefferon & Boniwell, 2011; Sofi et al., 2008). There are also certain types of foods like bananas, turkey, chocolate and cheese that can increase neurotransmitters (such as serotonin and dopamine) that are linked with lower levels of depression, stress and anxiety and improved mental health, sleep, and the experience of pleasure or subjective wellbeing (Hefferon & Boniwell, 2011). Switching to a diet that is rich in nutrients that support brain function such as the Mediterranean diet, which consists of fish, fruit and vegetables, olive oil, whole grain and legumes, can improve subjective mood (in particular vigour, contentment and alertness) in as little as ten days, while consuming at least seven serves of fruit and vegetables per day has also been found to enhance positive mood states (Blanchflower et al., 2013; McMillan et al., 2011).

Body based interventions: Practices such as body scanning, yoga and progressive muscle relaxation can help people to connect with their bodies reducing muscle tension and anxiety and leading to improved function, awareness, and use of their bodies (Hefferon, 2015).

Dealing with trauma and adversity: Illness or physical trauma can heighten body awareness and lead to post-traumatic growth, a situation in which adverse circumstances can promote psychological wellbeing as individuals are propelled to higher levels of functioning as they learn to adapt to a new set of circumstances (Hefferon, 2012).

Adapting traditional positive psychology interventions: Traditional positive psychology interventions such as 'expressing gratitude' or cultivating strengths tend to have a cognitive focus and are thus quite passive activities. These could be modified to incorporate more corporeal features and/or greater active participation. For example, a gratitude intervention might focus on what the body does well or, character strengths could be cultivated in relation to physical activity (Hefferon, 2015).

There are many suggestions for strengthening what works in positive psychology and lifestyle medicine to create combined perspectives, theories and interventions. As can be evidenced from some of the initial attempts at doing this by Heffron and her colleagues, as well as our own work, there is a growing interest to integrate mind and body work in our understanding of what makes individuals flourish.

Below are some interventions that integrate positive psychology, lifestyle medicine and broader systems approaches.

Integrated practice innovations

- **Mindful walking in nature**

Mindful nature walking is a form of 'meditation in motion' that involves walking in a natural environment, such as a forest or park, with the intention of being present and attentive to the experience of walking and to the natural surroundings. The practice involves cultivating mindfulness, which is the ability to be fully present and engaged in the current moment, without judgment or distraction. The goal of mindful nature walking is to deepen one's connection with nature, reduce stress and anxiety, improve focus and concentration, and promote overall wellbeing.

During mindful nature walking, one pays attention to the sensations in their body as they walk, the movements of their feet and legs, and the flow of their breath. They also observe the sights, sounds, and smells of nature around them, such as the rustling of leaves, the chirping of birds, feeling rain drops on your face and the scent of flowers. It is a simple and accessible practice that can be done alone or in groups. There is evidence to support mindful walking in nature can improve one's level of mindfulness and psychological state (Gotink et al., 2016).

- **Best possible physical self**

The Best Possible Self intervention (BPS) is a positive psychology technique that aims to help individuals envision their ideal future and increase optimism and wellbeing. Results from a systematic review and meta-analysis (Carrillo et al., 2019) found that the Best Possible Self intervention significantly improves wellbeing, optimism and positive affect relative to controls. In addition to promoting positive emotions and wellbeing, the BPS intervention can also increase goal attainment and performance on a task that required persistence and effort (Sheldon & Lyubomirsky, 2006).

This common positive psychology intervention can be modified to focus on the physical self. As an example, individuals are instructed to find a quiet and comfortable place and take a few deep breaths to calm their mind. They can close their eyes and imagine themselves at a future point in time (e.g., five or ten years from now) where everything has gone as well as it possibly could in relation to their physical health. They have accomplished all their physical health goals and aspirations, and you are living their best life. They then visualise the details of this ideal future, including how they feel, where they are, who they are with, and what they are doing. They are asked to use all their senses to make the experience as vivid and real as possible and then to spend about 10–20 minutes recording and going over these details. As they reflect on their vision, they are asked to identify the skills, strengths, and resources that they currently have that will help them achieve their best possible physical self. Next, they are invited to develop an action plan outlining the steps they need to take to make their vision a reality and to break the plan down into smaller, achievable goals and set a timeline for completing each one. Finally, they are encouraged to repeat the visualisation exercise weekly and to track their progress towards their goals.

- **Applying signature strengths to accomplishing lifestyle goals.**

  Signature strengths are the traits that come most naturally to a person and bring them happiness, energy and fulfilment when they use them. These can include character strengths such as creativity, humour, bravery, love and perseverance and honesty.

  Research in positive psychology has found that recognising and utilising one's signature strengths can lead to greater wellbeing and satisfaction in life (Seligman et al., 2005). This is because when individuals use their signature strengths, they are more likely to experience a sense of flow, meaning, and purpose in their daily lives. Taking the time to think about personal signature strengths and how these can be mobilised to accomplish specific lifestyle goals such keeping a food diary (e.g., honesty, self-regulation), or making an effort to connect with others (open-mindedness, love) can be beneficial. The aim is to connect personal strengths with the task at hand to instil hope and confidence in the individual's capacity to accomplish a specific lifestyle goal.

Conclusion

Ultimately, there is a need to ascertain if the combined health and wellbeing approaches are more robust than individual approaches in achieving desired outcomes related to healthy functioning and flourishing. However, it is important to point out that environmental factors also play a key role in health and wellbeing. For example, connecting with nature such as in green or blue spaces can enhance mental health (WHO, 2021) and physical health (Astell-Burt & Feng, 2019). The built environment which can range from having the right temperature, good air quality, functional physical spaces, and recreational and health facilities can influence health and wellbeing (European Environment Agency, 2020). It is important to consider specific strategies relating to making green spaces and parks highly accessible, designing spaces that will promote physical activity such as bike paths and sports fields, and creating safe and comfortable spaces that promote social interaction and community gatherings.

These interdisciplinary approaches at the individual mind, body level, as well as at the systems level, are critical if progress in this direction is to be achieved. Moreover, it is important that we build this mind and body intelligence as part of the core training of health professionals so that working at the intersection of the mind and body becomes the norm and not the exception.

Takeaways

- There is a bi-directional relationship between the mind and body that needs to be fully leveraged for stronger health and wellbeing benefits.

  - The process of flourishing involves more than eating and sleeping well and being physically active. Psychological states such as positive affect, meaning and optimism play an equally important role and need to be considered.
  - There are many lifestyle behaviours that are conducive to psychological wellbeing including regular physical activity, a nutritious diet, quality connections with others, and sufficient high-quality sleep.

- Education that includes feedback from physiological systems and psychological and emotional systems is important. This enables the development of body and mind intelligence that can improve self-managed care.
- Many mind-body interventions are emerging but their outcomes and longer-term impact need further scientific testing.
- An integrated and interdisciplinary approach to training health professionals is paramount to future collaborations and innovations.

Wicked questions

1 Are we asking too much of our health professionals to have extensive competencies in areas related to both the mind and body (e.g., for those in lifestyle medicine to learn about positive psychology)?
2 Which are the key disciplines that need to work well together to enhance healthy lifestyles for all?
3 What is the best way to embed important information regarding the mind-body connection across disciplines or fields of inquiry?
4 What would you suggest as an intervention integrating positive psychology and lifestyle medicine?

References

Aked, J., Marks, N., Cordon, C., & Thompson, S. (2008). *Five ways to wellbeing: The evidence*. New Economic Foundation (NEF).

Astell-Burt, T., & Feng, X. (2019). Association of urban green space with mental health and general health among adults in Australia. *JAMA Network Open, 2*(7), e198209-e198209. https//doi.org/10.1001/jamanetworkopen.2019.8209

Austad, C. S., & Gendron, M. S. (2018). Biofeedback: Using the power of the mind–body connection, technology, and business in psychotherapies of the future. *Professional Psychology: Research and Practice, 49*(4), 264–273. https://doi.org/10.1037/pro0000197

Australian Institute of Health and Welfare (2018). Physical activity across the life stages. Cat. no. PHE 225. Canberra: AIHW.

Blanchflower, D. G., Oswald, A. J., & Stewart-Brown, S. (2013). Is psychological wellbeing linked to the consumption of fruit and vegetables? *Social Indicators Research, 114*, 785–801. https://doi.org/10.1007/s11205-012-0173-y

Boehm, J. K., & Kubzansky, L. D. (2012). The heart's content: The association between positive psychological well-being and cardiovascular health. *Psychological Bulletin, 138*(4), 655–691. https://doi.org/10.1037/a0027448

Brani, O., Hefferon, K., Lomas, T., Ivtzan, I., & Painter, J. (2014). The impact of body awareness on subjective wellbeing: The role of mindfulness. *International Body Psychotherapy Journal, 13*(1), 95–107.

Briñol, P., Petty, R. E., & Wagner, B. (2009). Body posture effects on self-evaluation: A self-validation approach. *European Journal of Social Psychology, 39*(6), 1053–1064. https://doi.org/10.1002/ejsp.607

Butler, J., & Kern, M. L. (2016). The PERMA-profiler: A brief multidimensional measure of flourishing. *International Journal of Wellbeing, 6*, 1–48. https://doi.org/10.5502/ijw.v6i3.526

Carrillo, A., Rubio-Aparicio, M., Molinari, G., Enrique, Á., Sánchez-Meca, J., & Baños, R. M. (2019). Effects of the best possible self intervention: A systematic review and meta-analysis. *PloS one, 14*(9), e0222386. https://doi.org/10.1371/journal.pone.0222386

Cohen, S., Alper, C. M., Doyle, W. J., Treanor, J. J., & Turner, R. B. (2006). Positive emotional style predicts resistance to illness after experimental exposure to rhinovirus or influenza a virus. *Psychosomatic Medicine, 68*(6), 809–815. https://doi.org/10.1097/01.psy.0000245867.92364.3c

Dishman, R. K. (1997). The norepinephrine hypothesis. In W. P. Morgan (Ed.), *Physical activity and mental health* (pp. 199–212). Taylor & Francis.

European Environment Agency (2020). *Healthy environment, healthy lives: How the environment influences health and well being in Europe*, EEA Report No 21/2019, European Environment Agency.

Fancourt, D., & Steptoe, A. (2020). The longitudinal relationship between changes in wellbeing and inflammatory markers: Are associations independent of depression? *Brain, Behavior, and Immunity, 83*, 146–152. https://doi.org/10.1016/j.bbi.2019.10.004

Faulkner, G., Hefferon, K., & Mutrie, N. (2020). Putting positive psychology into motion through physical activity. In S. Joseph (Ed.), *Positive psychology in practice: Promoting human flourishing in work, health, education, and everyday life* (2nd ed., pp. 207–222). Wiley.

Foster, J. A., & McVey Neufeld, K. A. (2013). Gut-brain axis: How the microbiome influences anxiety and depression. *Trends in Neurosciences, 36*(5), 305–312. https://doi.org/10.1016/j.tins.2013.01.005

Fox, K. R. (2000). Self-esteem, self-perceptions and exercise. *International Journal of Sport Psychology, 31*(2), 228–240.

Friedman, H. S., & Kern, M. L. (2014). Personality, well-being, and health. *Annual Review of Psychology, 65*(1), 719–742. https://doi.org/10.1146/annurev-psych-010213-115123

Gotink, R. A., Hermans, K. S. F. M., Geschwind, N., De Nooij, R., De Groot, W. T., & Speckens, A. E. M. (2016). Mindfulness and mood stimulate each other in an upward spiral: A mindful walking intervention using experience sampling. *Mindfulness, 7*(5), 1114–1122. https://doi.org/10.1007/s12671-016-0550-8

Hefferon, K. (2012). Bringing back the body into positive psychology: The theory of corporeal posttraumatic growth in breast cancer survivorship. *Psychology, 3*(12A), 1238–1242. https://doi.org/10.4236/psych.2012.312A183

Hefferon, K. (2013). *Positive psychology and the body: The somatopsychic side to flourishing.* McGraw-Hill.

Hefferon, K. (2015). The role of embodiment in optimal functioning. In S. Joseph (Ed.), *Positive psychology in practice: Promoting human flourishing in work, health, education, and everyday life* (2nd ed., pp. 791–806). Wiley. https://doi.org/10.1002/9781118996874.ch45

Hefferon, K., & Boniwell, I. (2011). *Positive psychology: Theory, research and applications.* McGraw-Hill.

Hoffmann, P. (1997). The endorphin hypothesis. In W. P. Morgan (Ed.), *Physical activity and mental health* (pp. 163–177). Taylor & Francis.

Liang, S., Wu, X., Hu, X., Wang, T., & Jin, F. (2018). Recognizing depression from the microbiota–gut–brain axis. *International Journal of Molecular Sciences, 19*(6), 1592. https://doi.org/10.3390/ijms19061592

Lianov, L. S., Adamson, K., Kelly, J. H, Matthews, S., Palma, M., & Rea, B. L. (2022). Lifestyle medicine core competencies: 2022 update. *American Journal of Lifestyle Medicine, 16*(6), 734–739. https://doi.org/10.3390/ijms19061592

McDonald, A. (2022). Incorporating lifestyle medicine into practice: A prescription for better health. *American Family Physician, 106*(3), 229–230.

McMillan, L., Owen, L., Kras, M., & Scholey, A. (2011). Behavioural effects of a 10-day Mediterranean diet. *Appetite, 56*(1), 143–147. https://doi.org/10.1016/j.appet.2010.11.149

Meier, B. P., Schnall, S., Schwarz, N., & Bargh, J. A. (2012). Embodiment in social psychology. *Topics in Cognitive Science, 4*(4), 705–716. https://doi.org/10.1111/j.1756-8765.2012.01212.x

Norrish, J. M. (2015). *Positive education: The Geelong Grammar School journey.* Oxford University Press.

Norrish, J. M., Williams, P., O'Connor, M., & Robinson, J. (2013). An applied framework for positive education. *International Journal of Wellbeing,* 3(2), 147–161. https://www.internationaljournalofwellbeing.org/index.php/ijow/article/view/250/358

Peters, M. L. (2015). Emotional and cognitive influences on pain experience. *Modern Trends in Pharmacopsychiatry, 30,* 138–152. https://doi.org/10.1159/000435938

Petrie, K. J., Fontanilla, I., Thomas, M. G., Booth, R. J., & Pennebaker, J. W. (2004). Effect of written emotional expression on immune function in patients with human immunodeficiency virus infection: A randomized trial. *Psychosomatic Medicine, 66*(2), 272–275. https://doi.org/10.1097/01.psy.0000116782.49850.d3

Pressman, S. D., & Cohen, S. (2005). Does positive affect influence health? *Psychological Bulletin, 131*(6), 925–971. https://doi.org/10.1037/0033-2909.131.6.925

Robinson, P., Oades, L. G., & Caputi, P. (2015). Conceptualising and measuring mental fitness: A Delphi study. *International Journal of Wellbeing, 5*(1), 53–73. https://doi.org/10.5502/ijw.v5i1.4

Seligman, M. E. P. (2011). *Flourish: A visionary new understanding of happiness and well-being.* Free Press.

Seligman, M., Steen, T., Park, N., & Peterson, C. (2005). Positive psychology progress: Empirical validation of interventions. *The American Psychologist, 60,* 410–421. https://doi.org/10.1037/0003-066X.60.5.410

Sofi, F., Cesari, F., Abbate, R., Gensini, G. F., & Casini, A. (2008). Adherence to Mediterranean diet and health status. Meta-analysis. *British Medical Journal (Clinical Research ed.), 337,* a1344. https://doi.org/10.1136/bmj.a1344

Sheldon, K. M., & Lyubomirsky, S. (2006). Achieving Sustainable Gains in Happiness: Change Your Actions, not Your Circumstances. *Journal of Happiness Studies: An Interdisciplinary Forum on Subjective Well-Being, 7*(1), 55–86. https://doi.org/10.1007/s10902-005-0868-8

Steptoe, A., Wardle, J., & Marmot, M. (2005). Positive affect and markers of inflammation: Discrete positive emotions predict lower levels of inflammatory cytokines. *Brain, Behavior, and Immunity, 19*(4), 345–352. https://doi.org/10.1037/emo0000033

Vacharkulksemsuk, T., & Fredrickson, B. L. (2012). Strangers in sync: Achieving embodied rapport through shared movements. *Journal of Experimental Social Psychology, 48*(1), 399–402. https://doi.org/10.1016/j.jesp.2011.07.015

Vilvoskaya, A. (2021). Science, philosophy, and culture. In M. Walsh. *The body in coaching and training: An introduction to embodied facilitation* (pp. 32–62). Mc Graw Hill.

WHO (2021). *Green and blue spaces and mental health: New evidence and perspectives for action.* Copenhagen: WHO Regional Office for Europe; Licence: CC BY-NC-SA 3.0 IGO.

Witek-Janusek, L., Albuquerque, K., Chroniak, K. R., Chroniak, C., Durazo-Arvizu, R., & Mathews, H. L. (2008). Effect of mindfulness based stress reduction on immune function, quality of life and coping in women newly diagnosed with early stage breast cancer. *Brain, Behavior, and Immunity, 22*(6), 969–981. https://doi.org/10.1016/j.bbi.2008.01.012

5

CHARACTER STRENGTHS AND POSITIVE HEALTH

Dorota Weziak-Bialowolska, Piotr Bialowolski
and Ryan M. Niemiec

Trends in positive psychology and positive health prompted a shift of focus from reducing health risks and preventing ill health to promoting factors that contribute positively to health and well-being (Kubzansky et al., 2018; Seligman, 2008; Seligman et al., 2005). These factors are often referred to as health resources or health assets and have been central elements of salutogenesis and patient-centeredness (Forssén, 2007; Hollnagel & Malterud, 1995; Malterud & Hollnagel, 1997, 1998). Although the idea of salutogenesis and general resistance resources have long been present in the literature (Antonovsky, 1979, 1987, 1996; Lindström & Eriksson, 2005), the majority of public health and epidemiological research has focused predominantly on diseases, risk factors and exposures, rather than on the identification of personal health assets that may have a salutogenic effect on health, longevity and well-being. This has been changing recently, and not only have some scholars become more vocal in suggesting further scrutiny of positive health resources (Seligman, 2008; Seligman et al., 2005; VanderWeele et al., 2020) but also an even larger group of practitioners has become interested in adopting a salutogenic perspective while identifying health resources relevant for their target populations (Cloninger & Cloninger, 2011; Forssén, 2007; Malterud & Hollnagel, 1998). There is growing awareness that without the inclusion of positive health assets, the picture of both the distribution and determinants of health at the population level is likely to be distorted. It has been theoretically argued and empirically demonstrated that these positive health resources can both, positively affect health, and potentially alleviate negative consequences of health risk factors and harmful exposures (Boyle et al., 2009; Peterson & Seligman, 2004; VanderWeele et al., 2020; Weziak-Bialowolska et al., 2022).

The effect sizes of positive health impacts emerging from the research are of comparable magnitude to those observed with conventional risk factors (VanderWeele et al., 2020). However, the underlying mechanisms are

DOI: 10.4324/9781003378426-7

believed to be different than those involved in the prevention of ill health, as there is increasing evidence that the absence of disease does not necessarily imply the presence of good health (Keyes, 2002). A classification of saluto-genic health resources has been proposed (Adler & Matthews, 1994; Brown et al., 2017). This distinguishes between contextual and personal health factors. The former comprise of inter alia environmental factors, charac-teristics of workplace settings, or other social environments. Regarding the latter, among the personal salutogenic health resources, psychosocial and behavioral factors are included. One of the most often examined personal resources is character strengths. Although the science of character strengths in the last 20 years is particularly robust, their study in positive health is more emergent.

Virtues and character strengths

Since antiquity, moral philosophers, religious thinkers, and scholars in gen-eral have argued that acting in accordance with virtue and having an excellent character, reflected in engagement in good deeds and affirmation for integrity and moral behavior, not only may contribute to health and well-being, but are indispensable to attain the state of complete well-being (Aristotle, 2009; Cloninger & Cloninger, 2011). A similar perspective has been recently adopted by positive psychology (Huber et al., 2019; Peterson & Seligman, 2004; Schmidt, 1980; Seligman et al., 2005).

Virtues and character strengths are psychological constructs, with virtues being the higher-order category made up of lower-order character strengths. Virtues are presented as the essential characteristics valued and accentuated by moral philosophers and religious thinkers. Character strengths are defined as positive personality traits comprising moral valence that are fundamental to identity and produce positive outcomes for oneself/others. They are argued to play an important role in both enhancing the impact of positives in life and protecting against adversities (Niemiec, 2018, 2020; Park & Peterson, 2009; Peterson & Seligman, 2004; VanderWeele, 2017).

It should be noted that character strengths and positive personality traits are similar concepts. However, character strengths are associated with moral valence, while personality traits are valued neutrally. Nevertheless, character strengths and positive personality traits are associated with the expression of feelings and thoughts and are believed to contribute to one's goodness reflected in being authentic and consistent with one's strengths, as well as doing good and acting morally (Dametto & Noronha, 2021).

The most popular and most studied, science-based conceptualization of char-acter strengths is the VIA Classification of character strengths and virtues. It is a system of 24 character strengths grouped into six virtues and was the result of cross-cultural studies, analyses across countries, and a review of virtue/strengths texts across time and cultures dating back 2,600 years (Peterson & Seligman, 2004). See Table 5.1 for details

Table 5.1 Classification of virtues and character strengths -
VIA inventory of strengths and virtues

Virtue	Character strength
Wisdom	Creativity
	Curiosity
	Judgement
	Love of learning
	Perspective
Courage	Bravery
	Honesty
	Perseverance
	Zest
Humanity	Kindness
	Love
	Social intelligence
Justice	Fairness
	Leadership
	Teamwork
Temperance	Forgiveness
	Humility
	Prudence
	Self-regulation
Transcendence	Appreciation of beauty & excellence
	Gratitude
	Hope
	Humor
	Spirituality

Assessment of character strengths

The most utilized instrument to measure character strengths is the VIA Inventory of Strengths (VIA-IS, or "VIA Survey"). The VIA-IS measures the 24 character strengths and six virtues (VIA Institute, 2023). This instrument is psychometrically validated and freely available. The assessment has been completed by approximately 27 million people, the questionnaire has been translated into 51 languages, and an assessment is completed by someone in the world every 10 seconds (Niemiec, 2019a). This VIA Classification and VIA Inventory have been widely applied in a range of fields (e.g., business, education, medicine, coaching) and topic areas (e.g., peace studies, happiness, relationships, achievement, resilience) amounting to over 800 peer-reviewed articles as of the end of 2022 (VIA Institute, 2023). Derivative measures used by scientists across the globe are described online and in a technical manual (McGrath, 2019).

Various other instruments designed to measure character strengths and virtues have also been developed. These include (i) the Character Assessment Scale proposed by Schmidt (1980); (ii) the Character Strengths Rating Form by Ruch et al. (2014); (iii) the Applicability of Character Strengths Rating Scales by Harzer and Ruch (2013); (iv) the Temperament and Character Inventory (TCI) by Cloninger et al. (1993, 2011); (v) the Self-Rated Character Strengths; (vi) the Character and Virtue measure by VanderWeele (2017), among others. While some of them [i.e., (ii), (iii), and (v)] used Peterson's and Seligman's (2004) conceptualization, others used different conceptual frameworks. For example, (v) was developed based on studies of personality development, social, cognitive and developmental psychology, as well as neuropharmacological and neurobehavioral studies of learning; (i) drew upon Christian virtues and is morally oriented, similarly (vi), which is also morally oriented, originated from the concept of human flourishing (VanderWeele, 2017) and focuses on one's contribution to the good of oneself and others.

These instruments, despite being different, serve as useful tools not only to examine the character strengths one has oneself, but also to identify those that rank the highest in the character strengths profile of the person. These character strengths are called signature character strengths and are hypothesized to contribute to greater fulfillment, sense of self, identity and authenticity (Peterson & Seligman, 2004)

A distinction should be made between possessing a certain level of character strengths and their use (Wood et al., 2011). These two concepts are still often confused in empirical research. A similar confusion can be found in the notions of strengths and character strengths that are also frequently used interchangeably, despite the former being rather an umbrella term for the latter. Researchers have called for stronger distinctions between different kinds of strengths, namely talents (also called abilities or intelligences), skills (also called competencies), interests (also called passions), resources (also called external supports), and the focus of this chapter, character strengths (Niemiec, 2018). Character strengths are viewed as the core that supports the expression of each of the other categories. For example, one must use tremendous levels of the character strengths of perseverance, self-regulation, hope and prudence in order to operationalize and make substantial progress with one's talent/ability for sport (e.g., tennis) or music (e.g., guitar) (Niemiec & Pearce, 2021). Each of these strength categories warrants its own sophisticated scientific body of knowledge and, in turn, scientific study of the interaction of these strength categories is needed.

Despite this need, specific instruments to measure character strengths use are limited. However, the Strength Use Scale (van Zyl et al., 2021; Wood et al., 2011) and Applicability of Character Strengths Rating Scales (Harzer & Ruch, 2013) have been developed and applied to fill in the void in this area.

Evidence on the well-being and health impacts of character strengths

There is substantial empirical evidence supporting the impact on health and well-being of character strengths-based interventions both in life and at work. These interventions aim to raise awareness and enhance the regular application of character strengths for individual and societal benefits (Ruch et al., 2020). In this regard, previous research has shown that interventions comprising signature character strengths (the strengths occupying the top ranks in the individual's character strengths profile), as well as kindness-based, gratitude-based interventions substantially contribute to greater happiness, life satisfaction, and well-being in general, as well as to the amelioration of depressive symptoms (Curry et al., 2018; Khanna & Singh, 2019; Rowland & Curry, 2019; Schutte & Malouff, 2019; Seligman et al., 2005). The findings of a structured literature review showed that other types of strengths interventions also contribute favorably to well-being, work engagement, personal growth, and favorable group and team outcomes, with the character strength of hope being shown to be a mediator of the relationship between strengths intervention and increased personal growth (Ghielen et al., 2018). These conclusions were also corroborated by a meta-analysis of the effectiveness of positive psychology interventions reporting small to medium effects (lasting up to three months) on well-being, quality of life, depression, anxiety, and stress (Carr et al., 2020).

Although there is agreement on the effectiveness of character strengths-based interventions for health and well-being, the evidence on whether the interventions aiming to increase the level of character strengths or to enhance the more frequent use of strengths-concordant behavior is limited (Ruch et al., 2020). However, there are some indications of the existence of such a mechanism in a short-term perspective (Gander et al., 2021).

In the workplace setting, the application of mindfulness-based strengths practice (MBSP) has been shown to bring about positive effects in terms of task performance and work satisfaction (Pang & Ruch, 2019) as well as numerous other well-being factors over and above mindfulness-alone (Monzani et al., 2021). An application of signature character strengths was found to be associated with subsequent increases in job satisfaction, work engagement, meaning fostered by one's job, and socio-moral climate at work (Harzer & Ruch, 2013; Höge et al., 2020; Huber et al., 2019). In particular, the use of character strengths of fairness, honesty, judgment, and love was found to be beneficial for psychological well-being and work engagement among hospital physicians (Huber et al., 2019). Supervisor support, but not necessarily support from colleagues on a given day, was associated with an increased strength use on the following day (Lavy et al., 2017) and socio-moral climate at work was shown to improve the applicability of signature character strengths even six months later (Höge et al., 2020).

The importance of character strengths for the alleviation of specific diseases has been indicated for the treatment of chronic pain (Graziosi et al., 2020). For patients suffering from chronic illnesses, character strengths-based interventions have been shown to reduce depression, improve self-efficacy and increase psychological well-being (Yan et al., 2020) and, for those with multiple sclerosis and cardiovascular diseases, to improve their quality of life (Huffman et al., 2016; Smedema, 2020). In a study examining the links between fibromyalgia and depression, character strengths were indicated as an important health promoting factor (Hirsch et al., 2020). For patients with chronic health conditions and disabilities, it was found that character strengths moderated the relationship between COVID-19 stress and well-being (Umucu et al., 2021).

Favorable associations have also been identified between character strengths and physical fitness (Proyer et al., 2013), self-reported health conditions (Proyer et al., 2013), self-assessed physical and mental health (Hausler et al., 2017; Weziak-Bialowolska, Bialowolski, et al., 2023; Weziak-Bialowolska, Bialowolski, VanderWeele, et al., 2021), subjective well-being (Dulin & Hill, 2003; Martínez-Martí & Ruch, 2014; Shoshani & Slone, 2013) and human flourishing (Niemiec, 2014, 2020; Schutte & Malouff, 2019). Prior research also documented a prospective association between a tendency to act according to moral standards and ethical behaviors and lower risks of incident cognitive impairment not dementia, depression, lower limitations in mobility, and less difficulty in instrumental activities of daily living among middle-aged and older adults (Bogg & Roberts, 2004; Sutin et al., 2018; Weziak-Bialowolska, Bialowolski, & Niemiec, 2021). In addition, positive longitudinal associations have been reported between living a life according to high moral standards and lower odds of clinically diagnosed depression and between the use of character strengths to help others and reduced odds of clinically diagnosed cardiovascular disease (Weziak-Bialowolska, Lee, et al., 2023).

Character strengths and health behaviors

Prior research showed that various character strengths are favorably associated with positive health behaviors. For example, zest, which is reflected in energy and enthusiasm for life, has been found to be associated with healthy eating and diet quality (Jackson & DiPlacido, 2020; Weziak-Bialowolska, Bialowolski, et al., 2023). Self-regulation - an attitude of discipline and resistance to temptations - has been reported to be associated with exercising, reduced smoking, and limited alcohol consumption (De Boer et al., 2011; Weziak-Bialowolska, Bialowolski, et al., 2023) as well as adherence to chronic disease medications (Wilson et al., 2020).

The character strength of forgiveness was found to be associated with obtaining sufficient sleep and perseverance was associated with healthy exercise (Weziak-Bialowolska, Bialowolski, et al., 2023). Regarding the former, it has been argued that an ability to let go of thoughts and difficulties allows the body and mind to rest. Regarding the latter, the ability to overcome various mental and physical challenges plays a role in maintaining a habit of physical activity. Furthermore, people who scored high on kindness, love of learning, prudence, and self-regulation were found to have a reduced risk of concurrent smoking and drinking, while people who scored high on creativity were found to have a reduced risk of excessive drinking and an increased risk of smoking (Weziak-Bialowolska, Bialowolski, et al., 2023). Since the study used cross-sectional data, it was not explained whether smoking positively affects creativity or the other way around, or whether there is a latent factor contributing to both. To explain the underlaying mechanism, further research is needed.

Optimal use of character strengths

Previous empirical evidence has also indicated that high level and/or application of some character strengths does not necessarily imply positive health effects. For example, prior research conducted on a large sample of individuals from more than 100 countries indicated that the strengths of appreciation of beauty, humor, perseverance, and social intelligence were associated with an increased concurrent risk of smoking and excessive drinking (Weziak-Bialowolska, Bialowolski, et al., 2023). These findings are consistent with research on character strengths imbalances and suboptimal use of character strengths (Niemiec, 2019a). Niemiec (2019a) argued that each character strength can be located on a continuum ranging between too much and too little. Similar arguments apply to the use of strengths. Concepts of underuse and overuse of character strengths were introduced to signal possible conflicts with expected positive outcomes. For example, an overuse of the character strength of judgment, which involves displaying critical and detailed thinking and analysis, is considered as being rigid, cynical, narrow-minded, and lost in one's head (Niemiec, 2019a). Such overuse may contribute to being excessively critical (i.e., judgmental) towards oneself and others, and getting lost in negative vicious cycles of thinking and feeling that characterize common mental disorders. An overuse of kindness, reflected in being overly focused on others and thus neglecting self-care and self-compassion, can make one feel overextended, drained, and compassion fatigued (Niemiec, 2019a; Weziak-Bialowolska, Bialowolski, et al., 2023).

The reasons for overuse and underuse of character strengths are numerous. Practical strategies for the optimal use of character strengths and the management of overuse and underuse include: direct questioning, mindfulness, strengths spotting, eliciting feedback from others, tempering overused strengths, and use of a leading strength to boost an underused one (Niemiec, 2019a).

Mechanisms

Although the associations between character strengths and broadly understood well-being and health are well documented, relatively little is known about the paths through which this impact is transmitted. However, some mechanisms have been proposed on the basis of theoretical considerations and fragmented empirical evidence. Firstly, evolutionary theory suggests that cooperation increases the chances of survival and facilitates adaptation to environmental changes. Cooperation is believed to be facilitated by the application of the character strengths of kindness, generosity and altruistic behaviors in general. The same strengths are also understood to enhance positive and pleasurable emotions which, in turn, lead to greater emotional well-being (Aknin et al., 2013; Lyubomirsky et al., 2005), and are prospectively associated with longevity (Lee et al., 2019; Rozanski et al., 2019). Secondly, neuroimaging data show that the moral decision-making processes and emotions related to moral judgements activate the same part of the human brain – the ventromedial prefrontal cortex (Garrigan et al., 2016; Greene et al., 2001). This implicitly suggests that mental health is likely to be connected to one's reaction when faced with moral dilemmas. Thirdly, specific mechanisms concerning preferences for delayed gratification and consequently decisions made while faced with immediate versus delayed outcomes, have been shown to be related to the application of character strengths. Prior research documented human preferences for present versus delayed gratification (Kirby & Marakovic, 1996) but some evidence indicates positive effects of delayed gratification on positive health outcomes (Weziak-Bialowolska, Lee, et al., 2023) and health related choices (Daugherty & Brase, 2010) including health behaviors (Weziak-Bialowolska, Bialowolski, et al., 2023). If one can refrain from immediate pleasurable, but potentially harmful, activities such as smoking, excessive alcohol intake, or compulsive eating, one may not get instant relief from stress or a craving, but one can expect a healthier outcome later on (e.g., lower risk of a disease such as diabetes, lung cancer, or obesity, among others) (Daugherty & Brase, 2010). It has been argued that the possession of character strengths may not be sufficient to generate positive health outcomes. Such positive outcomes are possible only if these strengths are used in an optimal way and lead to the feeling of accomplishment and meaning (Aristotle, 2009; Seligman & Csikszentmihalyi, 2000).

Conclusion

Although much evidence on the associations between character strengths and health/well-being is available, it is mostly based on cross-sectional data. Some longitudinal evidence is also available, but since it is based on observational (and not experimental) studies, causal interpretations should be formulated with caution. More studies on the causal impacts of character strengths are urgently needed. To this end, intervention studies examining the effects of character strengths and use of character strengths on various pillars of health [conceptualized in the framework of either five pillars of health (Niemiec, 2019b) or six pillars of lifestyle medicine (Frates et al., 2021)] as well as on primary prevention, health promotion, and lifestyle adjustment are pivotal for the future of character strengths and health research. In particular, more evidence on how to increase optimal health (in people who are already relatively healthy) and manage sub-optimal/poor health (such as the various chronic diseases) through character strengths interventions could help develop new tools for individuals and for healthcare policy makers.

Character strengths appear to be a largely untapped set of tools and resources for healthcare. Their deliberate use with physicians, nurses, medical staff, and patients – as well as their integration within existing healthcare structures – holds substantial promise for improving wellness and preventing disease at the individual level, systems level, and societal level.

Takeaways

- The science of character strengths measurement is robust; however, evidence on their health effects is more emergent.
- Character strengths, that is positive personality traits comprising moral valence, are fundamental to one's identity, producing positive outcomes for oneself and others by enhancing the impact of positives in life and protecting against adversities.
- Signature character strengths are the character strengths that rank highest in the character strengths profile of a person.
- Evidence of salutogenic effects of possessing and utilizing character strengths has been on the rise.
- Suboptimal use of character strengths can lead to unfavorable health and well-being outcomes.

Wicked questions

1 In what situations is it more important for a person to deploy a signature strength as opposed to focusing on building up a lower strength in their profile?
2 What are the best interventions that can be used for any of the 24 character strengths and which interventions are unique to each strength?
3 Can a person improve their overall health and manage physical illnesses/diseases and disabilities by optimally expressing their signature strengths regularly across contexts?

Funding

Dorota Weziak-Bialowolska's work has been funded by the Norwegian Financial Mechanism 2014–2021 (UMO-2020/37/K/HS6/02772).

References

Adler, N., & Matthews, K. (1994). Health psychology: Why do some people get sick and some stay well? *Annual Review of Psychology*, 45, 229–259. https://doi.org/10.1146/annurev.ps.45.020194.001305

Aknin, L. B., Dunn, E. W., Helliwell, J. F., Biswas-Diener, R., Nyende, P., Barrington-Leigh, C. P., Burns, J., Kemeza, I., Ashton-James, C. E., & Norton, M. I. (2013). Prosocial spending and well-being: Cross-cultural evidence for a psychological universal. *Journal of Personality and Social Psychology*, 104(4), 635–652. https://doi.org/10.1037/a0031578

Antonovsky, A. (1979). *Health, stress and coping.* Jossey-Bass Inc.

Antonovsky, A. (1987). *Unraveling the mystery of health: How people manage stress and stay well.* Jossey-Bass Inc.

Antonovsky, A. (1996). The salutogenic model as a theory to guide health promotion. *Health Promotion International*, 11(1), 11–18. https://doi.org/10.1093/heapro/11.1.11

Aristotle. (2009). *The Nicomachean Ethics* (W. D. Rose (1877–1971) & L. Brown (eds.)). Oxford University Press.

Bogg, T., & Roberts, B. W. (2004). Conscientiousness and health-related behaviors: A meta-analysis of the leading behavioral contributors to mortality. *Psychological Bulletin*, 130(6), 887–919. https://doi.org/10.1037/0033-2909.130.6.887

Boyle, P. A., Barnes, L. L., Buchman, A. S., & Bennett, D. A. (2009). Purpose in life is associated with mortality among community-dwelling older persons. *Psychosomatic Medicine*, 71(5), 574–579. https://doi.org/10.1097/PSY.0b013e3181a5a7c0

Brown, D. J., Arnold, R., Fletcher, D., & Standage, M. (2017). Human thriving: A conceptual debate and literature review. *European Psychologist*, 22(3), 167–179. https://doi.org/10.1027/1016-9040/a000294

Carr, A., Cullen, K., Keeney, C., Canning, C., Mooney, O., Chinseallaigh, E., & O'Dowd, A. (2020). Effectiveness of positive psychology interventions: A systematic review and meta-analysis. *Journal of Positive Psychology*, 1–21. https://doi.org/10.1080/17439760.2020.1818807

Cloninger, C. R., & Cloninger, K. M. (2011). Person-centered therapeutics. *The International Journal of Person Centered Medicine*, 1(1), 43–52.

Cloninger, C. R., Svrakic, D. M., & Przybeck, T. R. (1993). A psychobiological model for temperament and character. *Archives of General Psychiatry*, 50, 975–990.

Curry, O. S., Rowland, L. A., Van Lissa, C. J., Zlotowitz, S., McAlaney, J., & Whitehouse, H. (2018). Happy to help? A systematic review and meta-analysis of the effects of performing acts of kindness on the well-being of the actor. *Journal of Experimental Social Psychology*, 76, 320–329. https://doi.org/10.1016/j.jesp.2018.02.014

Dametto, D. M., & Noronha, A. P. P. (2021). Study between personality traits and character strengths in adolescents. *Current Psychology*, 40(5), 2067–2072. https://doi.org/10.1007/s12144-019-0146-2

Daugherty, J. R., & Brase, G. L. (2010). Taking time to be healthy: Predicting health behaviors with delay discounting and time perspective. *Personality and Individual Differences*, 48(2), 202–207. https://doi.org/10.1016/j.paid.2009.10.007

De Boer, B. J., Van Hooft, E. J., & Bakker, A. B. (2011). Stop and start control: A distinction within self-control. *European Journal of Personality*, 25, 349–362. https://doi.org/10.1002/per.796

Dulin, P. L., & Hill, R. D. (2003). Relationships between altruistic activity and positive and negative affect among low-income older adult service providers. *Aging and Mental Health*, 7(4), 294–299. https://doi.org/10.1080/1360786031000120697

Forssén, A. S. k. (2007). Humour, beauty, and culture as personal health resources: Experiences of elderly Swedish women. *Scandinavian Journal of Public Health*, 35(3), 228–234. https://doi.org/10.1080/14034940601160680

Frates, B., Bonnet, J. P., Joseph, R., & Peterson, J. A. (2021). *Lifestyle medicine handbook: An introduction to the power of healthy habits*. Healthy Learning.

Gander, F., Wagner, L., Amann, L., & Ruch, W. (2021). What are character strengths good for? A daily diary study on character strengths enactment. *Journal of Positive Psychology*, 17(5), 718–728. https://doi.org/10.1080/17439760.2021.1926532

Garrigan, B., Adlam, A. L. R., & Langdon, P. E. (2016). The neural correlates of moral decision-making: A systematic review and meta-analysis of moral evaluations and response decision judgements. *Brain and Cognition*, 108, 88–97. https://doi.org/10.1016/j.bandc.2016.10.002

Ghielen, S. T. S., van Woerkom, M., & Christina Meyers, M. (2018). Promoting positive outcomes through strengths interventions: A literature review. *Journal of Positive Psychology*, 13(6), 573–585. https://doi.org/10.1080/17439760.2017.1365164

Graziosi, M., Yaden, D. B., Clifton, J. D. W., Mikanik, N., & Niemiec, R. M. (2020). A strengths-based approach to chronic pain. *Journal of Positive Psychology*. https://doi.org/10.1080/17439760.2020.1858337

Greene, J. D., Sommerville, R. B., Nystrom, L. E., Darley, J. M., & Cohen, J. D. (2001). An fMRI investigation of emotional engagement in moral judgment. *Science*, 293, 2105–2108. https://doi.org/10.1126/science.1062872

Harzer, C., & Ruch, W. (2013). The Application of Signature Character Strengths and Positive Experiences at Work. *Journal of Happiness Studies*, 14(3), 965–983. https://doi.org/10.1007/s10902-012-9364-0

Hausler, M., Strecker, C., Huber, A., Brenner, M., Höge, T., & Höfer, S. (2017). Associations between the Application of Signature Character Strengths, Health and Well-being of Health Professionals. *Frontiers in Psychology*, 8(1307), 1–11. https://doi.org/10.3389/fpsyg.2017.01307

Hirsch, J. K., Treaster, M. K., Kaniuka, A. R., Brooks, B. D., Sirois, F. M., Kohls, N., Nöfer, E., Toussaint, L. L., & Offenbächer, M. (2020). Fibromyalgia impact and depressive symptoms: Can perceiving a silver lining make a difference? *Scandinavian Journal of Psychology*, 61, 543–548. https://doi.org/10.1111/sjop.12598

Höge, T., Strecker, C., Hausler, M., Huber, A., & Höfer, S. (2020). Perceived socio-moral climate and the applicability of signature character strengths at work: A study among hospital physicians. *Applied Research in Quality of Life*, 15(2), 463–484. https://doi.org/10.1007/s11482-018-9697-x

Hollnagel, H., & Malterud, K. (1995). Shifting attention from objective risk factors to patients' self-assessed health resources: A clinical model for general practice. *Family Practice*, 12(4), 423–429. https://doi.org/10.1093/fampra/12.4.423

Huber, A., Strecker, C., Hausler, M., Kachel, T., Hoge, T., & Hofer, S. (2020). Possession and applicability of signature character strengths: What is essential for well-being, work engagement, and burnout? *Applied Research Quality Life*, 15, 415–436. https://doi.org/10.1007/s11482-018-9699-8

Huffman, J. C., Millstein, R. A., Mastromauro, C. A., Moore, S. V., Celano, C. M., Bedoya, C. A., Suarez, L., Boehm, J. K., & Januzzi, J. L. (2016). A positive psychology intervention for patients with an acute coronary syndrome: Treatment development and proof-of-concept trial. *Journal of Happiness Studies*, 17, 1985–2006. https://doi.org/10.1007/s10902-015-9681-1

Jackson, C. E., & DiPlacido, J. (2020). Vitality as a mediator between diet quality and subjective wellbeing among college students. *Journal of Happiness Studies*, 21, 1617–1639. https://doi.org/10.1007/s10902-019-00150-6

Keyes, C. L. M. (2002). The mental health continuum: From languishing to flourishing in life. *Journal of Health and Social Behavior*, 43(2), 207–222. https://doi.org/10.2307/3090197

Khanna, P., & Singh, K. (2019). Do all positive psychology exercises work for everyone? Replication of Seligman et al.'s (2005) Interventions among adolescents. *Psychological Studies*, 64(1), 1–10. https://doi.org/10.1007/s12646-019-00477-3

Kirby, K. N., & Marakovic, N. N. (1996). Delay-discounting probabilistic rewards: Rates decrease as amounts increase. *Psychonomic Bulletin and Review*, 3, 100–104.

Kubzansky, L. D., Huffman, J. C., Boehm, J. K., Hernandez, R., Kim, E. S., Koga, H. K., Feig, E. H., Lloyd-Jones, D. M., Seligman, M. E. P., & Labarthe, D. R. (2018). Positive psychological well-being and cardiovascular disease: JACC health promotion series. *Journal of the American College of Cardiology*, 72(12), 1382–1396. https://doi.org/10.1016/j.jacc.2018.07.042

Lavy, S., Littman-Ovadia, H., & Boiman-Meshita, M. (2017). The Wind Beneath My Wings: Effects of Social Support on Daily Use of Character Strengths at Work. *Journal of Career Assessment*, 25(4), 703–714. https://doi.org/10.1177/1069072716665861

Lee, L. O., James, P., Zevon, E. S., Kim, E. S., Trudel-Fitzgerald, C., Spiro, A., Grodstein, F., & Kubzansky, L. D. (2019). Optimism is associated with exceptional longevity in 2 epidemiologic cohorts of men and women. *Proceedings of the National*

Academy of Sciences of the United States of America, 116(37), 18357–18362. https://doi.org/10.1073/pnas.1900712116

Lindström, B., & Eriksson, M. (2005). Salutogenesis. *Journal of Epidemiology and Community Health*, 59(6), 440–442. https://doi.org/10.1136/jech.2005.034777

Lyubomirsky, S., Sheldon, K. M., & Schadke, D. (2005). Pursuing happiness: The architecture of sustainable change. *Review of General Psychology*, 9(2), 111–131.

Malterud, K., & Hollnagel, H. (1997). Women's self-assessed personal health resources. *Scandinavian Journal of Primary Health Care*, 15(4), 163–168. https://doi.org/10.3109/02813439709035021

Malterud, K., & Hollnagel, H. (1998). Talking with women about personal health resources in general practice: Key questions about salutogenesis. *Scandinavian Journal of Primary Health Care*, 16(2), 66–71. https://doi.org/10.1080/028134398750003188

Martínez-Martí, M. L., & Ruch, W. (2014). Character strengths and well-being across the life span: Data from a representative sample of German-speaking adults living in Switzerland. *Frontiers in Psychology*, 5(NOV), 1–10. https://doi.org/10.3389/fpsyg.2014.01253

McGrath, R. E. (2019). *Technical report: The VIA assessment suite for adults: Development and initial evaluation* (rev. ed.). VIA Institute on Character.

Monzani, L., Escartín, J., Ceja, L., & Bakker, A. B. (2021). Blending mindfulness practices and character strengths increases employee well-being: A second-order meta-analysis and a follow-up field experiment. *Human Resource Management Journal*, 31(4), 1025–1062. https://doi.org/10.1111/1748-8583.12360

Niemiec, R. M. (2014). *Mindfulness and character strengths: A practical guide to flourishing*. Hogrefe Publishing.

Niemiec, R. M. (2018). *Character strengths interventions. A field guide for practitioners*. Hofgrefe Publishing.

Niemiec, R. M. (2019a). Finding the golden mean: The overuse, underuse, and optimal use of character strengths. *Counselling Psychology Quarterly*, 32(3–4), 453–471. https://doi.org/10.1080/09515070.2019.1617674

Niemiec, R. M. (2019b). *The strengths-based workbook for stress relief*. New Harbinger.

Niemiec, R. M. (2020). Six functions of character strengths for thriving at times of adversity and opportunity: A theoretical perspective. *Applied Research in Quality of Life*, 15, 551–572. https://doi.org/10.1007/s11482-018-9692-2

Niemiec, R. M., & Pearce, R. (2021). The practice of character strengths: Unifying definitions, principles, and exploration of what's soaring, emerging, and ripe with potential in science and in practice. *Frontiers in Psychology*, 11(January). https://doi.org/10.3389/fpsyg.2020.590220

Pang, D., & Ruch, W. (2019). Fusing character strengths and mindfulness interventions: Benefits for job satisfaction and performance. *Journal of Occupational Health Psychology*, 24(1), 150–162. https://doi.org/10.1037/ocp0000144.supp

Park, N., & Peterson, C. (2009). Character strengths: Research and practice. *Journal of College and Character*, 10(4), 1–10. https://doi.org/10.2202/1940-1639.1042

Peterson, C., & Seligman, M. E. P. (2004). *Character strengths and virtues. A Handbook and Classification*. New York: Oxford University Press; Washington DC: American Psychological Association.

Proyer, R. T., Gander, F., Wellenzohn, S., & Ruch, W. (2013). What good are character strengths beyond subjective well-being? The contribution of the good character on self-reported health-oriented behavior, physical fitness, and the subjective health status. *Journal of Positive Psychology*, 8(3), 222–232. https://doi.org/10.1080/17439760.2013.777767

Rowland, L., & Curry, O. S. (2019). A range of kindness activities boost happiness. *Journal of Social Psychology*, 159(3), 340–343. https://doi.org/10.1080/0022454 5.2018.1469461

Rozanski, A., Bavishi, C., Kubzansky, L. D., & Cohen, R. (2019). Association of optimism with cardiovascular events and all-cause mortality: A systematic review and meta-analysis. *JAMA Network Open*, 2(9), e1912200. https://doi.org/10.1001/jamanetworkopen.2019.12200

Ruch, W., Martínez-Martí, M. L., Proyer, R. T., & Harzer, C. (2014). The Character Strengths Rating Form (CSRF): Development and initial assessment of a 24-item rating scale to assess character strengths. *Personality and Individual Differences*, 68, 53–58. https://doi.org/10.1016/j.paid.2014.03.042

Ruch, W., Niemiec, R. M., McGrath, R. E., Gander, F., & Proyer, R. T. (2020). Character strengths-based interventions: Open questions and ideas for future research. *Journal of Positive Psychology*, 1–5. https://doi.org/10.1080/17439760.2020.1789700

Schmidt, P. F. (1980). The character assessment scale: A new tool for the counselor. *Journal of Pastoral Care*, 34(2), 76–83. https://doi.org/10.1177/002234098003400202

Schutte, N. S., & Malouff, J. M. (2019). The impact of signature character strengths interventions: A meta-analysis. *Journal of Happiness Studies*, 20(4), 1179–1196. https://doi.org/10.1007/s10902-018-9990-2

Seligman, M. E. P. (2008). Positive health. *Applied Psychology*, 57, 3–18. https://doi.org/10.1111/j.1464-0597.2008.00351.x

Seligman, M. E. P., & Csikszentmihalyi, M. (2000). Positive psychology. An introduction. *The American Psychologist*, 55(1), 5–14. https://doi.org/10.1037/0003-066X.55.1.5

Seligman, M. E. P., Steen, T. A., Park, N., & Peterson, C. (2005). Positive psychology progress: Empirical validation of interventions. *The American Psychologist*, 60(5), 410–421. https://doi.org/10.1037/0003-066X.60.5.410

Shoshani, A., & Slone, M. (2013). Middle school transition from the strengths perspective: Young adolescents' character strengths, subjective well-being, and school adjustment. *Journal of Happiness Studies*, 14(4), 1163–1181. https://doi.org/10.1007/s10902-012-9374-y

Smedema, S. M. (2020). An analysis of the relationship of character strengths and quality of life in persons with multiple sclerosis. *Quality of Life Research*, 29, 1259–1270. https://doi.org/10.1007/s11136-019-02397-1

Sutin, A. R., Stephan, Y., & Terracciano, A. (2018). Facets of conscientiousness and risk of dementia. *Psychological Medicine*, 48, 974–982. https://doi.org/10.1017/S0033291717002306

Umucu, E., Tansey, T. N., Brooks, J., & Lee, B. (2021). The protective tole of vharacter dtrengths in COVID-19 dtress and eell-being in individuals with chronic conditions and disabilities: An exploratory study. *Rehabilitation Counseling Bulletin*, 64(2), 67–74. https://doi.org/10.1177/0034355220967093

van Zyl, L. E., Arijs, D., Cole, M. L., Gliśka-Newes, A., Roll, L. C., Rothmann, S., Shankland, R., Stavros, J. M., & Verger, N. B. (2021). The strengths use scale: Psychometric properties, longitudinal invariance and criterion validity. *Frontiers in Psychology*, 12(June), 1–17. https://doi.org/10.3389/fpsyg.2021.676153

VanderWeele, T. J. (2017). On the promotion of human flourishing. *Proceedings of the National Academy of Sciences of the United States of America*, 114(31), 8148–8156. https://doi.org/10.1073/pnas.1702996114

VanderWeele, T. J., Chen, Y., Long, K., Kim, E. S., Trudel-Fitzgerald, C., & Kubzansky, L. D. (2020). Positive epidemiology? *Epidemiology*, 31(2), 189–193. https://doi.org/10.1097/EDE.0000000000001147

VIA Institute. (2023). *What the research says about character strengths*. https://www.viacharacter.org/research/findings

Weziak-Bialowolska, D., Bialowolski, P., Lee, M. T., Chen, Y., VanderWeele, T. J., & McNeely, E. (2022). Prospective associations between social connectedness and mental health. Evidence from a longitudinal survey and health insurance claims data.

International Journal of Public Health, 67, 1604710. https://doi.org/10.3389/ijph.2022.1604710

Weziak-Bialowolska, D., Bialowolski, P., & Niemiec, R. M. (2021). Being good, doing good: The role of honesty and integrity for health. *Social Science & Medicine*, 291, 114494. https://doi.org/10.1016/j.socscimed.2021.114494

Weziak-Bialowolska, D., Bialowolski, P., & Niemiec, R. M. (2023). Character strengths and health-related quality of life in a large international sample. *Journal of Research in Personality*, 103, 104338. https://doi.org/10.1016/j.jrp.2022.104338

Weziak-Bialowolska, D., Bialowolski, P., VanderWeele, T. J., & McNeely, E. (2021). Character strengths involving an orientation to promote good can help your health and well-being. Evidence from two longitudinal studies. *American Journal of Health Promotion*, 35(3), 388–398. https://doi.org/10.1177/0890117120964083

Weziak-Bialowolska, D., Lee, M. T., Bialowolski, P., Chen, Y., VanderWeele, T. J., & McNeely, E. (2023). Prospective associations between strengths of moral character and health. Longitudinal evidence from survey and insurance claims data. *Social Psychiatry and Psychiatric Epidemiology*, 58, 163–176. https://doi.org/10.1007/s00127-022-02344-5

Wilson, T. E., Hennessy, E. A., Falzon, L., Boyd, R., Kronish, I. M., & Birk, J. L. (2020). Effectiveness of interventions targeting self-regulation to improve adherence to chronic disease medications: A meta-review of meta-analyses. *Health Psychology Review*, 14(1), 66–85. https://doi.org/10.1080/17437199.2019.1706615

Wood, A. M., Linley, P. A., Maltby, J., Kashdan, T. B., & Hurling, R. (2011). Using personal and psychological strengths leads to increases in well-being over time: A longitudinal study and the development of the strengths use questionnaire. *Personality and Individual Differences*, 50(1), 15–19. https://doi.org/10.1016/j.paid.2010.08.004

Yan, T., Chan, C. W. H., Chow, K. M., Zheng, W., & Sun, M. (2020). A systematic review of the effects of character strengths-based intervention on the psychological well-being of patients suffering from chronic illnesses. *Journal of Advanced Nursing*, 76, 1567–1580. https://doi.org/10.1111/jan.14356

6

DO OUR RELATIONSHIPS MAKE US HEALTHIER?

Physiological correlates of social connections and close relationships

Çağla Sanri and Aaron Jarden

Good quality relationships are not a typical suggestion we get from a doctor, either to recover from a disease, or to live longer, yet evidence suggests that good relationships are as effective as well-established behavioural factors. Over the last decade, accumulating research indicates that the number and quality of people's relationships have direct implications for their physical health and psychological wellbeing. Such research highlights effects on mortality, with greater effect sizes equating to, or exceeding, those of well-established risk factors, such as alcohol abuse, smoking, lack of exercise, sleep, or a nutritious diet (Berkman et al., 2000; Holt-Lunstad et al., 2010).

In a seminal paper, House and colleagues (1988) reviewed the first epidemiological studies that investigated the link between stronger social ties and greater longevity. Appraising data from five prospective studies, they concluded that greater quality and quantity of social ties predicted longevity, and that lack of good quality relationships constitutes a major risk factor for physical health, rivalling the effects of well-established risk factors such as smoking, high blood pressure, obesity, and physical inactivity. More recently, Holt-Lunstad and colleagues (2010) supported these claims in a meta-analysis of 148 studies, involving over 300,000+ participants, indicating that people with stronger social bonds have greater longevity. Our relationships and interactions with others alter how we think, feel, and behave, and consequently, these changes have physiological impacts, including changes in endocrine, cardiovascular, and immune system functioning (Kiecolt-Glaser, 2018). In this chapter, we outline and describe the theories, mechanisms, and relationship processes to understand the links between positive health and personal relationships. We start this journey with attachment theory.

DOI: 10.4324/9781003378426-8

Attachment theory

There are theoretical reasons as to why relationships are important for physical health. According to Attachment Theory, connecting socially is a universal biological need (Bowlby, 1969). This theory was influenced by earlier work showing that attachment among animals, including rhesus monkeys (Harlow, 1959), was an innate tendency. Harlow (1959) observed that young rhesus monkeys had a need for physical contact that was as strong as biological needs such as thirst or hunger. Bowlby (1969) extended this observation to humans arguing that there is an innate tendency to form a secure attachment to a primary attachment figure in all humans, which has an evolutionary value for survival. When left alone, human infants tend to require proximity and display signs of distress, which in turn draws the attention of caregivers to the needs of vulnerable infants (Ainsworth et al., 1978).

Based on the responsiveness of the caregiver to an infant, humans tend to develop an attachment orientation; of which there are four types – secure, anxious, avoidant, or fearful. An anxious or avoidant attachment orientation develops when infants receive a pattern of inconsistent care from their attachment figure, and they become unsure regarding the availability of their caregiver (Ainsworth et al., 1978). Unmet needs for social bonding and acceptance early in life cause bonding systems to develop abnormally, and lead to social dysfunction later in life (Pedersen, 2004). Early family environment is therefore a key source for learning about emotion regulation, and parents who are responsive and empathetic play a critical role in their children's ability for emotion regulation (Eisenberg et al., 1996; Morris et al., 2017). Maternal responsiveness leads to changes in the functioning of the body's major emotion-regulation system, the hypothalamic-pituitary-adrenocortical (HPA) axis, and its hormonal product cortisol, during childhood (Gunnar & Quevedo, 2008). Experimental research with rats, for example, shows that greater maternal early caregiving behaviours lead to less fearful behavioural responding, and less HPA responding, than rat pups with lower early caregiving (Liu et al., 1997).

Adult attachment

Given that better emotion regulation is associated with secure attachment in infancy and adolescence (Gilliom et al., 2002; Kobak & Sceery, 1988), is it possible to change our attachment orientation and the long-term fine-tuning of the HPA system in adulthood? Fortunately for those with less responsive caregivers, and even though attachment orientations develop in infancy, attachment orientations are continually shaped through later relationship experiences (typically with romantic partners in adulthood) informing cognition, affect, and behaviour across the life span (Shaver & Mikulincer, 2002). A longitudinal study on couples found that partner responsiveness predicted steeper declines in daytime cortisol a decade later (Slatcher et al., 2015), suggesting that adult romantic relationships lead to long-term changes in the HPA axis.

Individuals are known to vary along two dimensions of attachment insecurity: Anxiety and avoidance (Shaver & Mikulincer, 2002). People high in attachment anxiety need higher reassurance that their attachment figures love them and will stay with them. Such individuals tend to perceive relationship situations as more threatening than they truly are and ruminate on negative interactions. Alternatively, people high in attachment avoidance tend to be resistant to emotional intimacy and to being vulnerable, thus engaging in self-reliant deactivating strategies in which they minimize or suppress their emotional experiences. Secure individuals, who score low on both dimensions, typically display the most constructive relationship behaviours (Mikulincer et al., 2003). Individual differences in attachment anxiety and avoidance involve relative predispositions to engage in specific emotion-regulatory strategies (Mikulincer & Shaver, 2019) which influence how effectively individuals seek support in relationships (Ehrlich et al., 2016). Higher attachment anxiety is correlated with greater affect reactivity, which explains increased general negativity and interpersonal problems often experienced by anxiously attached individuals (Mikulincer & Shaver, 2019). Both attachment insecurities (high anxiety, high avoidance) increase the likelihood of later physical health problems (Pietromonaco & Beck, 2019). We now turn from attachment to the area of social support.

Social support

Social support refers to being part of a reciprocally supportive network in which one is loved, cared for, and esteemed (Cassel, 1976; Cobb, 1976). The importance of social support resources is not only emphasized for managing stressful life events (Seeman, 1996), but also as a protective factor for better health outcomes. For over four decades, social support has been known to modify health-relevant bodily processes, such as blood pressure and endocrine activity, as well as potentially pathogenic effects of stress (Cassel, 1976; Cobb, 1976).

Regular social contact is associated with reduced stress reactivity via modulating long-term physiological and neural reactivity to social threat. Using functional magnetic resonance imaging (fMRI), Eisenberger and colleagues (2007) assessed participants' neurocognitive reactivity to a social stressor. They found that participants who had regular interactions with supportive individuals across a ten-day period showed reduced cortisol reactivity to a social stressor. More specifically, regular social support was associated with diminished activity in the brain regions whose activity has previously been tied to social distress, including the dorsal anterior cingulate cortex (dACC) and Brodmann Area 8. These neuroendocrine processes were shown to mediate the pathway between social support and cortisol reactivity in response to stressful events (Eisenberger et al., 2007). Relatedly, the progression of cardiovascular diseases is also associated with low-quality social support (Barth, Schneider, & von Kanel, 2010) as well as social isolation (Heffner, Waring, Roberts, Eaton, & Gramling, 2011).

In summary, we can see from the above that both attachment styles and social support have direct impacts on physiological functioning. We now turn to more direct application of these theories.

Practice

Mechanisms linking relationships and health

Since hormones and neurotransmitters significantly alter cardiovascular and immune functioning, neuroendocrine functioning is an important mediator to understand the connection between relationships and health. Hormones travel in the bloodstream and are picked up by receptors all over the body, with their effects often relatively slow and long lasting. Neurotransmitters, on the other hand, are released in the brain into synapses, and produce fast responses linked to activity in specific brain regions (Fletcher et al., 2019). Some substances, like oxytocin or epinephrine, can be either hormones or neurotransmitters, but because of the blood–brain barrier they exert their effects differently either in the brain or the body, depending on where they are released.

During times of stress, the body goes into a fight or flight response, which triggers changes in the cardiovascular and endocrine system. The body releases the catecholamines epinephrine and norepinephrine, involving the release of corticosteroids including cortisol (Taylor, 2006). These changes release more stored glucose which has the effect of suppressing the immune system (Fletcher et al., 2019). These responses mobilize the body to meet the demands of pressing situations and are critical to provide protection against stressful situations. For example, exposed to a snake in the wild, we have a higher chance of survival if we stop everything else and focus on escaping the immediate danger. However, chronic or recurrent activation of the sympathetic nervous system of repeated stress is associated with detrimental long-term health effects (Uchino et al., 1996). Excessive discharge of epinephrine or norepinephrine, as a result of repeated stress, leads to a weaker immune system, development of hypertension and coronary artery disease, and neurochemical imbalances that may also lead to psychiatric disorders (Herbert & Cohen, 1993; Seeman et al., 2001).

The HPA axis is a crucial component of the neuroendocrine system that is involved in stress regulation, as well as regulating metabolism, immunity, and digestion (Carter et al, 2003; Coan et al., 2006). The body and brain work together using the HPA axis to regulate these hormones in stressful times, and our social relationships have a big impact on the functioning of HPA (Meaney, 2001). Comforting a distressed individual reduces the activation of the HPA axis, which is a core attachment process (Coan, 2008; Meaney, 2001). Even though there are many factors influencing stress regulation (e.g., individual differences in personality, knowledge, experience), one of the most consistent influences of stress regulation is the quality and quantity of our relationships (Cacioppo et al., 2015; Fletcher et al., 2019).

Relationship quality

Social support theory suggests that loneliness and social isolation can have detrimental health effects (Cacioppo & Patrick, 2008). However, simply having a relationship is not enough, as negative interactions can do harm. Distressed relationships are shown to deplete the self-regulatory resources needed to engage in more effortful health-enhancing behaviours. For example, poor social support is associated with excessive alcohol consumption (Peirce et al., 2000), and marital distress increases the risk of smoking behaviours (Bourassa et al., 2019). Distressed relationships with high levels of conflict and hostility use up self-regulatory resources that are needed to commit good health behaviours (Smith et al., 2011).

Researchers have argued that both positive and negative intense emotions happen most frequently in the context of ongoing close relationships, such as romantic relationships, parent–child, and close friendships (Berscheid & Ammazzalorso, 2004). Close relationships, such as during infancy and while mating, are associated with significant hormonal and physiological changes (Maroun & Wagner, 2016). Close relationships, therefore, have an outsized impact on health, and investigating the quality of these relationships informs us about the psychological processes by which relationships are linked to physical health.

Relationship processes

Some specific relationship processes have a higher impact on physical health than others. For example, interpersonal conflict is among the most common and disturbing daily stressor individuals encounter (Bolger et al., 1989). People who have persistent conflicts with family or friends are more likely to contract colds (Cohen et al., 1998), and people in distressed romantic relationships are more likely to become ill (Wickrama et al., 1997). Particularly relationship conflict with a romantic partner can significantly undermine health (Kiecolt-Glaser et al., 1993). For example, criticism from a partner was found to produce poorer cognitive functioning among people suffering from Alzheimer's type dementia (Vitaliano et al., 1993). Greater hostility during conflict between romantic partners is associated with greater blood pressure reactivity (Miller et al., 1999), slower wound healing, and greater production of pro-inflammatory cytokines (Kiecolt-Glaser et al., 2005). Longitudinal studies show that relationship-elicited negative emotions can have lasting effects. For example, Haase and colleagues (2016) found that hostility during conflict discussions with a romantic partner predicted cardiovascular and musculoskeletal complications 20 years later.

Although most research has investigated the detrimental effects of negative interactions and stress buffering effects in relationships, more recent research has investigated the effects of positive interactions. Affiliation processes within close relationships, such as disclosing thoughts and feelings, and providing/receiving social support, help relieve anxiety and reduce negative affect (Jakubiak & Feeney, 2017). Greater perceived partner responsiveness predicts healthier cortisol profiles (Slatcher et al., 2015) and lower mortality risk (Stanton et al., 2019). Positive and supportive couple interactions predict better cardiovascular health on a daily basis (e.g., lower cortisol and blood pressure; Gump et al., 2001; Holt-Lunstad et al., 2003). Experimental laboratory-based studies show supportive couple interactions buffer the psychophysiological effects of stressors (Ditzen et al., 2007; Grewen et al., 2003). For example, verbal expressions of social support or warm touch with a partner buffers stress responses (Holt-Lunstad et al., 2008), create more appropriate conditions to foster immunological response and healing (Gouin et al., 2010), and increases pain tolerance (Cano & Williams, 2010). These positive health effects are specific to interactions with an intimate partner. Coan and colleagues (2006) found that wives in satisfied marriages had higher resilience for a physical threat while holding their partners' hand, compared to participants in a no handholding condition or those holding a stranger's hand. Individuals in a couple relationship with high relationship satisfaction have lower threat-related neural activation than those in less satisfying relationships (Coan et al., 2006).

Perception of higher partner support has been associated with higher oxytocin levels (Grewen et al., 2005), which is also associated with better stress regulation and cardiovascular functioning. Oxytocin is a key neuroendocrine hormone that plays a crucial role in social bonding, both in mating and in infant–caregiver behaviours, that has benefits for physical health (Vargas-Martínez et al., 2014). Higher physical affection among couples, such as hugging or kissing, which is also known to increase oxytocin, predicted lower cortisol levels over a one-week period (Ditzen et al., 2008). Affectionate touch within the context of a close relationship influences several physiological mechanisms, including the HPA axis (Ditzen et al., 2007), neural functioning (Coan et al., 2006), as well as activation of autonomic pathways (Grewen et al., 2003). Technological developments and globalisation have dramatically changed the way in which people interact (Sanri & Goodwin, 2014) and made it possible to have interactions without physical contact. There is ongoing research on whether online interactions have equivalent or other unique benefits compared to face-to-face interactions.

Towards a more nuanced understanding of relationship quality

Although different relationship interactions are likely to lead to different outcomes, what constitutes positive and negative processes in relationships might vary by context. For example, McNulty and Russell (2010) investigated the long-term effects of a range of negative behaviours. They found that in the context of relationships and when facing minor problems, spouses' tendencies to blame, command, and reject their partners predicted sharp declines in their relationship satisfaction. However, the same behaviours benefited relationship satisfaction in the long term for relationships facing more serious problems, as some negative behaviours such as criticism can motivate partners to change their behaviours (McNulty & Russell, 2010; Overall et al., 2009).

On the other hand, seemingly positive interactions may not lead to positive outcomes if enacted with the wrong intent. For example, daily experience studies have shown that on days when individuals made sacrifices or engaged in sexual activity for approach goals, they reported greater feelings of satisfaction, but on days when they did so for avoidance goals, they reported less relationship satisfaction (Impett et al., 2005). More specifically, a partner engaging in sex to avoid disappointing their partner (an avoidance motive) may not feel as close and satisfied in the relationship as a partner who initiates sex with a desire to be close to their partner (an approach motive; Impett et al., 2005). We therefore need a more nuanced understanding of relationship quality.

Relationship flourishing and positive health

A recurrent observation of research on couple's relationship quality is that it has focused on factors differentiating distressed and satisfying relationships without attention to what might make for a truly positive relationship (Fincham & Beach, 2010). For example, focus of research has been on the negative aspects of couple's interactions, such as conflict and inter-partner violence, and how they relate to satisfaction or distress (e.g., Bradbury et al., 2012; Halford et al., 2010). These are important topics that inform conceptualisation of satisfying relationships, and provide guidelines for couple therapy to address relationship distress (Halford & Snyder, 2012). However, these topics do not necessarily inform what might constitute a flourishing relationship.

Relatedly, most research has looked into the link between satisfied relationships and their stress buffering effects on relationships. Yet a deeper understanding of high quality, flourishing relationships would give us a more complete understanding of the link between physical health and relationships, potentially uncovering whether being in a flourishing relationship generates positive outcomes beyond those attributable to being in a satisfying relationship.

To move beyond satisfying relationships, we need to develop a better understanding of high functioning, *flourishing relationships*. Relationship satisfaction is usually defined as a partners' global evaluation of their intimate relationship, and the content of measures of satisfaction typically focus on the absence of behaviours associated with distress in the relationship, such as conflict and negative feelings between the couple (e.g. Funk & Rogge, 2007; Spanier, 1976). Adapting a positive psychology approach and drawing from the theories of individual flourishing, Sanri (2018) conceptualised flourishing relationships as a combination of both hedonic and eudamonic elements, including high positive affect, self-growth within a relationship, partner compassion, and shared meaning.

Relationship flourishing, assessed by the Couple Flourishing Measure (CFM; Sanri et at., 2021, Sanri, 2018) was associated with individual wellbeing, including vitality, positive affect, and individual flourishing above and beyond relationship satisfaction. These findings support the potential value of relationship flourishing beyond relationship satisfaction in individual wellbeing. High positive affect and individual flourishing predict longevity and better health

(Chida & Steptoe, 2008; Cohen et al., 2016; Diener & Chan, 2011), hence a better understanding of flourishing relationships can unpack a wider potential of relationships for positive health.

Although more research is needed given there is not much on the link between flourishing relationships and health, it may well be the case that individuals in flourishing relationship benefit physiologically much more so than those in satisfied relationships. Based on the above review, and drawing from this evidence base, it could be hypothesized that flourishing relationships may positively improve the HPA axis (thus lowering cortisol), lower blood pressure, improve endocrine activity, increase optimal brain functioning (e.g., decreased dACC, and Brodmann Area 8 activity), and lower cardiovascular diseases. Additionally, flourishing relationships may improve immune functioning (e.g., less discharge of epinephrine or norepinephrine), less development of hypertension and coronary artery disease, lower production of pro-inflammatory cytokines, and aid in faster wound healing. Aspects such as these, and the degree of impact of each, are yet to be tested with regard to flourishing relationships in particular, and hold promise based on the above review.

Takeaways

General

- Social relationships have an equal or greater impact on longevity then risk factors such as stopping smoking or physical inactivity.
- Improvement in relationship quality can play a role in addressing negative physical health states.
- Inquiring about social relationships of all kinds can provide valuable information in a case formulation for a physical health problem.

Practical

- Learn more about the developing field of Positive Health.
- Consider psychological and psychosocial interventions in treatment formulations of physical health problems.
- Inquiring about social relationships of all kinds can provide valuable information in a case formulation for a physical health problem.

Wicked questions

1 To what degree can improved or flourishing relationships be a 'treatment' for physical health?
2 Should relationship quality and maintenance be prescribed? If so, how would this work, and how would it be monitored and evaluated?
3 What types of relationships, and at which stage in the life course, have the most impact on physiological correlates? (e.g., family, collegial, romantic, friendships)

References

Ainsworth, M. D. S., Blehar, M. C., Waters, E., & Wall, S. (1978). Strange situation procedure. *Clinical Child Psychology and Psychiatry.* https://doi.org/10.1037/t28248-000

Barth, J., Schneider, S., & von Känel, R. (2010). Lack of social support in the etiology and the prognosis of coronary heart disease: a systematic review and meta-analysis. *Psychosomatic Medicine, 72*(3), 229–238. https://doi.org/10.1097/PSY.0b013e3181d01611

Berkman, L. F., Glass, T., Brissette, I., & Seeman, T. E. (2000). From social integration to health: Durkheim in the new millennium. *Social Science & Medicine, 51*(6), 843–857. https://doi.org/10.1016/S0277-9536(00)00065-4

Berscheid, E., & Ammazzalorso, H. (2001). Emotional experience in close relationships. Blackwell handbook of social psychology: Interpersonal processes, 308–330.

Bolger, N., Delongis, A., Kessler, R. C., & Schilling, E. A. (1989). Effects of daily stress on negative mood. *Journal of Personality and Social Psychology, 57*(5), 808–818. https://doi.org/10.1037/0022-3514.57.5.808

Bourassa, K. J., Ruiz, J. M., & Sbarra, D. A. (2019). Smoking and physical activity explain the increased mortality risk following marital separation and divorce: Evidence from the English longitudinal study of ageing. *Annals of Behavioral Medicine, 53*(3), 255–266. https://doi.org/10.1093/ABM/KAY038

Bowlby, J. (1969). *Attachment and Loss* (Vol. 1). Basic Books.

Bradbury, T. N., Fincham, F. D., & Beach, S. R. H. (2012). Research on the nature and determinants of marital satisfaction: A decade in review. *Journal of Marriage and Family, 62*(4), 964–980.

Cacioppo, J., & Patrick, W. (2008). *Loneliness: Human nature and the need for social connection.* WW Norton & Company, London.

Cacioppo, J. T., Cacioppo, S., Capitanio, J. P., & Cole, S. W. (2015). The neuroendocrinology of social isolation. *Annual Review of Psychology, 66*, 733. https://doi.org/10.1146/annurev-psych-010814-015240

Cano, A., & Williams, A. C. de C. (2010). Social interaction in pain: Reinforcing pain behaviors or building intimacy? *Pain, 149*(1), 9–11. https://doi.org/10.1016/j.pain.2009.10.010

Carter, J. B., Banister, E. W., & Blaber, A. P. (2003). Effect of endurance exercise on autonomic control of heart rate. *Sports Medicine* (Auckland, N.Z.), *33*(1), 33–46. https://doi.org/10.2165/00007256-200333010-00003

Cassel, J. (1976). The contribution of the social environment to host resistance: The Fourth Wade Hampton Frost Lecture. *American Journal of Epidemiology, 104*(2), 107–122.

Chida, Y., & Steptoe, A. (2008). Positive psychological well-being and mortality: A quantitative review of prospective observational studies. *Psychosomatic Medicine, 70*(7), 741–756. https://doi.org/10.1097/PSY.0B013E31818105BA

Coan, J. A. (2008). Toward a neuroscience of attachment. In J. Cassidy & P. R. Shaver (Eds.), *Handbook of attachment: Theory, research, and clinical applications* (pp. 241–265). The Guilford Press. NY.

Coan, J. A., Schaefer, H. S., & Davidson, R. J. (2006). Lending a hand: Social regulation of the neural response to threat. *Psychological Science, 17*(12), 1032–1039. https://doi.org/10.1111/j.1467-9280.2006.01832.x

Cobb, S. (1976). Social support as a moderator of life stress. *Psychosomatic Medicine, 38*, 300–314. https://journals.lww.com/psychosomaticmedicine/Citation/1976/09000/Social_Support_as_a_Moderator_of_Life_Stress.3.aspx

Cohen, R., Bavishi, C., & Rozanski, A. (2016). Purpose in life and its relationship to all-cause mortality and cardiovascular events: A meta-analysis. *Psychosomatic Medicine, 78*(2), 122–133. https://doi.org/10.1097/PSY.0000000000000274

Cohen, S., Doyle, W. J., Skoner, D. P., Frank, E., Rabin, B. S., & Gwaltney, J. M. (1998). Types of stressors that increase susceptibility to the common cold in healthy adults. *Health Psychology*, *17*(3), 214–223. https://doi.org/10.1037/0278-6133.17.3.214

Diener, E., & Chan, M. Y. (2011). *Happy people live longer: Subjective well-being contributes to health and longevity.* https://doi.org/10.1111/j.1758-0854.2010.01045.x

Ditzen, B., Hoppmann, C., & Klumb, P. (2008). Positive couple interactions and daily cortisol: On the stress-protecting role of intimacy. *Psychosomatic Medicine*, *70*(8), 883–889. https://doi.org/10.1097/PSY.0b013e318185c4fc

Ditzen, B., Neumann, I. D., Bodenmann, G., von Dawans, B., Turner, R. A., Ehlert, U., & Heinrichs, M. (2007). Effects of different kinds of couple interaction on cortisol and heart rate responses to stress in women. *Psychoneuroendocrinology*, *32*(5), 565–574. https://doi.org/10.1016/j.psyneuen.2007.03.011

Ehrlich, K. B., Miller, G. E., Jones, J. D., & Cassidy, J. (2016). Attachment and psychoneuroimmunology. In J. Cassidy & P. Shaver (Eds.), *Handbook of attachment: Theory, research, and clinical applications* (3rd ed., pp. 180–201). Guilford Press. NY.

Eisenberg, N., Fabes, R. A., & Murphy, B. C. (1996). Parents' Reactions to Children's Negative Emotions: Relations to Children's Social Competence and Comforting Behavior. *Child Development*, *67*(5), 2227–2247. https://doi.org/10.1111/J.1467-8624.1996.TB01854.X

Eisenberger, N., Taylor, S., Gable, S., & Hilmert, C. J. (2007). Neural pathways link social support to attenuated neuroendocrine stress responses. *Neuroimage*, *35*(4), 1601–1612. doi: 10.1016/j.neuroimage.2007.01.038

Fincham, F., & Beach, S. R. H. (2010). Of memes and marriage: Toward a positive relationship science. *Journal of Family Theory & Review*, *2*(1), 4–24. https://doi.org/10.1111/j.1756-2589.2010.00033.x

Fletcher, G., Simpson, J. A., Campbell, L., & Overall, N. C. (2019). The science of intimate relationships. *The Science of Intimate Relationships*. https://doi.org/10.1002/9781119519416

Funk, J. L., & Rogge, R. D. (2007). Testing the ruler with item response theory: increasing precision of measurement for relationship satisfaction with the Couples Satisfaction Index. Journal of family psychology, *21*(4), 572. https://doi.org/10.1037/0893-3200.21.4.572

Gilliom, M., Shaw, D. S., Beck, J. E., Schonberg, M. A., & Lukon, J. L. (2002). Anger regulation in disadvantaged preschool boys: Strategies, antecedents, and the development of self-control. *Developmental Psychology*, *38*(2), 222. https://doi.org/10.1037/0012-1649.38.2.222

Gouin, J.-P., Carter, C. S., Pournajafi-Nazarloo, H., Glaser, R., Malarkey, W. B., Loving, T. J., Stowell, J., & Kiecolt-Glaser, J. K. (2010). Marital behavior, oxytocin, vasopressin, and wound healing. *Psychoneuroendocrinology*, *35*(7), 1082–1090. https://doi.org/10.1016/j.psyneuen.2010.01.009

Grewen, K. M., Anderson, B. J., Girdler, S. S., & Light, K. C. (2003). Warm partner contact is related to lower cardiovascular reactivity. *Behavioral Medicine (Washington, D.C.)*, *29*(3), 123–130. https://doi.org/10.1080/08964280309596065

Grewen, K. M., Girdler, S. S., Amico, J., & Light, K. C. (2005). Effects of partner support on resting oxytocin, cortisol, norepinephrine, and blood pressure before and after warm partner contact. *Psychosomatic Medicine*, *67*(4), 531–538. https://doi.org/10.1097/01.psy.0000170341.88395.47

Gump, B. B., Polk, D. E., Kamarck, T. W., & Shiffman, S. M. (2001). Partner interactions are associated with reduced blood pressure in the natural environment: Ambulatory monitoring evidence from a healthy, multiethnic adult sample. *Psychosomatic Medicine*, *63*(3), 423–433.

Gunnar, M. R., & Quevedo, K. M. (2008). Early care experiences and HPA axis regulation in children: A mechanism for later trauma vulnerability. *Progress in Brain Research*, *167*, 137. https://doi.org/10.1016/S0079-6123(07)67010-1

Haase, C. M., Holley, S. R., Bloch, L., Verstaen, A., & Levenson, R. W. (2016). Interpersonal emotional behaviors and physical health: A 20-year longitudinal study of long-term married couples. *Emotion, 16*(7), 965–977. https://doi.org/10.1037/A0040239

Halford, W. K., Farrugia, C., Lizzio, A., & Wilson, K. (2010). Relationship aggression, violence and self-regulation in Australian newlywed couples. *Australian Journal of Psychology, 62*(2), 82–92. https://doi.org/10.1080/00049530902804169

Halford, W. K., & Snyder, D. K. (2012). Universal processes and common factors in couple therapy and relationship education. Guest Editors: W. Kim Halford & Douglas K. Snyder. *Behavior Therapy, 43*(1), 1–12. https://doi.org/10.1016/j.beth.2011.01.007

Harlow, H. F. (1959). Love in infant monkeys. *Scientific American, 200*(6), 68–75.

Heffner, K. L., Waring, M. E., Roberts, M. B., Eaton, C. B., & Gramling, R. (2011). Social isolation, C-reactive protein, and coronary heart disease mortality among community-dwelling adults. *Social Science & Medicine* (1982), *72*(9), 1482–1488. https://doi.org/10.1016/j.socscimed.2011.03.016

Herbert, T. B., & Cohen, S. (1993). Depression and immunity: A meta-analytic review. *Psychological Bulletin, 113*(3), 472–486. https://doi.org/10.1037/0033-2909.113.3.472

Holt-Lunstad, J., Birmingham, W. A., & Light, K. C. (2008). Influence of a "Warm Touch" support enhancement intervention among married couples on ambulatory blood pressure, oxytocin, alpha amylase, and cortisol. *Psychosomatic Medicine, 70*(9), 976–985. https://doi.org/10.1097/PSY.0b013e318187aef7

Holt-Lunstad, J., Smith, T. B., & Layton, J. B. (2010). Social relationships and mortality risk: A meta-analytic review. *PLoS Medicine, 7*(7). https://doi.org/10.1371/journal.pmed.1000316

Holt-Lunstad, J., Uchino, B. N., Smith, T. W., Olson-Cerny, C., & Nealey-Moore, J. B. (2003). Social relationships and ambulatory blood pressure: Structural and qualitative predictors of cardiovascular function during everyday social interactions. *Health Psychology: Official Journal of the Division of Health Psychology, American Psychological Association, 22*(4), 388–397. https://doi.org/10.1037/0278-6133.22.4.388

House, J. S., Landis, K. R., & Umberson, D. (1988). Social relationships and health. *Science, 241*(4865), 540–545. https://doi.org/10.1126/SCIENCE.3399889

Impett, E. A., Peplau, L., & Gable, S. L. (2005). Approach and avoidance sexual motives: Implications for personal and interpersonal well-being. *Personal Relationships, 12*(4), 465–482. https://doi.org/10.1111/j.1475-6811.2005.00126.x

Jakubiak, B. K., & Feeney, B. C. (2017). Affectionate touch to promote relational, psychological, and physical well-being in adulthood: A theoretical model and review of the research. *Personality and Social Psychology Review, 21*(3), 228–252. https://doi.org/10.1177/1088868316650307

Kiecolt-Glaser, J. K. (2018). Marriage, divorce, and the immune system. *American Psychologist, 73*(9), 1098–1108. https://doi.org/10.1037/AMP0000388

Kiecolt-Glaser, J. K., Loving, T. J., Stowell, J. R., Malarkey, W. B., Lemeshow, S., Dickinson, S. L., & Glaser, R. (2005). Hostile marital interactions, proinflammatory cytokine production, and wound healing. *Archives of General Psychiatry, 62*(12), 1377–1384. https://doi.org/10.1001/ARCHPSYC.62.12.1377

Kiecolt-Glaser, J. K., Malarkey, W. B., Chee, M., Newton, T., Cacioppo, J. T., Mao, H.-Y., & Glaser, R. (1993). Negative behavior during marital conflict is associated with immunological down-regulation. *Psychosomatic Medicine, 55*(5), 395–409.

Kobak, R. R., & Sceery, A. (1988). Attachment in late adolescence: Working models, affect regulation, and representations of self and others. *Child Development*, 135–146.

Liu, D., Diorio, J., Tannenbaum, B., Caldji, C., Francis, D., Freedman, A., Sharma, S., Pearson, D., Plotsky, P. M., & Meaney, M. J. (1997). Maternal care, hippocampal glucocorticoid receptors, and hypothalamic-pituitary-adrenal responses to stress. *Science, 277*(5332), 1659–1662. https://doi.org/10.1126/science.277.5332.1659

Maroun, M., & Wagner, S. (2016). Oxytocin and memory of emotional stimuli: Some dance to remember, some dance to forget. *Biological Psychiatry, 79*(3), 203–212. https://www.sciencedirect.com/science/article/pii/S0006322315006101

McNulty, J. K., & Russell, V. M. (2010). When "Negative" behaviors are positive: A contextual analysis of the long-term effects of problem-solving behaviors on changes in relationship satisfaction. *Journal of Personality and Social Psychology, 98*(4), 587–604. https://doi.org/10.1037/a0017479

Meaney, M. J. (2001). Maternal care, gene expression, and the transmission of individual differences in stress reactivity across generations. *Annual Review of Neuroscience, 24,* 1161–1192. https://doi.org/10.1146/ANNUREV.NEURO.24.1.1161

Mikulincer, M., & Shaver, P. R. (2019). Attachment orientations and emotion regulation. *Current Opinion in Psychology, 25,* 6–10. https://doi.org/10.1016/j.copsyc .2018.02.006

Mikulincer, M., Shaver, P. R., & Pereg, D. (2003). Attachment theory and affect regulation: The dynamics, development, and cognitive consequences of attachment-related strategies. *Motivation and Emotion, 27*(2), 77–102. https://doi.org/10.1023/A:1024515519160

Miller, G. E., Dopp, J. M., Myers, H. F., Stevens, S. Y., & Fahey, J. L. (1999). Psychosocial predictors of natural killer cell mobilization during marital conflict. *Health Psychology, 18*(3), 262–271. https://doi.org/10.1037/0278-6133.18.3.262

Morris, A. S., Criss, M. M., Silk, J. S., & Houltberg, B. J. (2017). The impact of parenting on emotion regulation during childhood and adolescence. *Child Development Perspectives, 11*(4), 233–238. https://doi.org/10.1111/CDEP.12238

Overall, N. C., Fletcher, G. J. O., Simpson, J. A., & Sibley, C. G. (2009). Regulating partners in intimate relationships: The costs and benefits of different communication strategies. *Journal of Personality and Social Psychology, 96*(3), 620–639. https://doi.org/10.1037/A0012961

Pedersen, C. A. (2004). Biological aspects of social bonding and the roots of human violence. *Annals of the New York Academy of Sciences, 1036,* 106–127. https://doi.org/10.1196/annals.1330.006

Peirce, R. S., Frone, M. R., Russell, M., Cooper, M. L., & Mudar, P. (2000). A longitudinal model of social contact, social support, depression, and alcohol use. Health Psychology, *19*(1), 28–38. https://doi.org/10.1037/0278-6133.19.1.28

Pietromonaco, P. R., & Beck, L. A. (2019). Adult attachment and physical health. *Current Opinion in Psychology, 25,* 115–120. https://doi.org/10.1016/j.copsyc. 2018.04.004

Sanri, Ç., & Goodwin, R. (2014). The influence of globalization and technological development on intimate relationships. In C. R. Agnew (Ed.), *Social influences on romantic relationships: Beyond the dyad* (pp. 11–32). Cambridge University Press. https://doi.org/10.1017/CBO9781139333610.003

Sanri, Ç., Halford, W. K., Rogge, R. D., & von Hippel, W. (2021). The couple flourishing measure. *Family Process, 60*(2), 457–476. https://doi.org/10.1111/FAMP.12632

Sanri, Ç. (2018). *Couple flourishing: Conceptualisation and psychological assessment.* https://doi.org/10.14264/UQL.2018.619

Seeman, T. E. (1996). Social ties and health: The benefits of social integration. *Annals of Epidemiology, 6*(5), 442–451. https://doi.org/10.1016/S1047-2797(96)00095-6

Seeman, T. E., Lusignolo, T. M., Albert, M., & Berkman, L. (2001). Social relationships, social support, and patterns of cognitive aging in healthy, high-functioning older adults: MacArthur studies of successful aging. *Health Psychology, 20*(4), 243–255. https://doi.org/10.1037/0278-6133.20.4.243

Shaver, P. R., & Mikulincer, M. (2002). Attachment-related psychodynamics. *Attachment and Human Development, 4*(2), 133–161. https://doi.org/10.1080/14616730210154171

Slatcher, R. B., Selcuk, E., & Ong, A. D. (2015). Perceived partner responsiveness predicts diurnal cortisol profiles 10 years later. *Psychological Science, 26*(7), 972–982. https://doi.org/10.1177/0956797615575022

Smith, T. W., Cribbet, M. R., Nealey-Moore, J. B., Uchino, B. N., Williams, P. G., MacKenzie, J., & Thayer, J. F. (2011). Matters of the variable heart: Respiratory sinus arrhythmia response to marital interaction and associations with marital quality. *Journal of Personality and Social Psychology, 100*(1), 103–119. https://doi.org/10.1037/A0021136

Spanier, G. B. (1976). Dyadic Adjustment Scale (DAS). *Journal of Marriage and the Family, 38*(1), 15–28. https://doi.org/10.1080/00926237908403730

Stanton, S. C. E., Selcuk, E., Farrell, A. K., Slatcher, R. B., & Ong, A. D. (2019). Perceived partner responsiveness, daily negative affect reactivity, and all-cause mortality: A 20-year longitudinal study. *Psychosomatic Medicine, 81*(1), 7. https://doi.org/10.1097/PSY.0000000000000618

Taylor, S. E. (2006). Tend and befriend: Biobehavioral bases of affiliation under stress. *Current Directions in Psychological Science, 15*(6), 273–277. https://doi.org/10.1111/j.1467-8721.2006.00451.x

Uchino, B., Cacioppo, J. T., & Kiekolt-Glaser, J. K. (1996). The relationship between social support and physiological processes: A review with emphasis on underlying mechanisms and implications for health. *Psychological Bulletin, 119*(3), 488–531. https://doi.org/10.1037/0033-2909.119.3.488

Vargas-Martínez, F., Uvnäs-Moberg, K., Petersson, M., Olausson, H. A., & Jiménez-Estrada, I. (2014). Neuropeptides as neuroprotective agents: Oxytocin a forefront developmental player in the mammalian brain. *Progress in Neurobiology, 123*, 37–78. https://doi.org/10.1016/J.PNEUROBIO.2014.10.001

Vitaliano, P. P., Young, H. M., Russo, J., Romano, J., & Magana-Amato, A. (1993). Does expressed emotion in spouses predict subsequent problems among care recipients with Alzheimer's disease? *Journal of Gerontology, 48*(4), P202–P209. https://doi.org/10.1093/GERONJ/48.4.P202

Wickrama, K. A. S., Lorenz, F. O., Conger, R. D., & Elder, G. H. (1997). Marital quality and physical illness: A latent growth curve analysis. *Journal of Marriage and the Family, 59*(1), 143. https://doi.org/10.2307/353668

7

THE POWER OF POSITIVE EMOTIONS

Trudy Meehan

Positive emotions play a significant role in enhancing wellbeing, personal growth, physical health and resilience. In this chapter, we will explore the theoretical background of positive emotions, practical applications in daily life, key takeaways, and pose thought-provoking questions to deepen our understanding. Before we consider the subtle power of positive emotions, it may help to juxtapose them to the significant power of so called negative emotions. The negativity bias (Baumeister, Bratslavsky, Finkenaure & Vohs, 2001) ensures that negative emotional experiences are more salient and lingering. We need to remember dangerous events and can avoid them in the future. These negative emotions are essential, especially in the fight-flight-freeze response. Since they are often recruited in life preserving moments, or moments when our ancient reptilian brain considers life threatening, negative emotions tend to close us down (we curl our body inward, round our shoulders in a protective posture, brace ourselves) and narrow our focus. They preserve our life in times of threat by narrowing our focus and helping us pay attention to threat and when we can't escape or avoid the threat to blocking out, removing us psychologically from danger. We are wired to pay attention to the negative, respond to these emotions and to remember the emotional tone and context of the eliciting events. So next to the "Velcro" sticking power and apparent significance of negative emotions, positive emotions are the Cinderella of the emotional world, they have been hiding in plain sight, largely ignored because they were considered short lived and insignificant. However, the pioneering work of Barbara Fredrickson and colleagues has shown that while the impact of positive emotions is smaller than that of negative emotions, it is cumulative, and most certainly not insignificant. This chapter will focus on Barbara Fredrickson's Broaden and Build Theory of Positive Emotions and look briefly at the potential for applying this theory in the field of Positive Health.

 DOI: 10.4324/9781003378426-9

Broaden and build theory of positive emotions

Theoretically, the field of positive emotions is rooted in positive psychology, a branch of psychology that focuses on the positive aspects of human life, including happiness, well-being, and thriving. Positive psychology emerged as a response to the traditional focus of psychology on mental illness and dysfunction. The Broaden and Build Theory, proposed by Barbara Fredrickson, outlines the transformative effects of positive emotions. Fredrickson's work is significant because she gives value to the previously unnoticed potential of positive emotions. Unlike negative emotions which narrow our responses, positive emotions broaden our cognitive and behavioural repertoire, allowing us to think more flexibly, explore new possibilities, and build psychological resources. Fredrickson identified ten positive emotions: joy, gratitude, serenity, interest, hope, pride, amusement, inspiration, awe and love.

Positive emotions

- Joy
- Gratitude
- Serenity
- Interest
- Hope
- Pride
- Amusement
- Inspiration
- Awe
- Love

Out of the ten positive emotions Fredrickson's theory considers, love is the most complex of these. It tends to contain many of the other positive emotions, and so is essentially a collective of positive emotions rather than a single emotional experience. Fredrickson has written extensively about love and her research focuses on love as small moments of mutual care and connection that she calls micromoments of positivity resonance. For Fredrickson positivity resonance does not require a historical relationship across time, it is a small positive emotional experience that can be felt even between strangers at times when there is mutual positive regard. We will explore Fredrickson's work on positivity resonance further along in the chapter.

Broaden and Build has empirical support, and its implications are far-reaching, particularly in interventions aiming to improve psychological wellbeing. However, the theory also faces critiques concerning the generalisation of positive emotions (Griskevicius, Shiota, & Neufeld, 2010), the need to consider cultural context (Tsai, 2007), and potential adverse consequences of excessive positive emotions such as over optimism contributing to underestimating risks (Johnson & Carver, 2006). The Broaden and Build Theory has been criticised for its silence on the potential maladaptive outcomes of excessive hedonic positive emotions, when people underestimate risks for example. The hedonic perspective (short-term pleasure) is often contrasted with the eudemonic perspective, which is rooted in realising one's true potential and living in accordance with one's values and virtues (Ryan & Deci, 2001). However, if we look at the list of positive emotions put forward by Fredrickson, the majority of the emotions sit in the eudemonic side of positive wellbeing. Joy and amusement are perhaps the only two emotions that are frankly hedonistic, short lived and momentary. The other emotions listed (gratitude, serenity, interest, hope, pride, inspiration, love) can feed into eudemonic wellbeing through their being experienced when we are connected or sharing experiences with other people or things, or tapping into our sense of meaning and purpose. Positive emotions not only enhance momentary experiences of but also have an impact on our overall wellbeing. By supporting resilience and learning, they help us expand our personal intellectual, social, physical and psychological resources making us more able to negotiate varying contexts. In essence, while negative emotions serve to protect us from immediate dangers, positive emotions enhance and build our long-term resources and capabilities.

Broaden

Positive emotions expand our focus and allow us to notice more things, so they help us be more inclusive and be more open minded and inclusive in our thinking. When we're in a positive emotional state, our mind opens up, our cognitive processes become more expansive. We're better able to think outside the box. So we get better at problem solving. We become more creative and innovative and more able to generate solutions. We're also more receptive to alternatives. This also means that we are more open to diversity. So we're more inclusive, not just in our thinking but in our ability to include people who are different from us. Positive emotions contribute not just to our personal health and wellbeing but allow us to move towards a more inclusive and community oriented society. Positive emotions support us to broaden our thinking and horizons of possible behaviours and responses and in providing this solid base, give a foundation for building new cognitive, social and behavioural skills.

Build

The other thing about positive emotions is that they help us build resources, which is really exciting. What Fredrickson means by this is that we literally can develop new skills by being open to learning. We gather new skills as we go, and add to our behavioural repertoire and emotional and cognitive development. In the realm of cognition, we get better problem solving, more open to learning. We get better at visualising things in the physical space. Supporting the building potential of positive emotions, research has shown that experiencing positive emotions increases our brain dopamine levels, particularly in this prefrontal cortex and the anterior cingulate (Ashby, Isen, & Turken, 1999; Schultz, 2007). These areas are really important in underlying our cognitive performance and making sure that our thinking processes work well. We broaden and build cognitive resources when we're in a positive emotional state, our mind opens up, our cognitive processes become more expansive (Fredrickson & Branigan, 2005). We're better able to think outside the box. So we get better at problem solving. We become more creative and innovative and more able to generate solutions. We're also more receptive to alternatives, and we have enhanced creativity, especially for verbal creativity tasks. In the area of physical health, there's promise that positive emotions can contribute to improving cardiovascular health (Kok et al., 2013) and contribute to improved physical coordination. In the social space, Fredrickson talks about creating and maintaining relationships and developing skills in that area. In the psychological realm, Fredrickson describes the ways in which this broadening and building can give us tools to support resilience, optimism, sense of identity and goal orientation. A positive emotion according to Fredrickson, can loosen the hold of a negative emotion and it dismantles the preparation effect of that negative emotion. As discussed above, negative emotions tend to close or narrow our focus, preparing us for fight or flight or freeze. This fight, flight, freeze response turns on physiological responses that are helpful but can feel uncomfortable and if they linger too long can be detrimental. Experiencing a positive emotion can undo some of these effects (Fredrickson, Mancuso, Branigan, & Tugade, 2000). By experiencing positive emotions, we can expand the range of emotions and the range of behaviours that we have available to us. We experience this in a positive feedback loop whereby as we develop more skills, we are more likely to feel positive emotions. Fredrickson calls this the upward spiral of positive emotion, which broaden and builds our emotional and behavioural repertoire.

Collective positive emotions – micromoments of positivity resonance

In general, we know the positive emotions are good for our brain and they give us a broad, flexible cognitive organisation, an ability to integrate diverse material interests they need. This also means that we are more open to diversity. So we're more inclusive, not just in our thinking, but in our ability to include people who are different from us. So it's important for a broader society that we experience positive emotions as well as for us as individuals. An interesting aspect of positive emotions is not just that they make us more likely to move from 'me' to 'we' in our thinking, but also that they are emotions that are shared, collectively experienced. Dacher Keltner and colleagues write about collective effervesce in describing the experience of awe within a collective group body experience (Bai et al., 2017; Piff, Dietze, Feinberg, Stancato & Keltner, 2015). Others in the arts and health field write about the role of the arts in creating situations in which we collectively experience shared positive emotions (Darewych, & Riedel Bowers, 2018; Verneert, Nijs, & De Baets, 2021). Christopher Bailey (2022) the

Arts and Health Lead for the World Health Organisation speaks about the role of art in bringing more compassion into the world and he describes compassion as a shared emotion appealing to the Latin definition of the word which means 'to suffer together'. Fredrickson and colleagues also speak about a collective experience of positive emotions expanding on the Broaden and Build Theory by focusing on positive emotions in the context of social relationships. Waugh & Fredrickson (2006) argue that positive emotions play a crucial role in building social resources, enhancing social bonds, and promoting wellbeing within social interactions.

Positive social connections have numerous benefits for individuals' mental and physical health. Strong social support networks have been associated with lower rates of mental health problems, such as depression and anxiety (Cohen & Wills, 1985). Positive social interactions have also been linked to increased longevity, better immune functioning, and reduced risk of chronic diseases (Uchino, 2006). Furthermore, positive social connections are not limited to personal relationships but also extend to broader social networks and communities. Building positive social connections at the community level can contribute to the development of social capital, which refers to the resources and support available within a community (Kawachi et al., 2004). Social capital enhances collective wellbeing, fosters social cohesion, and promotes community resilience.

It is important to note that the quality of social connections matters. Positive social connections characterised by trust, empathy, and reciprocity have more significant benefits compared to superficial or negative relationships (Fredrickson, 2003). Therefore, nurturing and maintaining authentic and meaningful relationships will foster stronger and more impactful social connections. However, we cannot lose sight of the value of small moments of positive connection and this may be an area where many of us have the most agency to change and activate in our daily lives. Love or social connection, for Fredrickson is not solely a romantic love between two individuals with an intense bond or familial love shared because of kinship bonds. Instead she talks about love as "micro moments of positivity resonance" and emphasises that this feeling can be experienced between strangers and is not reliant only on shared bonds or history together. Fredrickson's work is important because it opens an opportunity to make positive change even when long-term bonding is not an option for us. She uses the beautiful term "turning towards" to describe a process or mutual recognition and synchronisation that results in a momentary feeling of mutual care. Her description of 'turning to' has echoes of John Gottman's (Navarra & Gottman, 2019). description of interpersonal bids for connection in romantic relationships and reminds us of the power and potential of small moments of mutual recognition and connection. Her work too is aligned with the thinking of interpersonal neuropsychiatrist Dan Siegel (2001) who describes the process of developing "mindsight" so that we can have 'we' maps as well as 'me' maps in our thought, feeling and behavioural repertoire. Her work is also significant as she draws on a range of empirical research which points to some of the possible mechanisms underlying this process of connection, "one feeling across two bodies" (Fredrickson, 2013b). This feeling of micromoments of positivity reso-nance occurs for Fredrickson across two bodies through synchronisation of bio-logical processes in our brain activity, cardiovascular system and neurochemistry.

Brain synchronisation

Neurologist Uri Hasson and his colleagues' have conducted intriguing research showing of brain-to-brain coupling across two individuals during shared story telling (Hasson, Ghazanfar, Galantucci, Garrod, & Keysers, 2012). Hasson et al. (2012) used Functional MRI to look at brain activity in two individuals when one was telling a story and the other one was listening. The research found alignment of neural activity in regions of the brain implicated in empa-thy and emotional processing (e.g. the insula). This synchronised activity in such brain regions may be why we not only share information but also par-take in a shared positive emotional experiences. Hasson's work suggests that the positivity resonance experienced during social communication is a joint act performed by two brains, highlighting the importance and value of active listening and presence in our social interactions with the goal of creating and sharing a social experience. For Fredrickson this work is significant because the neural synchrony observed in brain-to-brain coupling provides a plausible neu-ral basis for positivity resonance. The observation of individuals' brain activity aligning during social interactions, serves as a foundational mechanism for the experience of positivity resonance and is supported and complimented by other empirical studies (Kenreich, Djalovski, Kraus, Louzoun, & Feldman, 2017; Leong, Byrne, Clackson, Georgieva, Lam & Wass, 2017; Stephens, Silbert, & Hasson, 2010).

Heart rate variability synchronisation and the vagus nerve

Fredrickson talks about the importance of the vagus nerve in our capacity to love and connect and be in relationship with other people. Why is that the case? We know that the vagus nerve is an important for the fight or flight response, but it's also used for the connect response. When we connect with others the vagus nerve acts to slow down a racing heart and brings soothing to us. It acts in conjunction with oxytocin, which we'll explore below. The higher our vagal tone, the better we are able to utilise this calm and connect response. Fredrick-son argues that moments of positivity resonance improve vagal tone and are supported by good vagal tone. She argues that people with higher vagal tone are more socially skilled and able to forge positive relationships. When you en-gage in positive social interactions (positivity resonance), your body responds by, among other things, stimulating the vagus nerve. The good feeling that happens when we have positive social interactions engages the vagus nerve. The vagus nerve, in turn, helps to slow down the heart rate and increase Heart Rate Variability (HRV) (Kok et al., 2013). Fredrickson's thinking is complemented by the work of Polyvagal Theorists such as Stephen Porges (2007) who show that the vagus nerve plays a central role in emotional regulation, social engagement and interpersonal connection. Polyvagal theory is not without criticisms and Fredrickson's work although resting on a strong empirical study (Kok et al., 2013), is relatively new and the field continues to evolve. However despite these caveats, there is an inspiring vision in Fredrickson's work. She argues that we can improve vagal tone by experiencing more positivity resonance micro moments and that love or positivity resonance operates on a 'use it or lose it' mechanism. If we don't exercise it regularly, if we don't practice positive social connection and mutual care, we lose our vagal tone, and diminish our capacity to love. Positive emotions and positivity resonance can be fostered and practiced, much like exercising muscles, and this practice can have cascading benefits for individuals and their social environments (Fredrickson, 2013a; Kok et al., 2013).

Neurochemical synchronisation

As mentioned above, the vagus nerve acts in concert with oxytocin to induce feelings of love, calm and connection. Oxytocin colloquially understood at 'the cuddle hormone'. It's released in various social situations, especially during moments of positive connection, such as hugging, touching, or bonding and as such is implicated in social bonding and trust (Uvnäs-Moberg, Bruzelius, Alster, & Lundeberg, 1993). Oxytocin helps to calm fears and bring us closer, but also making us better judges of whether the other person is indeed trustworthy or not, therefore also making the prospect of connection safer. Fredrickson points out that there is synchrony in oxytocin levels among individuals during moments of positivity resonance, further strengthening the bonds (Fredrickson, 2013a). The release of oxytocin during these moments is thought to be one of the physiological underpinnings of positivity resonance (Fredrickson, 2013a; Grewen, Girdler, Amico, & Light, 2005; Kosfeld, Heinrichs, Zak, Fischbacher, & Fehr, 2005; Shamay-Tsoory & Abu-Akel, 2016).

Barbara Fredrickson's Broaden and Build Theory, when integrated with the concept of positivity resonance and the supporting research on brain coupling, HRV and oxytocin, offers a promising view of the mechanics and impact of shared positive emotions. It encourages the view that love can be seen as micro moments of connection that can be fostered, thus having far-reaching implications for individuals' wellbeing and social coherence. Positive emotions play a vital role in fostering healthy and fulfilling relationships. Engaging in positive emotional experiences with our partners, friends, and family members deepens emotional bonds and strengthens the quality of our relationships. Expressing love, appreciation, and affection can generate positive emotions and build a strong foundation of emotional intimacy. Furthermore, positive emotions are contagious, and when shared within relationships, they create a positive feedback loop, strengthening the emotional connection and increasing relationship satisfaction (Gable, Reis, Impett, & Asher, 2004).

Application

Further research examining alternative theories and assessing the critiques of Broaden and Build Theory is essential for the ongoing development of this theoretical framework and continuing to develop a more nuanced understanding of positive emotions. However, despite these ongoing limitations, there are promising applications of positive emotions as conceptualised and harnessed by the Broaden and Build Theory which we will discuss in the rest of this chapter.

Positive emotional regulation strategies

Incorporating positive emotion regulation strategies into daily life can significantly enhance wellbeing and overall life satisfaction. Savouring positive experiences is one such strategy that involves fully engaging with and appreciating positive moments, allowing them to linger and deepen our positive emotional state (Bryant & Veroff, 2017). By savouring experiences, individuals can extract more meaning and enjoyment from even the simplest of activities. Expressing gratitude, either through gratitude journaling or expressing appreciation to others, has been shown to increase positive emotions and overall happiness (Armenta, Fritz, & Lyubomirsky, 2017). Regular practice of gratitude can shift our attention towards the positive aspects of life, leading to improved wellbeing (Emmons & McCullough, 2003).

Mindfulness practices, such as meditation and mindful breathing, help cultivate present moment awareness and promote a positive outlook (Lindsay et al., 2018). By training our minds to focus on the present moment without judgment, mindfulness allows us to fully experience positive emotions as they arise. Engaging in meaningful activities that align with personal values and interests can also generate positive emotions and a sense of fulfilment. By pursuing activities that bring us joy and purpose, we can tap into a wellspring of positive emotions and enhance our overall wellbeing. Finally, fostering positive social connections through acts of kindness, active listening, and empathy can amplify positive emotions both in ourselves and in others (Nelson, Layous, Cole, & Lyubomirsky, 2016).

Positive emotions and mental health

The relationship between positive emotions and mental health is a growing but complex area of research. In clinical research, interventions fostering positive emotion have been used to reduce symptoms of depression and anxiety (Seligman et al., 2005). Despite these promising results, delineating direct causal pathways and mechanisms are challenging in this area as many interventions have increasing positive emotion as a secondary effect regardless of whether this was the intention or not. Gratitude exercises, acts of kindness and meditation that supports positive emotion have shown promising results in impacting on symptoms of depression and anxiety as well as improving overall wellbeing. Practicing gratitude can help individuals focus on positive aspects of their lives, which can increase happiness and reduce depressive symptoms (Emmons & McCullough, 2003). Cultivating gratitude through practices such as gratitude journaling, writing thank-you notes, or engaging in gratitude exercises has been found to significantly enhance positive emotions and wellbeing (Wood et al., 2010). These practices shift individuals' focus towards the positive aspects of their lives, fostering feelings of appreciation and contentment. Acts of kindness have similar effects. Performing kind acts for others can lead to increased wellbeing and decreased symptoms of depression (Otake, Shimai, Tanaka-Matsumi, Otsui, & Fredrickson, 2006). Building and maintaining positive connections through acts of kindness, active listening, and expressions of gratitude and appreciation to others enhance positive emotions within relationships (Fredrickson, 2013a). Cultivating positive relationships not only fosters a sense of belonging but also promotes overall life satisfaction and psychological wellbeing and reduces loneliness.

As mentioned above, meditation, particularly mindfulness, and loving-kindness meditation, have also shown promising results in fostering positive emotions and improving wellbeing (Fredrickson, Cohn, Coffey, Pek, & Finkel 2008). These practices foster a non-judgmental awareness of the present moment and promote positive attitudes toward oneself and others which is posited to contribute to reducing symptoms of depression and anxiety (Fredrickson et al., 2008). By cultivating non-judgmental awareness of the present moment, individuals develop a deeper appreciation for positive experiences and emotions, leading to increased happiness and improved emotional regulation (Garland et al., 2015; Keng et al., 2011) which may support good mental health.

Perhaps most interesting is the value of positive emotions as a buffer against stress and promoting adaptive coping and resilience by reducing latency in recovery from negative emotions (Sin & Lyubomirsky, 2009). One of the mechanisms through which positive emotions may buffer against mental health issues is by promoting psychological resilience. According to Tugade and Fredrickson (2004), positive emotions can help individuals to bounce back from negative emotional experiences and adapt to stressful situations. When people are able to use positive emotions to put negative experiences into perspective, they can recover more rapidly from adversity and stress. Importantly, positive emotions have been found to have physiological effects that can contribute to mental health. For example, Fredrickson and Levenson (1998) found that positive emotions can 'undo' the cardiovascular effects of negative emotions, which may partially explain their role in promoting psychological resilience. In addition to resilience, positive emotions can improve social support, which is an essential component of mental health. Positive emotions can foster social bonds and improve interpersonal skills (Waugh & Fredrickson, 2006). Having a strong social support system in turn is associated with lower levels of depression and anxiety.

Positive emotions and physical health

In addition to their psychological benefits, positive emotions have been linked to improved physical health outcomes. Research suggests that experiencing positive emotions on a regular basis can strengthen the immune system, lower the risk of cardiovascular disease, reduce inflammation, and enhance overall resilience against illness (Sin & Lyubomirsky, 2009). Positive emotions promote healthier lifestyle choices, such as engaging in regular exercise, maintaining a balanced diet, and getting sufficient sleep. Furthermore, positive emotions have been associated with faster recovery from illness or surgery and increased longevity (Pressman & Cohen, 2005). The integration of positive emotions within lifestyle medicine interventions can contribute to improved physical health outcomes and overall wellbeing.

As discussed above, Fredrickson and colleagues (Kok et al., 2013) have argued that increasing our perception of positive social connections can improve vagal tone. They use vagal tone as a proxy indicator for physical health. The vagus nerve is one of the longest nerves in the body, connecting the brain to the heart and other organs. Thayer and Lane (2007) argue that the vagus nerve is a crucial component of the brain-heart connection, deeply involved in emotional regulation. They suggest that a high vagal tone, which means the vagus nerve is functioning efficiently, is associated with better emotional regulation and cardiovascular health (Thayer & Lane, 2007). Porges' (2007) work on Polyvagal Theory argues that positive social engagement, can stimulate the vagus nerve, contributing to emotional and physiological wellbeing. This connection is crucial because it lays the foundation for understanding how positive emotions and social interactions are linked to vagal activity and, consequently, to heart health. HRV is the variation in time between heartbeats and is considered a marker of heart health and vagal function. When we experience positivity resonance, our positive emotions are amplified, and we feel more connected to others. This process can stimulate the vagus nerve and increase HRV, thereby promoting heart health. Kemp et al. (2012) explored the relationship between depression, HRV, and social connectedness. They discovered that positive social interactions are associated with higher HRV, implying better cardiovascular health and vagus nerve function. Furthermore, as discussed above oxytocin works in conjunction with the vagus nerve to underpin positivity resonance. The release of oxytocin during positive connections not only helps to establish social bonds but also has beneficial physiological effects, including those related to cardiovascular health (Uvnäs-Moberg et al., 1993). This is pivotal in understanding how positivity resonance, through its fostering of positive emotions and connections, can directly impact cardiovascular health (Kemp et al., 2012).

Drawing on the evidence for using vagal tone as a proxy indicator for physical health Kok, Fredrickson and colleagues (Kok et al., 2013) state that there is a "self-sustaining upward-spiral dynamic" (p. 1123) at play between social interactions, positive emotions and physical health. They argue that they have demonstrated "a causal link between positive emotions and improved vagal tone" (p. 1129). The work is significant because vagal tone was generally seen as stable but they have demonstrated that we can impact on our autonomic health by improving social connections. Secondly, the research supports this causal mechanisms for the health promoting benefits found in other studies that have linked positive social connections with good physical health (Kemp, Quintana, Felmingham, Matthews & Jelinek, 2012; Porges, 2007; Thayer & Lane, 2007).

Recent studies emphasise the role of positive emotions in reducing the risk of chronic diseases and improving psychological resilience. For instance, research highlights that positive emotions are associated with reduced inflammatory responses, improved immune function, and decreased risk of cardiovascular disease (Kok et al., 2013; Stellar et al., 2015). Furthermore, individuals who experience positive emotions tend to report lower levels of stress and exhibit better coping mechanisms in the face of adversity (Tugade & Fredrickson, 2004)

The application of positive emotions in the positive health field

In clinical or coaching practice, leveraging the utility of positive emotions is crucial for helping individuals live healthy lives. Positive emotions have a profound impact on overall wellbeing, and incorporating them into positive health interventions can enhance health outcomes and support sustainable lifestyle changes. By leveraging the utility of positive emotions our their practice, we can support individuals in adopting and sustaining healthy lifestyle behaviours. Positive emotions serve as powerful resources that promote wellbeing, resilience, and motivation. Integrating positive emotion-focused interventions into our practice can enhance patient outcomes, through supporting motivation and facilitating behaviour change, Here are some ways to effectively leverage positive emotions in clinical/coaching practice:

1 Cultivate Positive Emotional States: Encourage our clients to engage in activities that evoke positive emotions, such as practicing gratitude, engaging in enjoyable hobbies, spending time with loved ones, and engaging in acts of kindness. By consciously cultivating positive emotional states, individuals can experience increased motivation, resilience, and satisfaction, which can support their commitment to healthy behaviours and positive lifestyle changes (Kashdan et al., 2017; Parks et al., 2012). Fredrickson and colleagues (Fredrickson & Losada, 2005) have advocated for the "positivity ratio," wherein individuals are encouraged to experience about three positive emotions for every negative emotion, as a guide for improving emotional wellbeing. Fredrickson has been criticised and answered criticisms on the specific calculation and accuracy of the ratio (Fredrickson, 2013c) However, remains plausible, based on other positive interaction ratios such as the prediction that successful marriages tend to have a ratio of 5:1 positive

to negative interactions (Gottman, 1993, 1994) that we need to have more positive than negative emotions if we are to benefit from the magic of positive emotions.

2 Promote Positive Self-Talk: Work with our clients to develop positive self-talk and cultivate self-compassion. Encourage them to replace negative self-statements with positive affirmations and supportive thoughts. Positive self-talk can enhance self-efficacy, self-confidence, and optimism, facilitating healthier choices and behaviours (Sirois & Wood, 2017).

3 Meditation and Positive Emotional Regulation: Integrate mindfulness practices into positive health interventions to promote present-moment awareness and positive emotion regulation. By cultivating mindfulness, individuals can develop a greater capacity to savour positive experiences, regulate negative emotions, and make healthier choices (Garland et al., 2015). Loving Kindness Meditation (Fredrickson et al., 2008) involves meditating on compassionate thoughts and feelings toward oneself and others and has been shown to improve self-compassion.

4 Strengths based approaches: Utilise a strengths-based approach that focuses on identifying and building upon individuals' unique strengths and positive qualities. Help clients recognise and utilise their personal strengths in pursuit of their health goals. This approach fosters self-efficacy, optimism, and a sense of empowerment, which can enhance motivation and engagement in healthy behaviours (Proyer et al., 2019).

5 Incorporate Positive Psychology Interventions: Integrate evidence based positive psychology interventions into our positive health practice. These interventions, such as positive journaling, three good things exercise, and positive reframing, have shown promising results in enhancing wellbeing and promoting healthier behaviours. They provide individuals with practical tools to cultivate positive emotions, resilience, and overall psychological flourishing (Sin & Lyubomirsky, 2009).

6 Foster Positive Social Connections: Recognise the importance of social connections in promoting positive emotions and overall health. Encourage our clients to engage in meaningful relationships, join support groups, or participate in community activities that foster positive social interactions. Positive social connections can provide emotional support, motivation, and a sense of belonging, which contribute to overall wellbeing and healthy living (Holt-Lunstad et al., 2010).

7 Tailor Interventions to Individual Needs and Context: Remember that individuals may have different preferences and responses to positive emotions. Tailor interventions to meet each person's unique needs, considering their cultural background, personality traits, and personal values. By personalising interventions, we can maximise their effectiveness and relevance for individuals seeking to live healthy lives.

8 Support Behaviour Change and Adherence: Positive emotions are leveraged to facilitate behaviour change and improve adherence to healthy lifestyle practices. Positive emotions act as powerful motivators in pursuing and achieving

goals. When individuals experience positive emotions, they are more likely to approach challenges with enthusiasm, persistence, and creativity. Positive emotions increase intrinsic motivation and enhance the belief in one's ability to succeed, leading to higher levels of goal attainment. By intentionally incorporating positive emotions into the goal setting process, our clients can cultivate a positive mindset, boost motivation, and increase their chances of success (Sheldon & Lyubomirsky, 2004). By creating positive emotional experiences associated with healthy behaviours, individuals are more motivated and inclined to adopt and maintain those behaviours. Lifestyle medicine programs incorporate strategies to evoke positive emotions and reinforce positive associations with healthy habits, thereby increasing long-term adherence (Rippe, 2018).

Summary

Incorporating positive emotions into our lives can have transformative effects on our wellbeing, health, personal growth, and resilience. By understanding the theoretical background and exploring practical applications we can move towards an appreciation of the power of positive emotions. Embracing positive emotions as an integral component of positive health can optimise physical and mental health outcomes, leading to a healthy and thriving life.

Takeaways

- Positive emotions broaden our cognitive and behavioural repertoires, enhancing creativity, problem-solving, health, wellbeing and resilience.
- Positive emotional regulation strategies such as savouring, gratitude, meditation, and meaningful activities can be incorporated into daily life to promote wellbeing.
- Cultivation positive emotions within relationships deepens emotional bonds and strengthens the quality of our relationships.
- We can experience micromoments of connection with strangers and do not need the shared history of an intimate or kinship relationship to experience positivity resonance.
- Positive emotions show promise in impacting both physical and mental health and promoting adaptive coping.
- Positive emotions support motivation, intrinsic motivation and resilience.

Wicked questions

1 How can individuals cultivate positive emotions in the face of adversity or challenging life circumstances? If it fair to expect them to do this?
2 How do personal preferences and cultural factors influence what counts as something that evokes a positive emotion? How can we design universal interventions when one persons 'awe' might be another person's 'awful'?

3 How can we sensitively incorporate positive emotion interventions into situations of suffering and despair while ensuring that we acknowledge and make space for suffering?
4 How can we best study the mechanisms and impact of an emotional experience that is one emotion shared across two bodies (e.g. positivity resonance)?

References

Armenta, C. N., Fritz, M. M., & Lyubomirsky, S. (2017). Functions of positive emotions: Gratitude as a motivator of self-improvement and positive change. *Emotion Review*, 9(3), 183–190.
Ashby, F. G., Isen, A. M., & Turken, A. U. (1999). A neuropsychological theory of positive affect and its influence on cognition. *Psychological Review*, 106(3), 529.
Bai, Y., Maruskin, L. A., Chen, S., Gordon, A. M., Stellar, J. E., McNeil, G. D.,... & Keltner, D. (2017). Awe, the diminished self, and collective engagement: Universals and cultural variations in the small self. *Journal of Personality and Social Psychology*, 113(2), 185. https://doi.org/10.1037/pspa0000087
Bailey, C. (2022). The Vanishing Point - Performance. https://www.youtube.com/watch?v=QDe-EGMaWgY
Baumeister, R. F., Bratslavsky, E., Finkenauer, C., & Vohs, K. D. (2001). Bad is stronger than good. *Review of General Psychology*, 5(4), 323–370.
Bryant, F. B., & Veroff, J. (2017). *Savoring: A new model of positive experience*. Psychology Press.
Cohen, S., & Wills, T. A. (1985). Stress, social support, and the buffering hypothesis. *Psychological Bulletin*, 98(2), 310–357.
Darewych, O. H., & Riedel Bowers, N. (2018). Positive arts interventions: Creative clinical tools promoting psychological well-being. *International Journal of Art Therapy*, 23(2), 62–69. https://doi.org/10.1080/17454832.2017.1378241
Emmons, R. A., & McCullough, M. E. (2003). Counting blessings versus burdens: An experimental investigation of gratitude and subjective well-being in daily life. *Journal of Personality and Social Psychology*, 84(2), 377–389. https://doi.org/10.1037/0022-3514.84.2.377
Fredrickson, B. L. (2003). The value of positive emotions: The emerging science of positive psychology is coming to understand why it's good to feel good. *American Scientist*, 91(4), 330–335.
Fredrickson, B. L. (2013a). *Love 2.0: How our supreme emotion affects everything we feel, think, do, and become*. Penguin.
Fredrickson, B. L. (2013b). Positive emotions broaden and build. In E. L. Deci & R. M. Ryan (Eds.), *Handbook of self-determination research* (pp. 143–156). The University of Rochester Press.
Fredrickson, B. L. (2013c). Updated thinking on positivity ratios. *American Psychologist*, 68(9), 814–822. https://doi.org/10.1037/a0033584
Fredrickson, B. L., & Branigan, C. (2005). Positive emotions broaden the scope of attention and thought-action repertoires. *Cognition & Emotion*, 19(3), 313–332.
Fredrickson, B. L., Cohn, M. A., Coffey, K. A., Pek, J., & Finkel, S. M. (2008). Open hearts build lives: Positive emotions, induced through loving-kindness meditation, build consequential personal resources. *Journal of Personality and Social Psychology*, 95(5), 1045–1062.
Fredrickson, B. L., & Levenson, R. W. (1998). Positive emotions speed recovery from the cardiovascular sequelae of negative emotions. *Cognition & Emotion*, 12(2), 191–220.

Fredrickson, B. L., & Losada, M. F. (2005). Positive affect and the complex dynamics of human flourishing. *American Psychologist*, 60(7), 678.

Fredrickson, B. L., Mancuso, R. A., Branigan, C., & Tugade, M. M. (2000). The undoing effect of positive emotions. *Motivation and Emotion*, 24(4), 237–258.

Gable, S. L., Reis, H. T., Impett, E. A., & Asher, E. R. (2004). What do you do when things go right? The intrapersonal and interpersonal benefits of sharing positive events. *Journal of Personality and Social Psychology*, 87(2), 228.

Garland, E. L., Farb, N. A., Goldin, P. R., & Fredrickson, B. L. (2015). Mindfulness broadens awareness and builds eudaimonic meaning: A process model of mindful positive emotion regulation. *Psychological Inquiry*, 26(4), 293–314. https://doi.org/10.1080/1047840X.2015.1064294

Gottman, J. M. (1993). The roles of conflict engagement, escalation, or avoidance in marital interaction: A longitudinal view of five types of couples. *Journal of Consulting and Clinical Psychology*, 61, 6–15.

Gottman, J. M., (1994). *What predicts divorce?* Lawrence Erlbaum Associates.

Grewen, K. M., Girdler, S. S., Amico, J., & Light, K. C. (2005). Effects of partner support on resting oxytocin, cortisol, norepinephrine, and blood pressure before and after warm partner contact. *Psychosomatic Medicine*, 67(4), 531–538.

Griskevicius, V., Shiota, M. N., & Neufeld, S. L. (2010). Influence of different positive emotions on persuasion processing: A functional evolutionary approach. *Emotion*, 10(2), 190–206.

Hasson, U., Ghazanfar, A. A., Galantucci, B., Garrod, S., & Keysers, C. (2012). Brain-to-brain coupling: A mechanism for creating and sharing a social world. *Trends in Cognitive Sciences*, 16(2), 114–121. https://doi.org/10.1016/j.tics.2011.12.007

Holt-Lunstad, J., Smith, T. B., & Layton, J. B. (2010). Social relationships and mortality risk: A meta-analytic review. *PLOS Medicine*, 7(7), e1000316. https://doi.org/10.1371/journal.pmed.1000316

Johnson, S. L., & Carver, C. S. (2006). Extreme goal setting and vulnerability to mania among undiagnosed young adults. *Cognitive Therapy and Research*, 30(3), 377–395.

Kashdan, T. B., Biswas-Diener, R., & King, L. A. (2017). Reconsidering happiness: The costs of distinguishing between hedonics and eudaimonia. In L. G. Aspinwall & U. M. Staudinger (Eds.), *The Oxford Handbook of Human Motivation* (pp. 486–501). Oxford University Press.

Kawachi, I., Subramanian, S. V., & Kim, D. (2004). Social capital and health: A decade of progress and beyond. In S. V. Subramanian & I. Kawachi (Eds.), *Social capital and health* (pp. 1–26). Springer.

Kemp, A. H., Quintana, D. S., Felmingham, K. L., Matthews, S., & Jelinek, H. F. (2012). Depression, comorbid anxiety disorders, and heart rate variability in physically healthy, unmedicated patients: Implications for cardiovascular risk. *PloS One*, 7(2), e30777.

Keng, S. L., Smoski, M. J., & Robins, C. J. (2011). Effects of mindfulness on psychological health: A review of empirical studies. *Clinical Psychology Review*, 31(6), 1041–1056. https://doi.org/10.1016/j.cpr.2011.04.006

Kenreich, S., Djalovski, A., Kraus, L., Louzoun, Y., & Feldman, R. (2017). Brain-to-brain synchrony during naturalistic social interactions. *Scientific Reports*, 7(1), 1–12.

Kok, B. E., Coffey, K. A., Cohn, M. A., Catalino, L. I., Vacharkulksemsuk, T., Algoe, S. B.,... & Fredrickson, B. L. (2013). How positive emotions build physical health: Perceived positive social connections account for the upward spiral between positive emotions and vagal tone. *Psychological Science*, 24(7), 1123–1132.

Kosfeld, M., Heinrichs, M., Zak, P. J., Fischbacher, U., & Fehr, E. (2005). Oxytocin increases trust in humans. *Nature*, 435(7042), 673–676. https://doi.org/10.1038/nature03701

Leong, V., Byrne, E., Clackson, K., Georgieva, S., Lam, S., & Wass, S. (2017). Speaker gaze increases information coupling between infant and adult brains. *Proceedings of the National Academy of Sciences*, 114(50), 13290–13295.

Lindsay, E. K., Chin, B., Greco, C. M., Young, S., Brown, K. W., Wright, A. G.,... & Creswell, J. D. (2018). How mindfulness training promotes positive emotions: Dismantling acceptance skills training in two randomized controlled trials. *Journal of Personality and Social Psychology*, 115(6), 944.

Navarra, R. J., & Gottman, J. M. (2019). Bids and turning toward in Gottman Method Couple Therapy. In J. Lebow, A. Chambers, & D. C., Breunlin (Eds.). *Encyclopedia of couple and family therapy* (pp. 253–255). Springer International Publishing.

Nelson, S. K., Layous, K., Cole, S. W., & Lyubomirsky, S. (2016). Do unto others or treat yourself? The effects of prosocial and self-focused behavior on psychological flourishing. *Emotion*, 16(6), 850.

Otake, K., Shimai, S., Tanaka-Matsumi, J., Otsui, K., & Fredrickson, B. L. (2006). Happy people become happier through kindness: A counting kindnesses intervention. *Journal of Happiness Studies*, 7(3), 361–375.

Parks, A. C., Della Porta, M. D., Pierce, R. S., Zilca, R., & Lyubomirsky, S. (2012). Pursuing happiness in everyday life: The characteristics and behaviors of online happiness seekers. *Emotion*, 12(6), 1222–1234. https://doi.org/10.1037/a0028587

Piff, P. K., Dietze, P., Feinberg, M., Stancato, D. M., & Keltner, D. (2015). Awe, the small self, and prosocial behavior. *Journal of Personality and Social Psychology*, 108(6), 883. https://doi.org/10.1037/pspi0000018

Porges, S. W. (2007). The polyvagal perspective. *Biological Psychology*, 74(2), 16–143.

Pressman, S. D., & Cohen, S. (2005). Does positive affect influence health?. *Psychological Bulletin*, 131(6), 925.

Proyer, R. T., Gander, F., Wellenzohn, S., & Ruch, W. (2019). Strengths-based positive psychology interventions: A randomized placebo-controlled online trial on long-term effects for a signature strengths–vs. a lesser strengths–intervention. *Frontiers in Psychology*, 10, 456. https://doi.org/10.3389/fpsyg.2015.00456

Rippe, J. M. (2018). Lifestyle medicine: The health promoting power of daily habits and practices. *American Journal of Lifestyle Medicine*, 12(6), 499–512. https://doi.org/10.1177/1559827618785554. PMID: 30783405; PMCID: PMC6367881.

Ryan, R. M., & Deci, E. L. (2001). On happiness and human potentials: A review of research on hedonic and eudemonic well-being. *Annual Review of Psychology*, 52(1), 141–166.

Schultz, W. (2007). Multiple dopamine functions at different time courses. *Annual Review of Neuroscience*, 30, 259–288.

Seligman, M. E. P., Steen, T. A., Park, N., & Peterson, C. (2005). Positive psychology progress: Empirical validation of interventions. *American Psychologist*, 60(5), 410–421. https://doi.org/10.1037/0003-066X.60.5.410

Shamay-Tsoory, S. G., & Abu-Akel, A. (2016). The social salience hypothesis of oxytocin. *Biological Psychiatry*, 79(3), 194–202.

Sheldon, K. M., & Lyubomirsky, S. (2004). Achieving Sustainable New Happiness: Prospects, Practices, and Prescriptions. In P. A. Linley & S. Joseph (Eds.), *Positive psychology in practice* (pp. 127–145). John Wiley & Sons, Inc. https://doi.org/10.1002/9780470939338.ch8

Siegel, D.J. (2001). Toward an interpersonal neurobiology of the developing mind: Attachment relationships, "mindsight," and neural integration. *Infant Mental Health Journal*,22,67–94.https://doi.org/10.1002/1097-0355(200101/04)22:1<67::AID-IMHJ3>3.0.CO;2-G

Sin, N. L., & Lyubomirsky, S. (2009). Enhancing well-being and alleviating depressive symptoms with positive psychology interventions: A practice-friendly meta-analysis. *Journal of Clinical Psychology*, 65(5), 467–487. https://doi.org/10.1002/jclp.20593

Sirois, F. M., & Wood, A. M. (2017). Gratitude uniquely predicts lower depression in chronic illness populations: A longitudinal study of inflammatory bowel disease and arthritis. *Health Psychology*, 36(2), 122–132. https://doi.org/10.1037/hea0000436

Stellar, J. E., John-Henderson, N., Anderson, C. L., Gordon, A. M., McNeil, G. D., & Keltner, D. (2015). Positive affect and markers of inflammation: Discrete positive emotions predict lower levels of inflammatory cytokines. *Emotion*, 15(2), 129–133.

Stephens, G. J., Silbert, L. J., & Hasson, U. (2010). Speaker-listener neural coupling underlies successful communication. *Proceedings of the National Academy of Sciences*, 107(32), 14425–14430.

Thayer, J. F., & Lane, R. D. (2007). The role of vagal function in the risk for cardio-vascular disease and mortality. *Biological Psychology*, 74(2), 224–242. https://doi.org/10.1016/j.biopsycho.2005.11.013

Tsai, J. L. (2007). Ideal affect: Cultural causes and behavioural consequences. *Perspectives on Psychological Science*, 2(3), 242–259.

Tugade, M. M., & Fredrickson, B. L. (2004). Resilient individuals use positive emotions to bounce back from negative emotional experiences. *Journal of Personality and Social Psychology*, 86(2), 320–333. https://doi.org/10.1037/0022-3514.86.2.320

Uchino, B. N. (2006). Social support and health: A review of physiological processes potentially underlying links to disease outcomes. *Journal of Behavioral Medicine*, 29(4), 377–387.

Uvnäs-Moberg, K., Bruzelius, G., Alster, P., & Lundeberg, T. (1993). The antinociceptive effect of non-noxious sensory stimulation is mediated partly through oxytocinergic mechanisms. *Acta Physiologica Scandinavica*, 149(2), 199–204.

Verneert, F., Nijs, L., & De Baets, T. (2021). A space for collaborative creativity. How collective improvising shapes 'a sense of belonging'. *Frontiers in Psychology*, 12, 1080.

Waugh, C. E., & Fredrickson, B. L. (2006). Nice to know you: Positive emotions, self–other overlap, and complex understanding in the formation of a new relationship. *The Journal of Positive Psychology*, 1(2), 93–106.

Wood, A. M., Froh, J. J., & Geraghty, A. W. A. (2010). Gratitude and well-being: A review and theoretical integration. *Clinical Psychology Review*, 30(7), 890–905. https://doi.org/10.1016/j.cpr.2010.03.005

8

RESILIENT GRIEVING

How can the field of positive health better support those coping with loss?

Lucy C. Hone, Tiffani Clingin and Brigitte Lavoie

Given grieving is a multi-dimensional experience affecting health broadly – emotionally, psychologically, physically, behaviourally, socially, cognitively, practically, and spiritually – bereavement science has an important role to play in augmenting the understanding of grief and grieving. Similarly, health-practitioners also perform a key function supporting the bereaved towards healthy adaptation to loss. Unfortunately, however, there currently exists a breakdown in the translation of science to practice, with many myths and misconceptions widely practiced despite lack of empirical evidence. One such myth is that there are universally applicable set stages of grief. Popularised by Elisabeth Kübler Ross's Five Stage model and later perpetuated by other writers, researchers are now calling for stage theory to be discarded.

> Major concerns include the absence of sound empirical evidence, conceptual clarity, or explanatory potential. It lacks practical utility for the design or allocation of treatment services, and it does not help identification of those at risk or with complications in the grieving process. Most disturbingly, the expectation that bereaved persons will, even should, go through stages of grieving can be harmful to those who do not.
> *(report Stroebe, Schut, & Boerner, 2017)*

Contemporary grief theorists widely agree, deeming them "suspiciously simplistic models" (Neimeyer, 2000, p. 54). Even Kübler Ross and her co-author, David Kessler, later wrote "they are not stops on some linear timeline in grief. Not everyone goes through all of them or in a prescribed order" (2005, p. 7).

Most worryingly, there is also evidence from both empirical research and our own practice that stage theory can be harmful for the bereaved. Silver and Wortman summarise as follows:

DOI: 10.4324/9781003378426-10   122

A mistaken belief in the stage model... can have devastating consequences. Not only can it lead bereaved persons to feel that they are not coping appropriately, but it can also result in ineffective support provision by members of their social network as well as unhelpful and potentially harmful responses by healthcare professionals.

(2007, p. 2692)

Our own experiences mirror this, with clients often expressing concern that they are "not grieving right" because they are not going through the five stages.
As Brigitte Lavoie (one of this chapter's authors) says,

I stopped using the stages of grief 20 years ago, because of the importance of 'Do no harm' that is even more relevant in suicide prevention. In that field, we had already introduced the Solution Focused Brief Therapy tools to foster hope, identify something that was worth living for and pay attention to what was working for each person. It made sense to do the same with people who were grieving. Since then, when I train people, I ask who has already stopped using the stages of grief and most clinicians raise their hands. It is encouraging and yet, some don't know what to do instead.
(personal communication with Lucy Hone, 15th December 2022)

So what can health professionals use instead? With backgrounds in Solution Focused Brief Therapy, positive psychology, and exercise science, the authors (practitioners with decades of experience from different parts of the world) have all worked to identify and apply more strengths-based, hopeful, agentic tools to support healthy adaptation to loss. Below we describe the theories, insights, professional and personal experiences that have shaped our approach to loss, and its effects on the bereaved.

Application of theories

Introducing resilient grieving (by Lucy Hone)

Resilient Grieving (RG) is the name I use to describe the application of resilience research to the bereavement context. RG has evolved over the last six years to become a flexible, modular, training programme responding to demand from a diverse range of health and education professionals for a practical, research-informed approach to support healthy adaptation to loss among the non-clinical population.

The concept came from my own experiences of coping with loss when our 12-year-old daughter was killed in a car accident in 2014. As a researcher investigating the epidemiology of flourishing, I was well acquainted with the field of positive psychology and, having recently lived through a two-year period of destructive earthquakes in Christchurch (NZ), resilience was a particular interest. So, when Abi died, I was struck by the passive tone of the grief resources

123

and the pathologising focus of health professionals' advice. While we were told we should expect to write off five years to her loss by Victim Support, my own field provided a more hopeful picture. For instance, the most common response to loss is resilience, whereby the bereaved demonstrated an ability to sustain reasonably stable and adaptive levels of functioning despite their loss (Bonanno, 2004).

> Many people are exposed to loss or potentially traumatic events at some point in their lives, and yet they continue to have positive emotional experiences and show only minor and transient disruptions in their ability to function. Unfortunately, because much of psychology's knowledge about how adults cope with loss or trauma has come from individuals who sought treatment or exhibited great distress, loss and trauma theorists have often viewed this type of resilience as either rare or pathological.
>
> *(explains Bonanno, 2004, p. 20)*

Based on what I knew about resilience being the most common response to bereavement (Bonanno, 2004) and requiring very ordinary processes (Masten, 2001; Reivich & Shatté, 2002; Southwick & Charney, 2012), I was curious to test the application of positive psychology to the grief context, a construct I termed Resilient Grieving in my first presentation on the topic at IPPA's World Congress (Hone, 2015).

RG adopts a positive health model, seeking to understand the determinants and evidence-based strategies associated with healthy grieving. Since 2017, our team has created a comprehensive practice programme sharing RG practices widely via several different formats. Included among these are: publishing a non-fiction book for lay audiences, Resilient Grieving (Hone, 2017), and a programme outline for practitioners (Verma & Neimeyer, 2020); a top 20 TED talk (TED, 2020); online training programmes for helping professionals; a dedicated podcast series; an audible course on Insight Timer; asynchronous and synchronous courses for the bereaved; and guest appearances on over a dozen podcasts globally.

Just as Rashid and Seligman created Positive Psychotherapy as the 'opposite' of psychotherapy-as-usual, RG as a conceptual model encourages the bereaved (and the wide range of professionals supporting them) to focus on what is still right and good in their lives, to "deploy what is best about them" (Rashid and Seligman, 2019). This approach contrasts with standard grief interventions by introducing the generative potential of positive emotions, realistic optimism, hope, meaning-making, posttraumatic growth, strong supportive relationships, strengths, mindfulness, and self-compassion to support healthy adaptation to loss and posttraumatic growth among non-clinical populations.

Part of the RG ethos is encouraging each individual to understand that we all grieve differently and they therefore need to identify what helps and what harms them adapt to their loss. This aligns with Layous and Lyubomirsky's work demonstrating the importance of individual person-activity fit for positive interventions (Sheldon et al., 2014). We do this by using a jigsaw metaphor, explaining that losing someone we love can feel like our life has been smashed apart. However, over time each of us can find ways of thinking, acting, and being that help piece our life back together again. In this way, the jigsaw metaphor is helpful in building both hope for the future and agency. We've found the jigsaw metaphor to be extremely popular among practitioners, because of its adaptability and potential for personalisation. Jo Soldan, clinical psychologist at Maggie's cancer support centre in Cardiff, Wales, has been using RG and the jigsaw metaphor in their bereavement groups for the past three years (personal communication, 9 December, 2022).

"We introduced it after I read Resilient Grieving and was blown away (to my shame) that grief was the only clinical area where I was not applying resilience research and understanding. Lucy's book was literally an aha moment for me – why had I not? We run a six week bereavement group and introduce a blank jigsaw at the end of session one (after people share their stories). Each group then completes their own jigsaw – writing on pieces as we go as they pull out the Resilient Grieving themes and ideas we share with one another. The Resilient Grieving model helps embody the dual process model in our groups in a way that I had not managed before. It gives time for the loss-oriented processing but also gives time and place to the restoration-orientated approach. We often give the group a jigsaw piece keyring at the last session to remind them of taking it one piece at a time. Our visitors' feedback consistently suggests they find it helpful, describing it as 'helpful, safe, inspiring, uplifting, fun' not words I used to hear before using the RG model!"

Below are three comments from individual staff at a New Zealand hospice describing the impact the RG model has had on them and their work (S. Marshall, personal communication, 14 December, 2022):

"I enjoyed learning about positive emotions and the focus on grief and joy co-existing. I have found it useful for myself personally, and also to support those that are grieving, in that they are allowed to feel good emotions too, it doesn't take away from their pain, grief and loss."

"I have been making more effort to ask patients of their families about loved ones that they have lost and to share good memories they have of them. It is especially useful to focus on the good times when they were well compared to the current focus on their illness at the end of life."

"As well as for professional development and ongoing learning to assist the bereaved families we work with, I am hoping our staff can utilise the course material for their own resilience as it has been extremely challenging working with the terminally ill during a pandemic."

The content and supporting research from our RG sessions are outlined below in Table 8.1 Practitioners wanting to integrate the theories and practices of RG

Table 8.1 Session-by-session description of the resilient grieving modular programme

Theme	Suggested content/positive interventions	Examples of supportive research	Suggested reflection questions & resources
Session 1 Introduction to Resilient Grieving	Deliver hope by relaying that resilience is common and that they already have intrapersonal and interpersonal resources that will help them manage; personal resilience story.	Reivich & Shatté (2002); Bonanno (2004); Bonanno (2019); Rashid & Seligman (2019); Charney & Southwich (2012); Masten (2001).	Tell me about a challenging time you've experienced in the past and how you've managed that?
Session 2 Mental agility	Attention focus; gratitude; realistic optimism; and self compassion.	Baumeister et al. (2001); Schneider (2001); Seligman et al. (2005); Neff (2018).	What and who are still good in your world? Is what you are doing (the way you are thinking or the way you are acting) helping or harming you in your quest to get through this?
Session 3 Positive Emotions	Introduce Broaden & Build Theory and Verstaen et al.'s work on life enhancing activities so that they understand positive experiences are part of grief and have a key role to play.	Fredrickson et al. (2008); Verstaen et al. (2018); Folkman (2008) Stroebe & Schut (2008).	Have u experienced any positive emotions at any time in your grief? Are you aware that positive and negative emotions can co-occur during stressful periods? How can you take a rest from grief, what replenishes you?
Session 4 Relationships	Tree of Positive Relationships; avoiding Thinking Traps; Understanding the different types of help typically required of the bereaved and identifying who might help in different ways.	Rashid & Seligman (2019); Reivich & Shatté (2002).	Who might provide emotional support? Who might provide practical support? Who might keep their memory alive? Who might help with informational support?

(Continued)

Table 8.1 (Continued)

Theme	Suggested content/positive interventions	Examples of supportive research	Suggested reflection questions & resources
Session 5 Knowing and using your strengths	Introducing strengths theory and practice; Invite participants to take the VIA survey and reflect on the results.	Niemiec (2013); Niemiec & Wedding (2013); Rashid & Seligman (2019); Gillham, Rashid & Anjum (2020).	Which strengths can you see you are using currently to help you manage your grief? Are there any you could be using more?
Session 6 Growth and meaning	Benefit finding; interventions to promote meaning making and sense making; understanding prevalence, key aspects and determinants of posttraumatic growth and being an expert companion.	Frankl (1985); Neimeyer, Baldwin, & Gillies (2006); Neimeyer et al. (2010); Calhoun & Tedeschi (2014); Tedeschi & Moore (2016); Wu et al. (2019)	What are you left with? What have you learned about yourself through this whole experience? How have your priorities shifted because of this loss?
Session 7 Coping with big emotions	Mindfulness; self-compassion and vulnerability; identifying sources of potential 'grief ambush'; introducing and identifying secondary losses.	Kabat-Zinn (2003); Neff (2011); Brené Brown (2012)	Can you relate to the idea of a grief ambush? What different ways does your loss impinge on your life? How can you use your insights about secondary losses to help prepare for grief ambushes?
Session 8 Hope, rituals and legacy building	Maintaining connections with the deceased via rituals; developing legacy building.	Corr & Doka (2019); Feudtner (2009); Bonanno (2019); Norton & Gino (2014)	What are you hoping for now? What matters most to you as you look forward? What did they teach you? What is their legacy to you and those that they have left behind?

in to their work, without embarking upon a longer programme, can find practical summaries of the key concepts in the book, Resilient Grieving (Hone, 2017) or by contacting the lead author.

Below are two case studies of how RG has been incorporated into different health practices internationally.

Case study 1

CASE STUDY DEMONSTRATING CHANGE USING THE PERMA-PROFILER
(BY TIFFANI CLINGIN)

Evidence indicates that happiness is pliant, shaped by our intentional behaviours (Diener et al., 2009). Knowing that happiness is malleable, scholars developed a range of positive psychology interventions (PPIs), defined as volitional exercises to heighten wellbeing. Here, we characterise wellbeing as "feeling good and functioning well" (Aked et al., 2008, p. 6). Growing empirical evidence ratifies an assortment of PPI types, particularly gratitude, meaning, strengths, empathy, forgiveness, and savouring practices (Parks & Schueller, 2014). Over time, interventions have been administered in workplaces, schools, and community groups, as well as with individuals (Kern et al., 2020).

This case study explores the innovative application of a suite of well-regarded PPIs from the strengths, savouring and relationship literature to help a 55-year-old client, Gerry grieving the unexpected death of his adult child. Gerry's 24-year-old daughter was found dead in her parked car, and the coroner could not find a cause, which was a great stress source for him. The loss occurred seven months before Gerry scheduled an appointment with a mental health social worker. On his intake paperwork, Gerry said he felt flat every day and had fleeting thoughts of dying to make his emotional pain end.

Gerry completed the Kessler psychological distress scale, a ten-item questionnaire to measure distress based on questions about anxiety and depressive symptoms that a person has experienced in the most recent four-week period, and scored 28, indicating high levels of psychological anguish (Andrews & Slade, 2001). Gerry also completed a second self-assessment questionnaire, the PERMA Profiler (Butler & Kern, 2016). The PERMA profiler measures eudaimonic and hedonic features of wellbeing, with scores enabling each component of PERMA to be calibrated individually. Extending his earlier work on authentic happiness, Seligman published Wellbeing Theory (2011), declaring positive emotion, engagement, relationships, meaning, and accomplishment (PERMA) to be the quintessential elements of wellbeing. Gerry scored 9.2 or very high functioning for meaning, but 6.3 or less, sub-optimal functioning, for all remaining elements of PERMA. The chosen metrics were intended to quantify the impact of the PPIs with Gerry.

Based on several elements of PERMA, Gerry's goals included: increasing the frequency and intensity of positive emotions, nurturing relationships, and amplifying performance. These correlate with the P, R, and A in PERMA. However, it was plausible that PPIs might also buttress meaning (M) and engagement (E), as evidenced by Goodman and partners (2018), whose study of 517 adults found that enhancing one of the elements tends to raise the others to a comparable degree.

The worker invited Gerry to contemplate favourable sensations: curiosity, pride, awe, hope, inspiration, gratitude, serenity, humour, and love, and consider how he could find these in his day. Studies affirm a correlation between positive emotions and success in diverse areas of life (Lopez et al., 2018). According to Fredrickson and Kurtz (2011), positive emotions have adaptational benefits, extending peoples' capacity for managing various needs, widening their thought-action repertoire, and bolstering their ability to think and behave in a novel, helpful way. Positive sensations raise resilience and help people bounce back from disappointments (Cohn & Fredrickson, 2009). Negative sensations, on the other hand, narrow focus and behaviour (Boniwell, 2012). As such, it made sense for Gerry to increase the intensity and frequency of positive emotions, helping him foster psychological and behavioural flexibility, via a process known as savouring. Savouring is the deliberate process of attending to pleasant feelings and consciously augmenting them (Peterson, 2006). Bryant and Veroff (2007) outline three central actions linked with savouring: recalling pleasant past experiences, reflecting on here-and-now pleasure, and anticipating coveted upcoming adventures. Regardless of the temporal focus, savouring interventions may be useful for heightening positive emotions and, therefore, helpful to Gerry in his grieving (Smith et al., 2014).

Dovetailing nicely with positive emotions are relationships. Defined as positive connections, relationships promote adaptive functioning, with belonging described as a critical human need (Dutton & Heaphy, 2003). Personal ties buttress hope and gratitude, and collaboration has an uplifting influence on mood and achievement, findings aligned with research confirming the broader benefits of belonging (House et al., 1988). Relationships have beneficial consequences for mental and physical health, explaining the goal of nurturing social connection for Gerry as he comes to terms with losing his daughter (Taylor, 2011). Gerry operationalised the goal by listing three people who count most and contacting them each week.

Next, Gerry performed the Values in Action (VIA) survey, a strengths-based classification concerned with positive human traits and virtues, to increase his recognition of his psychological capacities (Peterson & Seligman, 2004). The VIA enhances awareness of what is most useful in ourselves and each other, encouraging people to adopt and practice their strengths, cultivating genuine connections, fulfilment, and aiding goal attainment (Linley et al., 2010). Gerry's top VIA strengths – bravery, leadership, and self-regulation – provided helpful information about his psychological landscape, suggesting it might be natural for Gerry to act on his convictions and get things done (Peterson & Seligman, 2004). With this in mind, Gerry was encouraged to be mindful of his strengths, choosing one or more to use over the week to augment accomplishments: intrinsically motivated successes tend to mean the most, and small subjective wins could be especially helpful for Gerry's grief journey (Locke & Latham, 2002).

Notably, the research cannot say whether a particular technique will work for every individual (Schueller, 2012). So Layous and Lyubomirsky (2014) propose a person-activity fit criterion to explain the factors that mediate the efficacy of PPIs, including the characteristics of activities and individuals and the match between them, with the authors affirming that fit moderately regulates program gains. Similarly, Schueller (2014), in a study of person-activity fit, found that strength exercises are suited to introverts, with extroverts profiting from savouring activities. This distinction motivated the practitioner to add both to Gerry's care plan, to support each viewpoint.

After six weeks of work, Gerry retook the initial evaluations; the K10 and the PERMA Profiler. Self-evaluations are prone to reduced fidelity and self-reporting bias (Althubaiti, 2016). As such, practitioners should be cautious of self-evaluation and, at the same time, appreciate their worth. Gerry's K10 score fell to 21, which is a mild disorder. The PERMA results showed an increase in all domains to 7 or more, in keeping with normal functioning, except for meaning, rising slightly to 9.3, highly functioning.

Case study 2

HEARTS – A PARADIGM SHIFT IN CLINICAL BEREAVEMENT PRACTICE (BY BRIGITTE LAVOIE)

One of the most important contributions of Hone's work is to help clinicians believe that their clients are likely to get better after a devastating lost. This belief helps them see resilience in their clients and it helps them see that they can be a tutor for resilience. For instance, I used to tell my clients that healing was a long process, and they had to go through all the stages before they could get better. This made the process longer. I saw a big change in client responses when I changed my beliefs and the focus of our conversations.

One of the first examples was a client whose infant son had just died. When I first talked to him, I asked him to notice the things that helped him get through his days, the moments and the people that made things easier for him. He told me he insisted on having a meal with his wife, and the two of them felt more connected. It made them feel more hopeful. He said, "It made a big difference that you told me I had the right to live, even if my son was dead." These were his words, I had not actually said that. But it was explicit in our conversation that he didn't need to wait to have moments of reprieve.

HEARTS, an acronym to replace the stages of grief

Love is at the centre of grieving, for the person who has passed away, for the people who are still there, and maybe for ourselves and for life itself, so I use the word heart to summarise the most important aspects of RG: hope, emotions, agency, relationships, tailored interventions, and self-compassion (Lavoie, 2020). Clinicians can explore these themes using solution-focused questions (Lavoie, 2017) to help clients uncover their own resilience. It is easier for clients to feel hopeful when they see RG already happening in their own lives. It becomes evidence-based, i.e., based on the evidence of their own experience. Below I describe a few practice examples and sample questions.

Hope

Considering what happened, what are you hoping from our conversation?

What signs in your life will show you that you are getting better?

These questions can help identify client's hopes and what we need to do to help their hopes to grow. Grieving clients have all lost someone, but that doesn't mean their hopes are all the same.

Emotions

We can help clients see that the ten positive emotions exist and are legitimate, even while grieving. Here is one way to bring up this idea.

People can be surprised by the presence of more pleasant emotions as they are grieving. Some mention they feel even more connected, they feel gratitude, they appreciate nature in a different way. These emotions may sound like whispers, and sadness can be louder. If you pay attention to these whispers, it can help you keep your head above water and give you the strength you need to face the most difficult moments.

Agency, direction

I once worked with a young man with a drinking problem whose best friend died in a car crash before his eyes. He said, "That could have been me in the coffin. I didn't want my friend to die, but it was a wake-up call. That was the moment I decided to take control of my life." We didn't talk much about his friend or his past mistakes. We talked about the life he wanted for himself going forward. If clients see what happened as sign that things need to change, the most important thing to do with them could be to help make these changes happen.

Relationships

The people around your clients may not know how to help. It is important that your clients don't confound their lack of skill with a lack of love. This makes it even more important for them to be specific in their requests and to give people around them a "job" they can do.

What exactly do you need from _____? How could you let them know the difference it would make if they _____?

What would this person do if they knew?

Tailored interventions

A lot of grieving groups have adopted more tailored interventions. They re-placed "how was your week" with coping questions:

What was the most helpful thing you did this week?

What gives you the strength to put one foot in front of the other?

Facilitators have reported that, when they use these questions, fewer people drop out. One comment summarises the change: "I was surprised that we talked about the different ways we coped. Some of the group members inspired me, and some told me I inspired them. I left the group energized."

Self-compassion

Clinicians can encourage self-compassion in clients with their reactions to strug-gles: "You did the best you could under the circumstances. If it was easy, you would have done it already." They can also have a direct conversation about the way clients talk to themselves about what happened:

What are the most helpful, caring phrases you have heard since the event? Can you repeat them, or post them somewhere where you will see them?

In my trainings, I see a lot of clinicians ready to embrace change and to work to support RG in their clients. Sometimes it is hard, because the material and activities that are printed in official binders in their organisation are still heavily influenced by older models. I know a determined practitioner who didn't let this stop her from making changes. She had planned a walking path in the woods. The walk was divided into stations, each one about a stage of grieving. The goal was for clients to identify where they were in the stages and the work they still had left to do. In 24 hours after learning about RG, she changed the activity. For each station, she had clients reflect on one theme from the HEARTS acronym. Clients said they were afraid it was going to be difficult and didn't want to come, but the walk left them hopeful and grateful, and they were proud of everything they were doing to cope. This is another example of how clinicians will see more resilience when they believe it exists and when they ask clients to look for the signs that it is already happening.

Take aways

Practical

- Print off a blank jigsaw puzzle template from the internet. Build hope and belief that the bereaved can survive this loss using the suggested questions from the HEARTS framework above. Encourage them to build up a person-alised picture of what's helping them to adapt to their loss, suggesting they fill in each of the blank jigsaw puzzle pieces with the different ways of thinking, acting, and being they've found.
- Revise unhelpful myths and misunderstandings about grief (such as the com-monly held view that there are Five Stages to Grief) which frequently makes

the bereaved question whether they are grieving 'right.' Emphasise that there is no one 'right' way to grieve; instead, everyone grieves differently, and they'll find their own way.

- Invite bereaved clients to share the adaptive strategies they've used to cope with their grief by completing the Coping Assessment for Bereavement and Loss Experiences (CABLE; Crunk et al. 2021). This will help advance the field of Positive Health by expanding the body of knowledge regarding coping strategies, as well as potentially introducing the bereaved to alternative coping strategies.

General

- Despite a lack of empirical evidence, health-practitioners continue to promote the idea that people grieve in stages. This practice not only contradicts the deeply personal nature of grief (grief is as individual as your fingerprint, we all grieve differently) but we've seen the harm expectations of set stages continue to cause the bereaved.
- Our collective research and practice suggests both positive psychology and thanatology offer insights and strategies that bereaved individuals who wish to take an active and constructive role in their grief journey find useful and helpful. We'd like to see all practitioners working with the bereaved respect the wishes of those who want to be active participants in their grief process by suggesting active coping skills.
- In our experience, bereaved individuals find the explicit identification of their internal capacities and external supports both comforting and empowering, providing a more hopeful prescription for their ability to manage their loss. They felt mostly relieved when they heard they didn't have to go through stages and were allowed to have good moments as they were going through the most difficult time.
- In contrast to the traditional focus on complicated grief and prolonged grief disorder, we call upon thanatology researchers to broaden the scope of their empirical studies to investigate the effectiveness of Resilient Grieving theories, findings, and interventions in future research.
- As practitioners, when we know about prevalence of resilience and post-traumatic growth, we can see it in our clients and reflect what is already happening. We therefore encourage health practitioners globally to stop using stage models and try using some of the tools described below instead.

Wicked questions

- What has helped you navigate the losses of your life? (If you haven't experienced a close bereavement, either think about loss more broadly, or find a trusted friend or family member and ask them this question).
- If your organisation continues to adopt the Five Stages of Grief model, what can you do to help them understand its limitations, and potential harm? What

evidence will you use to encourage them to update their grief literature, advice and practices? If you cannot change the whole system, what can you do?
- While the Five Stages of Grief left many feeling they had to put life on hold while they grieved, evidence suggests that post-traumatic growth (PTG) is surprisingly common - as much as 52% of the bereaved experience reported moderate to high levels of PTG, according to a recent meta-analysis of 26 studies (Wu et al., 2019). We do not report this to place additional on the bereaved, but to suggest that raising the possibility of growth (in relationships, new directions and possibilities, a new way of looking at life/the world, an appreciation of their personal strength and shifts in spiritual or existential beliefs) can also be appropriate and empowering for the bereaved.

References

Aked, J., Marks, N., Cordon, C., & Thompson, S. (2008). *Five ways to wellbeing: The evidence*. New Economics Foundation.

Althubaiti, A. (2016). Information bias in health research: Definition, pitfalls, and adjustment methods. *Journal of Multidisciplinary Healthcare*, 9, 211–217.

Andrews, G., & Slade, T. (2001). Interpreting scores on the Kessler psychological distress scale (K10). *Australian and New Zealand Journal of Public Health*, 25(6), 494–497.

Baumeister, R. F., Bratslavsky, E., Finkenauer, C., & Vohs, K. D. (2001). Bad is stronger than good. *Review of General Psychology*, 5(4), 323–370.

Bonanno, G. A. (2004). Loss, trauma, and human resilience: Have we underestimated the human capacity to thrive after extremely aversive events? *American Psychologist*, 59(1), 20.

Bonanno, G. A. (2019). *The other side of sadness: What the new science of bereavement tells us about life after loss*. Hachette.

Boniwell, I. (2012). Positive psychology. In *A nutshell: The science of happiness*. McGraw-Hill Education (UK).

Brown, B. (2012). The power of vulnerability: Teachings on authenticity, connection and courage.

Bryant, F. B., & Veroff, J. (2007). *Savoring: A new model of positive experience*. Psychology Press.

Butler, J., & Kern, M. L. (2016). The PERMA-Profiler: A brief multidimensional measure of flourishing. *International Journal of Wellbeing*, 6(3).

Calhoun, L. G., & Tedeschi, R. G. (Eds.). (2014). *Handbook of posttraumatic growth: Research and practice*. Routledge.

Cohn, M. A., & Fredrickson, B. L. (2009). Positive emotions. In S. J. Lopez & C. R. Snyder (Eds.), *The Oxford handbook of positive psychology* (2nd ed., pp. 13–24). Oxford University Press.

Corr, C. A., & Doka, K. J. (2019). Continuing bonds and resilience. In *Promoting Resilience* (pp. 177–184). Routledge.

Crunk, A. E., Burke, L. A., Neimeyer, R. A., Robinson, E. H. M., & Bai, H. (2021). The coping assessment for bereavement and loss experiences (CABLE): Development and initial validation. *Death Studies*, 45(9), 677–691. https://doi.org/10.1080/074811 87.2019.1676323

Diener, E., Lucas, R. E., & Scollon, C. N. (2009). Beyond the hedonic treadmill: Revising the adaptation theory of well-being. In E. Diener (Ed.), *The science of well-being: The collected works of Ed Diener* (pp. 103–118). Springer.

Dutton, J. E., & Heaphy, E. D. (2003). The power of high-quality connections. In Cameron, K., & Dutton, J. (Eds.), *Positive organizational scholarship: Foundations of a new discipline* (pp. 263–278). Berrett-Koehler Publishers.

Feudtner, C. (2009). The breadth of hopes. *New England Journal of Medicine*, 361(24), 2306–2307. https://doi.org/10.1056/NEJMp0906516

Folkman, S. (2008). The case for positive emotions in the stress process. *Anxiety, Stress, and Coping*, 21(1), 3–14.

Frankl, V. E. (1985). *Man's search for meaning*. Simon and Schuster.

Fredrickson, B. L., Cohn, M. A., Coffey, K. A., Pek, J., & Finkel, S. M. (2008). Open hearts build lives: positive emotions, induced through loving-kindness meditation, build consequential personal resources. *Journal of Personality and Social Psychology*, 95(5), 1045.

Fredrickson, B. L., & Kurtz, L. E. (2011). Cultivating positive emotions to enhance human flourishing. In S. I. Donaldson, M. Csikszentmihalyi, & J. Nakamura, (Eds.), *Applied positive psychology: Improving everyday life, health, schools, work, and society* (pp. 35–47). Psychology Press..

Gillham, J., Rashid, T., & Anjum, A. (2020). *Strengths-Based Resilience: A Positive Psychology Program*. Hogrefe Publishing.

Goodman, F. R., Disabato, D. J., Kashdan, T. B., & Kauffman, S. B. (2018). Measuring well-being: A comparison of subjective well-being and PERMA. *The Journal of Positive Psychology*, 13(4), 321–332.

Hone, L. (2015). When happiness has a bad day. *Symposium delivered at the International Positive Psychology Association World Congress*. Tampa, Florida, July 2015.

Hone, L. (2017). *Resilient grieving: Finding strength and embracing life after a loss that changes everything*. The Experiment.

House, J. S., Landis, K. R., & Umberson, D. (1988). Social relationships and health. *Science*, 241(4865), 540–545.

Kabat-Zinn, J. (2003). Mindfulness-based interventions in context: Past, present, and future. *Clinical Psychology: Science and Practice*, 10(2), 144–156. https://doi.org/10.1093/clipsy.bpg016

Kern, M. L., Williams, P., Spong, C., Colla, R., Sharma, K., Downie, A., Taylor, J. A., Sharp, S., Siokou, C. & Oades, L. G. (2020). Systems informed positive psychology. *The Journal of Positive Psychology*, 15(6), 705–715.

Kübler-Ross, E., & Kessler, D. (2005). *On grief and grieving: Finding the meaning of grief through the five stages of loss*. Simon and Schuster.

Lavoie, B. (2017, July 13–16). *Combining positive psychology and solution-focused Brief Therapy: A promising model for promoting post-traumatic growth* [Conference presentation]. Fifth World Congress on Positive Psychology, Montreal, Quebec, Canada.

Lavoie, B. (2020). *Resilient grieving: Easier on the HEARTS of the bereaved: Guides and accompanying material*. Available at https://www.lavoiesolutions.com/app/download/11130281252/HEARTS+%26+AFTER+Guides+and+material.pdf?t=1661178427

Layous, K., & Lyubomirsky, S. (2014). The how, why, what, when, and who of happiness. In Gruber, J., & Moskowitz, J. T. (Eds.). *Positive emotion: Integrating the light sides and dark sides*, 473–495. Oxford University Press.

Linley, P. A., Nielsen, K. M., Gillett, R., & Biswas-Diener, R. (2010). Using signature strengths in pursuit of goals: Effects on goal progress, need satisfaction, and well-being, and implications for coaching psychologists. *International Coaching Psychology Review*, 5(1), 6–15.

Locke, E. A., & Latham, G. P. (2002). Building a practically useful theory of goal setting and task motivation: A 35-year odyssey. *American psychologist*, 57(9), 705.

Lopez, S. J., Pedrotti, J. T., & Snyder, C. R. (2018). *Positive psychology: The scientific and practical explorations of human strengths*. Sage Publications.

Masten, A. S. (2001). Ordinary magic: Resilience processes in development. *American Psychologist*, 56(3), 227.

Neff, K. (2011). *Self compassion*. Hachette.

Neff, K., & Germer, C. (2018). *The mindful self-compassion workbook: A proven way to accept yourself, build inner strength, and thrive*. Guilford Publications.

Neimeyer, R. A. (2000). Searching for the meaning of meaning: Grief therapy and the process of reconstruction. *Death Studies*, 24(6), 541–558.

Neimeyer, R. A., Baldwin S. A., & Gillies, J. (2006). Continuing bonds and reconstructing meaning: Mitigating complications in bereavement. *Death Studies*, 30(8), 715–738.

Neimeyer, R. A., Burke, L. A., Mackay, M. M., & van Dyke Stringer, J. G. (2010). Grief therapy and the reconstruction of meaning: From principles to practice. *Journal of Contemporary Psychotherapy*, 40(2), 73–83.

Niemiec, R. M. (2012). VIA character strengths: Research and practice (The first 10 years). In H. Knoop, & Delle Fave, A. (Eds.). Well-Being and Cultures. *Cross-Cultural Advancements in Positive Psychology*, vol 3. Springer, Dordrecht. https://doi.org/10.1007/978-94-007-4611-4_2

Niemiec, R. M., & Wedding, D. (2013). *Positive psychology at the movies: Using films to build virtues and character strengths*. Hogrefe Publishing.

Norton, M. I., & Gino, F. (2014). Rituals alleviate grieving for loved ones, lovers, and lotteries. *Journal of Experimental Psychology: General*, 143(1), 266.

Parks, A. C., & Schueller, S. (Eds.). (2014). *The Wiley Blackwell handbook of positive psychological interventions*. John Wiley & Sons.

Peterson, C. (2006). *A primer in positive psychology*. Oxford University Press.

Peterson, C., & Seligman, M. E. (2004). *Character strengths and virtues: A handbook and classification* (Vol. 1). Oxford University Press.

Rashid, T., & Seligman, M. E. (2019). *Positive Psychotherapy WB*. Oxford University Press.

Reivich, K., & Shatté, A. (2002). *The resilience factor: 7 essential skills for overcoming life's inevitable obstacles*. Broadway books.

Schneider, S. L. (2001). In search of realistic optimism: Meaning, knowledge, and warm fuzziness. *American Psychologist*, 56(3), 250.

Schueller, S. M. (2012). Personality fit and positive interventions: Extraverted and introverted individuals benefit from different happiness increasing strategies. *Psychology*, 3(12), 1166.

Schueller, S. M. (2014). Person-activity fit. In A. C. Parks, & S. Schueller (Eds.), *The Wiley Blackwell handbook of positive psychological interventions* (pp. 385–403). John Wiley & Sons.

Seligman, M. E. (2011). *Flourish: A visionary new understanding of happiness and well-being*. Simon and Schuster.

Seligman, M. E., Steen, T. A., Park, N., & Peterson, C. (2005). Positive psychology progress: Empirical validation of interventions. *American Psychologist*, 60(5), 410.

Sheldon, K. M., Boehm, J., & Lyubomirsky, S. (2014). Variety is the spice of happiness: The hedonic adaptation prevention model. In S. A. David, I. Boniwell, & A. C. Ayers (Eds.), *The Oxford handbook of happiness* (pp. 901–914). Oxford University Press.

Silver, R. C., & Wortman, C. B. (2007). The stage theory of grief. *The Journal of the American Medical Association*, 297(24), 2692–2694.

Smith, J. L., Harrison, P. R., Kurtz, J. L., & Bryant, F. B. (2014). Nurturing the Capacity to Savor: Interventions to enhance the enjoyment of positive experiences. In A. C. Parks, & S. Schueller (Eds.), *The Wiley Blackwell handbook of positive psychological interventions* (pp. 42–65). John Wiley & Sons.

Southwick, S. M., & Charney, D. S. (2012). The science of resilience: Implications for the prevention and treatment of depression. *Science*, 338(6103), 79–82. https://doi.org/10.1126/science.1222942

Stroebe, M. S., & Schut, H. (2008). The dual process model of coping with bereavement: Overview and update. *Grief Matters: The Australian Journal of Grief and Bereavement*, 11(1), 4–10.

Stroebe, M., Schut, H., & Boerner, K. (2017). Cautioning health-care professionals: Bereaved persons are misguided through the stages of grief. *OMEGA-Journal of Death and Dying*, 74(4), 455–473.

Taylor, S. E. (2011). Social support: A review. In H. S. Friedman (Ed.), *The Oxford handbook of health psychology* (pp. 189–214). Oxford University Press.

Tedeschi, R. G., & Moore, B. A. (2016). *The posttraumatic growth workbook: Coming through trauma wiser, stronger, and more resilient.* New Harbinger Publications.

TED.com. (2020). *The most popular talks of 2020.* https://www.ted.com/playlists/780/the_most_popular_talks_of_2020

TED.com (2020). *3 secrets of resilient people.* https://www.ted.com/talks/lucy_hone_3_secrets_of_resilient_people?utm_campaign=tedspread&utm_medium=referral&utm_source=tedcomshare

Verma, N., & Neimeyer, R. A. (2020). Grief and growth: An appreciative journey. *Practitioner*, 22(2), 36–41.

Verstaen, A., Moskowitz, J. T., Snowberg, K. E., Merrilees, J., & Dowling, G. A. (2018). Life enhancing activities for family caregivers of people with dementia: Protocol for a randomized controlled trial of a positive affect skills intervention. *Open Access Journal of Clinical Trials*, 10, 1.

Wu, X., Kaminga, A. C., Dai, W., Deng, J., Wang, Z., Pan, X., & Liu, A. (2019). The prevalence of moderate-to-high posttraumatic growth: A systematic review and meta-analysis. *Journal of Affective Disorders*, 243, 408–415. https://doi.org/10.1016/j.jad.2018.09.023

9

OPTIMISM, A CONCEPTUAL COMPLEXITY BUT A HEALTH RESOURCE?

Charles Martin-Krumm

The world's populations are confronted with multiple crises that are becoming global in scope, whether they are health crises (COVID 19), environmental crises (e.g., land resource issues), natural disaster crises (e.g., earthquakes in Turkey in 2023), or political or geo-political crises (e.g., the war in Ukraine). Inevitably, these crises have an impact that sometimes sets some individuals on the path of various psychological pathologies, depression or eco-anxiety. However, other individuals seem to get through these events without being particularly affected. What are the variables that could explain these inter-individual differences? Is it the environment in which they live that sustains them? Or is it individual resources that play a protective role? If it is a question of individual resources, potentially developed in a supportive environment, which resources could it be?

It is possible to assume that the ability of individuals to continue to project themselves positively into the future despite adversity is a key. Indeed, once the person is able to project themselves into a future that is favourable to them, they are oriented towards the future and not towards the past, which they might be likely to interpret negatively and brood over. Instead of feeling helpless, instead of perceiving a lack of control over the environment, these people can be active and adopt appropriate behaviours to deal with the situations they face, particularly in the area of health. This ability to project positively into the future may correspond to optimism. In other words, optimism can reveal people's ability to project themselves positively into the future despite the adversity they face. It is very easy to talk about optimism and it can be seen as a protective psychological resource for example. But what exactly is it? Only a capacity to project oneself positively into the future? A particular way of seeing the world? Something else?

The purpose of this chapter is to provide some answers to these questions. Optimism is often mentioned in a trivial way in conversations between friends, for example. Generally speaking, it is a positive projection towards the future.

DOI: 10.4324/9781003378426-11   138

However, it is clear that optimism covers a range of concepts that need to be defined in order to be studied. It will then be possible to assess the level of optimism, identify its consequences and potential methods of intervention. Firstly, some preliminaries will be developed and then direct and indirect approaches will be discussed (e.g., Martin-Krumm, 2012). The different parts will be structured around a common outline, definition and assessment, health consequences, and intervention. Antecedents will not be addressed. A final section will conclude by outlining the perspectives in this field of research and the limitations.

Conceptual preliminaries

Optimism, therefore, refers to being confident in the positive outcome of an event, whereas pessimism is about expecting the worst. From a scientific point of view, how can we go further than this trivial way of looking at things?

First, it is necessary to differentiate optimism from related concepts. For example, for Chang (2001), the Locus of Control developed by Rotter (1966) could be a source of confusion. In the same vein, a number of studies have highlighted a tendency for individuals to expect positive events rather than negative ones, as if there is an optimism bias that leads them to 'see life as rosy' (Sharot, 2011, for a review). An optimism bias can go as far as unrealistic optimism, which can be defined as the erroneous belief that one's own risk of facing problems is lower than that of other people (Weinstein, 1980). At their core, the findings of Sharot et al. (2007) reveal how unrealistic optimism is maintained even when the person is confronted with reality. In particular, differences in information encoding are thought to play a role in the adjustment of beliefs that maintain unrealistic optimism. Underestimating the risk of being confronted with negative events may have an adaptive function, that is associated with. reduced stress and anxiety (e.g., Sharot, 2011). However, this belief is mistakenly labelled as unrealistic optimism. In a similar vein, individuals may expect to live longer than average and underestimate their chances of divorce (Weinstein, 1980), or overestimate their chances on the labour market (Hoch, 1984). What should be considered here as positive illusions, also known as comparative optimism, when moderated, have a beneficial impact on adaptive goal-achieving behaviour and have an effect on both mental (Taylor & Brown, 1988) and physical health (Scheier & Carver, 1987).

Is it a state linked to a particular situation or rather a general personality trait? It is clear that optimism is considered to be a personality variable common to people, all of whom possess it but to varying degrees. The work therefore falls within the framework of differential psychology. A certain uniformity in the published results is noted. These show that invariably, whatever the type of measure, optimism is associated with desirable characteristics such as happiness, perseverance, achievement and health (Peterson, 2000, p. 47), or as protective factors against adjustment disorders (Southwick et al., 2005). Is this always the case? Given that optimism is associated with many variables that are not explained,

Peterson describes it as a "velcro" construct on which everything hangs (2000, p. 47). It is therefore clear that optimism and pessimism can be considered from different angles, with various conceptualisations, without there necessarily being any marked disagreement between the different research streams. It is also possible to consider that the levels of generality and stability will depend on the definition adopted with regard to the object of the research. It is in the measurement of these variables that the differences are most apparent, although correlations or trends have been observed in the scores obtained from different questionnaires (Martin-Krumm, 2012). It is therefore possible to identify different conceptions of optimism and pessimism which will have varying levels of generality and stability. For each of them, measurement tools are associated, for defensive pessimism (e.g., Optimism-Pessimism Prescreening Questionnaire, OPPQ; Norem & Cantor, 1986a), for dispositional optimism (e.g., LOT-R; Scheier et al., 1994), for hope (e.g., Hope Scale; Snyder et al., 1991) or for explanatory styles (e.g., Attributional Style Questionnaire, ASQ; Seligman et al., 1979). For Chang (2001), on the one hand, the multiple angles of attack offer a richness for understanding what may be at play with this variable.On the other hand, the pooling of data and comparison of results are made more problematic.

While the contours of this construct are beginning to emerge, particularly with regard to certain virtues associated with it, the very nature of this variable must also be considered. Schematically, two types of conception co-exist. In one, described as the direct conception, optimism and pessimism are based directly on the individual's expectations. If these are rather positive (e.g., I believe in my chances of success; When I am going through difficult times, I always think that things will get better) the individual will be considered rather optimistic. In the other conception, described as indirect, optimism and pessimism are not measured directly, but through other indicators such as the individual's willingness to mobilise one's resources to achieve goals. Additional indicators are the individual's confidence to achieve them (e.g., I am actively seeking to achieve my goals; I always think it will get better, I actively seek to achieve my goals; Even when others show signs of discouragement, I know I can find a solution to the problem), and trait attributions, such as internal or external, stable or unstable, general or specific character.

The objective of this contribution is therefore to develop the direct conceptions of optimism, strategy optimism with its corollary, defensive pessimism, and more particularly that of Carver and Scheier. The latter have given rise to an abundant literature on two indirect conceptions, hope and the theory of Explanatory Styles. Evaluation tools will be presented with the potential consequences of the psychological construct evoked on health or illness. Finally, limitations and research perspectives will be proposed.

What are direct conceptions of optimism?

Several theories consider optimism from a direct approach. The most representative are probably those developed by Norem and Cantor (1986a, 1986b) or by Carver and Scheier (1982). By direct approach, it is understood that optimism is based here directly on the positive expectations of individuals. Pessimism, on the other hand, is based on negative expectations of the individual.

Strategic optimism and defensive pessimism

While trivially optimism is always associated with beneficial consequences for the individual and pessimism with deleterious consequences, the theoretical framework developed by Norem and Cantor (1986a, 1986b) reveals that caution is needed.

Definition and measurement

Optimism or defensive pessimism are strategies rather than stable and general personality traits.. They are used unconsciously and are specific to the domains in which the individual operates (Norem, 2001). According to Norem (1998), the individual may use one in a given context and the other in a different context. This does not necessarily guarantee success, however. Indeed, these strategies may not be used adequately, hence the need for adjustments according to a logic in which costs and benefits are taken into account. Strategies can contribute to the regulation of emotions and behaviour, and have emotional and motivational consequences. A measurement tool has been developed, the OPPQ (Norem & Cantor, 1986a). While most propositions in other theoretical frameworks suggest that an individual is either optimistic or pessimistic, here the authors consider that the individual may be one or the other depending on the context. The strategy of defensive pessimism reflects a strong anxiety of the individual who, in order to control it, needs to anticipate a set of obstacles on the way to success in order to prepare himself accordingly. It thus allows the individual to protect himself from anxiety, which is therefore rather beneficial for him. The strategic optimist, on the other hand, might appear to be overconfident, but in fact seeks to avoid anything that might generate anxiety.

Consequences

Defensive pessimism will enable the individual to protect himself against a possible failure by preparing for it, to cushion the effects if necessary, and to motivate himself by increasing the effort made in order both to succeed and to increase the pleasure experienced of having done well (Showers & Ruben, 1990).

Therefore, even if many studies attest that optimism is associated with beneficial consequences in terms of coping, satisfaction or well-being, it must be noted that this framework proposes an alternative. Indeed, defensive pessimism, while it certainly reflects a lack of self-confidence and a high level of anxiety, nevertheless allows for success or satisfactory performance thanks to the analysis of conditions and possible scenarios by the person who resorts to it, and protects against anxiety. Conversely, the optimistic strategy is not necessarily associated with success either, because of a possible overconfidence that would lead the individual to neglect certain aspects of the task. In summary, defensive pessimism does not necessarily result in self-fulfilling prophecies (Norem, 2001) because those who resort to it use their anxiety by focusing on the task at hand and their efforts. Optimists, on the other hand, seem to be content with their self-confidence, which would tend to do them a disservice. However, both strategies have the advantage of promoting success, whether or not anxiety is present. For those who use defensive pessimism, negative affect and anticipation are needed to strengthen their focus, whereas anticipating the course of events can be detrimental for those who use the optimism strategy, as reflection does not fit with their strategy (Norem, 2001). Finally, care should be taken if an individual may appear anxious about potentially deleterious aspects of their health, or overconfident. This confidence, which would translate into strategic optimism, would ultimately protect them from the negative effects of anxiety on their health. In other words, these strategies may serve as effective anxiety protection measures.

Intervention

If management were to be envisaged, it would probably not consist of seeking to reassure the person who displays this form of pessimism, but rather of naming the obstacles that he or she perceives in reaching the goal, prioritising them according to their risk of occurrence and accompanying the individual during preparation. The person who uses an optimistic strategy as a functional response intended to avoid anxiety, may need to be fully present in order to manage possible mistakes.

Carver and Scheier's dispositional optimism

Definition and measurements

According to Carver and Scheier (2001), "optimists are people who expect to have positive experiences in the future. Pessimists are those who expect to have negative experiences" (p. 31). Optimism is conceived here as a cognitive variable that consists of a general confidence in having positive outcomes. This confidence is based on a rational estimate of the person's likelihood of success and confidence in self-efficacy. Optimistic disposition based on the person's general expectations has consequences for how the person regulates their actions in the face of difficulties or stressful situations. These expectations can be generalised across a variety of situations that are stable over time. It is in this context that dispositional optimism is defined as the stable tendency of participants to believe that they will have more positive than negative experiences overall in their lifetime (Carver & Scheier, 1982). According to this perspective, when an individual begins to be aware of contradictions between his or her behavioural or standard goals and his or her present situation, an evaluation procedure is initiated. A feedback loop that would allow progress towards the goal. This loop has four sub-functions: an input, a reference value, a comparison and an output. According to Carver and Scheier (2009), 'a discrepancy, or discrepancy, detected between input and output through this comparison is often called an "error signal" and the output is then a response to the detected error' (p. 209). If the individual believes that the contradictions between one's goals and the present situation or the reference value are likely to be reduced, the individual will make a new effort to achieve them. An optimist will be able to stand up, face the IR problems, give it their best shot and persevere. Rather than ignoring difficulties, they will accept reality and focus on solving problems in order to find solutions. These problems will, in turn, have less physical and emotional impact than for a pessimistic individual. If the expectation is more negative, efforts are reduced or a cessation of further attempts to make efforts follows. According to this model, there is a disposition of individuals to be optimistic or pessimistic.

Several tools measure this disposition. The Life Orientation Test, created by Scheier and Carver (1985) and later revised (LOT-R; Scheier et al., 1994) has been adapted for children (Youth Life Orientation Test; Ey et al., 2005) and has a longer version, Extended Life Orientation Test (ELOT; Chang et al., 1997). The psychometric qualities of these different scales are satisfactory.

Consequences

When confronted with problems, the optimistic individual would develop coping strategies, whereas the pessimistic individual would adopt a more passive and fatalistic approach. More specifically, optimists would adopt "vigilant" strategies (i.e., non-defensive attitude, "active" coping, involvement) whereas pessimists would be more inclined to adopt "avoidant" strategies (i.e., avoidance, denial, fatalism, resignation). Scheier and Carver (1987) argue that the more effective the optimist's cognitive strategies are, the more this should reduce the potential negative effects of stressors on physical and emotional health. It is possible to believe that optimism serves as a protective factor when a person faces difficulties in their life (Scheier & Carver, 1985). Several studies have therefore established a link between optimism and health. It is thought to promote physical and psychological health (e.g., Scheier & Carver, 1987; Carver et al., 1993). Optimism shown to be an important predictor of positive adjustment or subjective well-being (Diener et al., 1985). Lai (1997) has also been shown to promote psychological and physical well-being. Those who are more optimistic about life are less prone to depression and loneliness. In the field of cancer management, specifically breast cancer, Bozo et al. (2009) have demonstrated the link between optimism and post-traumatic growth in patients in the post-chemotherapy period. High levels of optimism and social support predicted post-traumatic growth. With the same type of patients, Büyükaşik-Çolak et al. (2012) were able to show that the impact of optimism on post-traumatic growth was moderated by coping strategies. The role of problem-focused coping was mainly highlighted in relation to emotion-focused coping. The relationship between optimism and problem-focused coping has been demonstrated in the context of post-traumatic growth. During the coronavirus pandemic, Agbaria and Mokh (2022) were able to confirm this link between optimism and coping with stress. Research results often reveal that optimism interacts with other variables and is not a sole predictor of health benefits. For example, Prati and Pietrantoni (2009) found a positive relationship between social support, optimism, coping strategies and post-traumatic growth. These findings could largely be replicated by Cassidy (2013), particularly in relation to the importance of support and optimism. In terms of support, Chopik et al. (2018) highlighted the impact of living with a spouse with high levels of optimism. This research found beneficial effects on the health of the spouse without observing any change in the level of optimism itself. This beneficial effect of high optimism and low pessimism on the ageing of the individuals themselves has been demonstrated independently of the couple's relationship (Craig et al., 2023). Chopik et al. (2020). In general, the level of optimism changes over the life course independently of life events and that this change follows an inverted U-shaped curve. Similarly, Kubzansky et al. (2018). Optimism has a beneficial effect on a set of biological functions that mitigate the deleterious effects of a range of stressors and episodes of psychological distress. Optimism also protects against hypertension (Kubzansky et al., 2020). In fact, the detailed results reveal that the relationship is complex. People with high levels of optimism are found to be able to project themselves positively into the future and tend to adopt health behaviours. This relationship between optimism and health behaviours had already been observed for sleep or alcohol consumption (Trudel-Fitzgerald et al., 2019), or for health behaviours in general (Boehm et al., 2018). Recently, Pavani and Colombo (2023) showed that the effects of optimism on emotional well-being were mediated by ruminations and appreciation, but not by avoidance or problem solving. The value of optimism in the field of quality of life and health has been amply demonstrated, as revealed by the results of the study by Kavya and Sannet (2023) which focused on young adults. According to these researchers, optimism, happiness and life satisfaction are very largely correlated. Optimism also protects against burnout (Fabella & Dela Paz-Aler, 2023).

Overall, the results show a link between optimism and perceived health. When it comes to objective health, with indicators based on biomarkers, for example, the results are more mixed. This is the case in a study by Arbel et al. (2020) which shows that in elderly couples, optimism and pessimism do not play a significant role in the level of biomarkers of cardiovascular disease, either in the person him/herself or in the influence he/she has on his/her partner. Kretz (2019) warns that inappropriate optimism and overly positive messages can be as deleterious and discouraging as pessimism. The beneficial aspects of optimism should therefore be put into perspective, even if the results of a body of work converge in this sense.

Intervention

The fact that optimism is considered as a dispositional variable, and therefore stable, undoubtedly justifies the difficulty of identifying studies dealing with interventions. Indeed, if dispositional optimism turns out to have rather beneficial consequences for the individual, how can one accompany a patient who turns out to be rather pessimistic? The fact that it is difficult to identify publications dealing with intervention does not imply that it is impossible to consider them. Indeed, given that this is an expectancy-based approach, it is possible to assume that one can develop an approach that includes formulating goals, positive projections into the future, and identifying the means to achieve them in the same way as for hope, a framework that will be developed below. Such an approach would require the design of tools to measure the level of achievement of defined health goals. The approach is classically practised in the context of functional rehabilitation for achieving goals joint amplitude following surgery. Craig et al. (2023) suggest that interventions to promote health would in turn increase optimism and reduce pessimism. Indeed, health is often seen as a consequence of optimism, but the relationship may be the reverse. In other words, supporting a patient in health behaviours is likely to have an effect on his or her level of optimism, which in turn could support health behaviours. The authors suggest that these interventions can be conducted at the level of individuals (e.g., quitting smoking and engaging in physical activity), health professionals (e.g., caring for the elderly and providing access to existing health care facilities for all), and even the community as a whole (e.g., access to volunteer work or access to community service). This work is at the crossroads between the responsibility of health professionals, who should, for example, help their patients to stop smoking (e.g., hypnosis sessions, motivational talks, prescription of patches) or to practise physical activities (e.g., by teaching the principles of progressiveness, by helping patients to enjoy themselves, etc.) and the responsibility of a local policy in favour of the general interest. Other means exist. For example, Wahyuni et al. (2019) were able to show that a web-based intervention based on optimism, coping and life satisfaction increased the level of optimism.

Direct conceptions of optimism or pessimism have been defined and their consequences outlined. What about indirect conceptions; which theoretical frameworks can be used? The next section explores definitions, consequences and intervention strategies.

What are indirect conceptions of optimism?

Hope

It is customary to consider that "hope is life". Following Krafft's (2022) considerations, while 'an optimistic person' may be inclined not to take into account the seriousness or urgency of a situation, a person who is hopeful would be active in his or her search for a solution and confronting difficulties. They are likely to identify solutions and adjust their behaviour (Krafft, 2022, p. 101). Therefore, hope would have several advantages compared to optimism in terms of disposition. For Kadlac (2015), hope implies a realistic approach to the present and the future which in turn protects against excessive levels of optimism or pessimism.

Like optimism as presented, hope can also be broken down into direct and indirect approaches.

Hope from a direct approach

A new theoretical framework has emerged under the impetus of Krafft and particularly Krafft et al. (2017). The initial aim was to propose a short measurement scale and later led to a new reframing of the concept.

Definition and measurements

As part of the international study on hope developed by Krafft et al. (2018) and Krafft (2022), a new scale to measure people's perception of hope was developed. It is based on the hope and optimism subscale of the World Health Organization Quality of Life, Spirituality, Religion, and Personal Beliefs Questionnaire (WHOQOL-SRPB). Its value was tested by comparing it with the Adult Dispositional Trait Hope Scale (Snyder et al., 1991). The scale and this conceptualisation of hope are the result of the aggregation of different elements existing in different tools and allowing direct access to the perception that individuals have their own levels of hope. Several precautions have been taken in order to avoid confusion between the different potential theoretical constructs. The term hope was systematically used and not both hope and optimism. The items were therefore formulated in such a way as to directly access the perception of the individuals "i.e., I feel hopeful; I am hopeful with regard to my life; Hope improves the quality of my life; Even in difficult times I am able to remain hopeful; In my life, hope outweighs anxiety; My hopes are usually fulfilled". The results of the different stages of the validation procedure revealed the robustness of the scale and a convergent validity in line with the literature with regard to self-efficacy, resilience, gratitude for example (Krafft et al., 2017). In the end, a new conceptualisation of hope was developed from the point of view of the perception that people have individual levels of hope.

Consequences

The consequences of hope seen from this angle have essentially consisted of studying the predictive force of hope on the meaning of life, satisfaction or well-being in different types of populations, young, adult and ageing. Essentially, these are cross-cultural perspectives made possible by the nature of the mode of administration of the different scales making up the Hope Barometer. Indeed, as a whole, the sessions of this study since 2017 have been administered via a website, which makes it possible both to mobilise a large number of respondents and to solicit participants of many nationalities. On the other hand, to date, it does not appear that any studies have been carried out in the area of health or intervention. However, effects on well-being have been demonstrated (e.g. Krafft et al., 2021). It is an understanding of hope that is attracting increasing interest. It can be assumed that such studies will be carried out in the near future.

Hope from an indirect approach

The indirect approach to hope has a history of development, conceptualisation and study in general.

Definition and measurements

Snyder develops a model that is structured around two dimensions. For Snyder, Irving, and Anderson (1991) hope can thus be defined as "a positive motivational state based on an interaction between energy and motivation directed towards goals (agency), as well as the different ways of achieving them (pathways)". Goals are the cognitive component that forms the glue of hope theory (Snyder, 1994). They provide mental targets that are expressed as images or representations (Snyder, 2002). They vary in terms of their temporal structure, revealing the coexistence of short-term and long-term goals. For Snyder (2002), people get closer to their goals by thinking about viable solutions, "pathways", to reach them. The "agency" dimension concerns the motivational dimension of the theory of hope and refers to the confidence and will that one deploys to achieve an expected result.

In its formulation, this concept was considered at two levels, trait and state, with ad hoc measurement tools. The Trait Hope Scale was developed by Snyder et al. in 1991. It identifies the dispositional level of hope in adults. A specific scale has been developed for children (The Children's Hope Scale; Snyder et al., 1997). Several measures have been developed including scales for 'state' hope. Indeed, moving down the hierarchical system from the most general to the most specific, Feldman et al. (2009) propose a scale designed to measure the level of hope concerning specific and identified goals (A Goal-Specific Hope Scale). This scale is based on the trait questionnaire,but the items are readjusted to address specific rather than general goals. To measure hope in a specific situation, i.e. "here and now", a scale has been developed (Snyder et al., 1996). In the end, there are a large number of tools that can either measure hope as a trait variable or as a state for general or very specific contexts.

Consequences

Hope has effects on patient well-being, resilience (Munoz et al., 2019), acceptance of care and pathological consequences (e.g., Cheavens et al., 2006). Studies have mainly focused on the consequences of hope in people with severe conditions such as cancer (e.g., Ho et al., 2011) mental illnesses (e.g., Werner, 2012) as well as in individuals with severe trauma such as burn victims (Barnum et al., 1998) or war veterans (e.g., Gilman et al., 2012). Other studies have also looked specifically at the impact of hope on the health of older people (e.g., Moraitou et al., 2006). Hope is thought to promote the use of coping strategies (e.g., Berg et al., 2008). Hope is believed to promote the use of coping strategies (e.g. Berg et al., 2008), enabling the development of adaptive behaviours in terms of prevention, screening or management of symptoms relating to certain pathologies (e.g., Irving et al., 2004). In particular, hope would enable people with cancer to better cope with the invasive nature of certain treatments, as well as the pain and fatigue generated, through a process of decentring negative affects and focusing on more positive thoughts (e.g., Hood et al., 2012). Given its relevance, the antecedents of hope are also being studied and some have revealed the impact of Adverse Childhood Experiences (ACEs) and Post-traumatic Stress Disorder (PTSD). Munoz et al.'s (2018) study found that survivors of childhood trauma had high levels of PTSD, anxiety and low levels of hope, with the effects of ACEs on hope being mediated by PTSD and anxiety.

Intervention

The undeniable interest of this theoretical framework is that it offers intervention modalities that are simple to implement. They are based both on the definition of the goals that may animate the person, the way they achieve them and the energy they are willing to commit to their achievement. The last aspect undoubtedly points to functional connections with existential psychology (the meaning that these goals have for the person) as well as the theory of self-determination. Indeed, if the achievement of goals is likely to feed the person's basic needs (i.e., social closeness, autonomy and fulfilment), it is likely that they will harness all of the energy required for achievement. A range of potential strategies are presented in the literature (e.g., Lopez, 2013). Goal setting can be achieved through the number of physical activity sessions a person is willing to schedule. Intervening on the operative component will consist in imagining different ways to reach the goal through the choice of physical activity(ies), the duration of the sessions, their intensity, and the self-knowledge that can be acquired (e.g., connected watches). A return to the motivational component will consist of ensuring that the person is involved in a pleasurable practice rather than in a forced practice that would be solely focused on their health.

Another very popular theory considered part of the indirect approach to optimism is the theory of explanatory styles.

Explanatory styles

The theory of explanatory styles (Abramson et al., 1978) originates from the theories of control and acquired resignation (Overmier & Seligman, 1967; Seligman & Maier, 1967; Seligman, 1975), but it rapidly emancipated itself. This theory requires conceptual clarification, provided below, in terms of measurement and intervention.

Definition and measures

This last conceptualisation of optimism according to an indirect approach consists of taking into account the causal schemas of individuals which they use to explain in a recurrent manner the causes of the events they face. It is this pattern that will reveal the optimistic or pessimistic nature of the individual's worldview. According to this theory, when an individual fails in a situation in which they perceive no way to achieve the goal, they learn the futility of their efforts and may become resigned. Learned resignation corresponds to a perception of in-dependence between behaviours and results, which gives rise to an expectation of uncontrollability that can extend beyond the situation that generated the learning. Subsequently, elements borrowed from causal attribution theory (e.g., Weiner, 1974) led to a reformulation of learned resignation theory (Abramson et al., 1978). The reformulation emphasises the way in which the individual ex-plains the uncontrollability of the events they face. The concept of 'attributional style' or 'explanatory style' or 'worldview' was born. Research around this con-cept has gradually moved away from the strict problems of learned resignation and now contributes to issues of a person's optimistic or pessimistic orientation (e.g., Chang, 2001).

Abramson et al. (1978) therefore developed resignation theory by taking into account how the person explains or interprets his lack of control over a situa-tion. The nature of his response – the causal attribution he formulates – then provides the characteristics of the resignation that follows. If the causal attribu-tion is stable ("this is going to go on for a long time because no matter what I do, nothing will change"), it will induce chronic resignation; if it is unstable, then the resignation will be transitory. On the other hand, if the causal attribu-tion is global ("it's all the same"), then the symptoms of resignation will be likely to generalise to various domains (i.e. global learned resignation). On the other hand, if the causes are specific, then the symptoms will be confined to a particular domain (i.e., specific learned resignation). Finally, the perception of a lack of control attributed to an internal cause ("it's all my fault"), will lead to a decrease in self-esteem (i.e., personal learned resignation), which will not be the case, if the cause invoked is external ("it's very difficult") (i.e., universal learned resignation) At this point, a potentially problematic aspect can be noted. Indeed, considering that the theory of styles is linked to that of resignation, an external cause supposedly revealing an optimistic view of events when confronted with adversity ultimately reveals a lack of control over the environment. Indeed, when the cause is external, it potentially implies a lack of control over it. This is un-doubtedly one of the reasons that led Peterson (2000) to envisage that dimen-sions could be adjusted, in particular the removal of the locus of causality.

The first explanatory style measure to be developed was the ASQ (Seligman et al., 1979). Several variants were subsequently developed (e.g., Children's ASQ; Kaslow et al., 1978; Forced-Choice ASQ; Reivich & Seligman, 1991), for the academic environment (e.g., Academic ASQ; Peterson & Barrett, 1987) or the financial environment (e.g., Financial Service ASQ; Proudfoot et al., 2001), or even for sport for example (Sport Attributional Style Scale; SASS, Hanra-han et al., 1989). Another evaluation procedure has been proposed, based on a qualitative approach. This is the Content Analysis of Verbatim Explanations (CAVE; Peterson et al., 1992).

These different tools give a glimpse of the theoretical developments that have been proposed. Indeed, whereas initially it was a variable that was considered at a general level, the various studies that have been carried out have shown that it is more related to a context, which has led to a hierarchical organisation of this psychological construct (Martin-Krumm et al., 2006). Another advance was to consider that style was not situated on a continuum ranging from the least to the most optimistic or the least to the most pessimistic. An orthogonality of axes was considered (Martin-Krumm et al., 2006; Salama-Younes et al., 2006), coupled with a hierarchy that could go from the most general to the most specific. The consequences in terms of intervention are important to take into account and for some reinforce previous practices (e.g., Seligman, 1991). They will be discussed in the rest of this chapter. More recently, a new measurement scale based on hypothetical negative events has been validated (Travers et al., 2015).

Consequences

Initially, the consequences of style were considered in the area of health and more specifically mental health, or rather illness (i.e., depression), positioning the explanatory style as a risk factor if it is pessimistic. This type of style is associated with poorer mental health (e.g., Peterson & Bossio, 2000), more depressive symptoms (e.g., Gillham et al., 2000), lower immune system efficiency (Brennan & Charnetzsky, 2000), resilience (e.g., Martin-krumm et al., 2003), more injuries (Peterson et al., 2001) or irrational thoughts (Ziegler & Hawley, 2001) and anxiety (e.g., Mineka et al., 1995). For their part, the work of Jones and Rakovshik (2019) confirmed the impact of style on social anxiety disorder and on inflated sense of responsibility. However, the results of this research should be treated with caution, given that explanatory style was measured using the CDSII (McAuley et al., 1992), a scale initially designed to measure causal attributions. Other work has replicated this type of result to some extent, but by differentiating scores on the two subscales of explanatory style, the negative and positive hypothetical events of the ASQ (Peterson et al., 1982). Jose et al. (2018) were able to show that the optimism subscale predicted well-being and satisfaction and the pessimism subscale predicted depression and anxiety while revealing that these effects were mediated by the ability to enjoy life. The Paquet et al. study (2020) also found that having an optimistic style protected people from burnout and that intervening on style could have an effect on reducing the impostor phenomenon in the work environment, with all the deleterious health effects that may be associated with it (Zanchetta et al., 2020). Like other concepts related to optimism, style also has effects on well-being. For example, the study by Han et al. (2022) revealed effects on the well-being of tourism professionals. Specifically, an optimistic style was positively associated with well-being, while a pessimistic style was negatively associated. The effects of style were also found on diagnoses and subsequent behaviours (Douzenis & Seretis, 2015). Patients' explanations or attributions of feelings or somatic events have mostly been studied in relation to mental disorders such as panic disorder and hypochondria. This understanding is multifaceted and the way in which people perceive an external event (or bodily sensation) influences their reaction to that event and therefore has an effect on them. Explanatory style is considered a psychological attribute and is a term used alternatively to attributional style. This is sometimes confusing. Explanatory style, as defined, can influence diagnosis and treatment as well as illness behaviour. Beyond this cautionary note, it is important to be careful in analysing the procedures that researchers use. They themselves are likely to maintain this confusion, as in the study by Jones and Rakovshik (2019).

Intervention

Taken together, the various studies reveal the beneficial effects of an optimistic style on health in general and on mental illness in particular, as well as on well-being (e.g., Abramson et al., 2000). The corollary has also been demonstrated. A pessimistic style has a negative impact on health. Therefore, interventions designed to enable a person to switch from a pessimistic to an optimistic style make sense, especially as such interventions have been shown to optimise the management of depression in cognitive therapies. This is the case, particularly when the therapy iscombined with interventions on explanatory flexibility. The latter is defined as the variability of an individual's responses to stable and global negative event items of the ASQ (Peterson et al., 1982). Moore et al.'s (2017). The approach highlights the importance of interventions on these dimensions, whereas for everyday life or health in general, interventions could be made on all three dimensions, internality, stability and globality of styles (Seligman, 1991, 2011). In principle, it is a matter of the practitioner getting the patient to discuss the causes they spontaneously invoke for the events they faces. It is not about getting them to finally realise that they are wrong in the explanation given, determined by their explanatory style, but rather about enabling them to identify alternative causes and more specifically to challenge their internality, stability and level of wholeness. The practitioner can draw on past experiences, especially when they have been successful, to support the reflection.

In the military field, an intervention in which the explanatory style component has been integrated makes it possible to strengthen the resilience of military personnel with a view to preventing PTSD (e.g., Cornum et al., 2011). Depression prevention programmes were quickly developed, including the Penn Optimism Program for youth in a school setting (e.g., Jaycox et al., 1994). Since then, many other prevention or resilience-building programmes have been developed and their effectiveness tested. In terms of intervention, these essentially consist of identifying the perception of events that an individual may face, how they interpret them (i.e., to what causes they attribute them) and the consequences that follow in terms of emotions, behaviour or knowledge. The aim of the intervention is then to allow the person to discuss the causes they have spontaneously invoked, to find alternative causes, to identify the emotions they feel. This intervention can be optimised by strengthening the person's mindfulness. In the end, considering that the person's primary problem is the perception of they lack of control over events, the most important aspect to develop is probably their regaining control over their environment. Contrary to what was initially assumed from a theoretical point of view, this amounts to attributing the lack of control over situations to internal causes with the appropriate support, undoubtedly allowing the individual to start to act on said causes. More than the locus of causality, it is undoubtedly the dimension of personal control that is in question here, while taking up the recommendations of Moore et al. (2017) regarding the dimensions of stability and globality of the causes invoked.

Conclusion

The main theoretical frameworks related to optimism were discussed in a synthetic way. This was done on the basis of a classification which groups them in terms of direct approaches (i.e., defensive pessimism strategy, dispositional optimism) and indirect approaches (i.e., hope and explanatory styles) knowing that hope itself could be declined in terms of direct and indirect approaches (Figure 9.1). Conceptual elements were provided as well as evaluation modalities. Their impacts on health were described. Principles of intervention were discussed.

In view of these different perspectives, it is clear that while it seems easy to talk about optimism in the context of popular psychology, caution is called for when the discussion takes a scientific turn. There are two aspects to be considered, depending on whether it is a question of research or intervention.

In research, not all problems related to the measurement of constructs and their definition as developed here are resolved, for dispositional optimism and for explanatory styles for example. Eichner et al. (2014) had already warned the scientific community about this dichotomy, optimistic or pessimistic. They therefore sought to provide semantic points of caution, optimists or optimistic. Indeed, rather than considering a continuum going from pessimism to optimism, it is advisable to consider the constructs differently, which would better reveal the complexity of the human being who can consider themselves sometimes one and sometimes the other depending on the moment, the context or

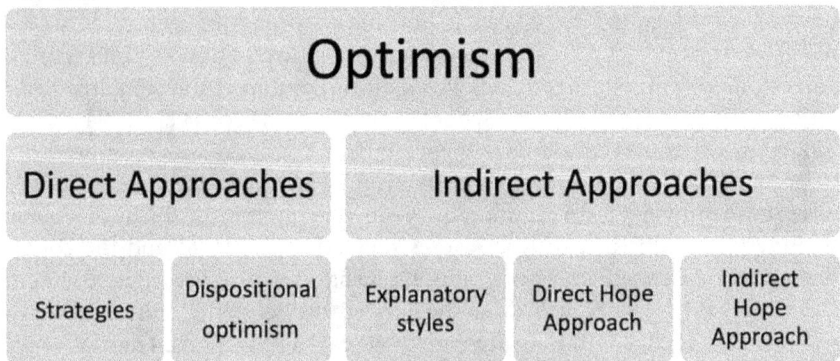

Figure 9.1 Different conceptions of optimism.

the situation. This had already been envisaged by Benyamini in patients suffering from arthritis (2005). This possibility has also been considered in the context of the study of explanatory styles. Work has revealed positive correlations between the two subscales, optimism style and pessimism style, whereas the correlations should theoretically be negative. This has led to a theoretical development highlighting the orthogonality of the axes with the possibility of identifying four profiles (e.g., Salama-Younès et al., 2009). Therefore, if it is conceivable that different profiles can be identified, whatever the theoretical frameworks, dispositional optimism or explanatory styles, high pessimism and low optimism (i.e., true pessimism), high optimism low pessimism (i.e., true optimism), high for both (i.e., realistic), low for both, which profile is the most protective? Which has the most deleterious effects? These questions open up promising perspectives to which cluster analyses would undoubtedly provide some answers. Another question concerns the calibration of the scales. What are the thresholds above which a person can be considered to be at risk of developing depression, for example? Furthermore, if optimism has its virtues, at what threshold does it become unrealistic to fall into what would be considered positive illusions or even illusions of control as mentioned by Bortolotti (2018)? At what thresholds is there a bias (Sharot, 2011)? At what point does a switch from resource to illusion occur (Chopik, 2021)? These questions as a whole also lead to philosophical reflections (see Milona, 2020, for a review). In terms of research, there is an entire section dealing with antecedents that have not been addressed here, although a number of questions arise. How much of this is genetic, for example? Or interactions with the psychosocial environment, education, life events?

In terms of intervention, it is ultimately just as necessary to be cautious. If optimism has an overall positive impact on people's health, it is not directly but often through complex processes. What are these processes? What are the variables that interact with optimism? Indeed, studies show a cascade of interactions that ultimately benefit the individual. Therefore, intervening is completely justified, but at what level exactly? On the level of optimism directly, like certain interventions on styles or on hope? On behaviours about the assumption that there will be effects on optimism in return? Which interventions precisely? How sustainable are the effects? What added value? These questions reveal not only how difficult it is to intervene, but also how difficult it is to evaluate the effectiveness of an intervention in order to differentiate between the quality of the therapeutic alliance with the patient and the effectiveness of the intervention itself.

This contribution reveals how complicated it is to talk about a concept that is so popular. Of course, it is not the only one! It could be the same for resilience or motivation. Talking about optimism does not necessarily mean thinking about the opposite of pessimism. Both may deserve special attention. In the end, optimism has not only beneficial effects and pessimism deleterious effects. Their respective effects on health are indirect. They are variables that are not general, but rather specific to certain contexts. They may fluctuate even if their evolution seems to follow an inverted U-shaped curve. It may be unrealistic, biased or even an illusion of control. In terms of intervention, the practitioner must inevitably ask himself the question of the nature of the optimism or pessimism that drives his patient. He must know that he can intervene mainly on the explanations given for negative events and their levels of internality, stability, globality and controllability. An alternative is to intervene on the patient's level of hope, the goals they set for themselves, the means they perceive to achieve them, and their level of motivation.

Overall, the ability to project positively into the future has proven to be crucial for people's health during the successive containment phases that populations have faced in the pandemic (e.g., Martin-Krumm et al., 2020) and therefore deserves the attention it has received in this chapter.

Takeaways

- Optimism is a simple concept to discuss at first glance, but it is in fact complex.
- While the consequences of optimism are generally beneficial to the individual and those of pessimism deleterious, care must be taken because optimism can be unrealistic, giving rise to illusions that do not encourage the person to act. Pessimism, on the other hand, can have positive aspects, particularly when, in terms of strategy, it enables individuals to protect themselves from anxiety.
- It is possible to intervene but the intervention must be based on the appropriate theoretical framework in order to identify the levers on which to act. The practitioner must therefore quickly take an option in order to identify the problem (i.e., defensive pessimism or true pessimism) and to intervene on the prioritisation of presumed difficulties, the explanations given in the face of adversity or the level of hope.

Wicked questions

1 How is optimism evolving?
2 What can be done to influence levels of optimism?
3 Is optimism innate or acquired?

References

Abramson, L. Y., Alloy, L. B., Hankin, B. L., Clements, C. M., Zhu, L., Hogan, M. E., & Whitehouse, W. G. (2000). Optimistic congnitive styles and invulnerability to depression. In J. Gillham (Ed.), *The science of optimism and hope: Research essays in honor of Martin E. P. Seligman* (pp. 75–98). Templeton Foundation Press.

Abramson, L. Y., Seligman, M. E. P., & Teasdale, J., (1978). Learned helplessness in humans: Critique and reformulation. *Journal of Abnormal Psychology*, (87)1, 49–74.

Agbaria, Q., & Abu Mokh, A. A. (2022). Self-efficacy and optimism as predictors of coping with stress as assessed during the coronavirus outbreak. *Cogent Education*, 9, 2080032. https://doi.org/10.1080/2331186X.2022.2080032

Arbel, R., Segel-Karpas, D., & Chopik, W. (2020). Optimism, pessimism, and health biomarkers in older couples. *British Journal of Health Psychology*. https://doi.org/10.1111/bjhp.12466

Barnum, D. D., Snyder, C. R., Rapoff, M. A., Mani, M. M., & Thompson, R. (1998). Hope and social support in psychological adjustment of children who have survived burn injuries and their matched controls. *Children's Health Care*, 27(1), 15–30.

Benyamini, Y. (2005). Can high optimism and high pessimism co-exist? Findings from arthritis patients coping with pain. *Personality and Individual Differences*, 38, 1463–1473.

Berg, C. J., Snyder, C. R., & Hamilton, N. (2008). The effectiveness of a hope intervention in coping with cold pressor pain. *Journal of Health Psychology*, 13(6), 804–809. https://doi.org/10.1177/1359105308093864

Boehm, J. K., Chen, Y., Koga, H., Mathur, M. B., Vie, L. L., & Kubzansky, L. D. (2018). Is optimism associated with healthier cardiovascular-related behavior? Meta-analyses of 3 health behaviors. *Circulation Research*, 122, 1119–1134.

Bortolotti, L. (2018). Optimism, agency, and success. *Ethical Theory and Moral Practice* 21(3), 521–535.

Bozo, Ö, Gündoğdu-Aktürk, E., & Büyükaşik-Çolak, C. (2009). The moderating role of different sources of perceived social support on the dispositional optimism - posttraumatic growth relationship in postoperative breast cancer patients. *Journal of Health Psychology*, 14(7), 1009–1020. https://doi.org/10.1177/1359105309342295

Brennan, F. X., & Charnetzsky, C. J. (2000). Explanatory style and immunoglobulin A (IgA). *Integrative Physiological and Behavioral Science*, 35(4), 251–255.

Büyükaşik-Çolak, C., Gündoğdu-Aktürk, E., & Bozo, Ö (2012). Mediating role of coping in the dispositional optimism-posttraumatic growth relation in breast cancer patients. *The Journal of Psychology: Interdisciplinary and Applied*, 146(5), 471–483. https://doi.org/10.1080/00223980.2012.654520

Carver, C. S., Pozo, C., Harris, S. D., Noriega, V., Scheier, M. F., Robinson, D. S., Ketcham, A. S., Moffat, F. L., & Clark, K. C. (1993). How coping mediates the effect of optimism on distress: A study of women with early stage breast cancer. *Journal of Personality and Social Psychology*, 65, 375–390.

Carver, C. S., & Scheier, M. F. (1982). Control theory: A useful conceptual framework for personality-social, clinical, and health psychology. *Psychological Bulletin*, 92, 111–135.

Carver, C. S., & Scheier, M. F. (2001). Optimism, pessimism, and self-regulation. In E. C. Chang (Ed.), *Optimism and pessimism; Implication for theory, research, and practice* (pp. 31–51). American Psychological Association.

Carver, C. S., & Scheier, M. F. (2009). Control processes, self-regulation and affect. In Y. Paquet (Ed.), *Psychology of control: Theories and applications* (pp. 207–225). De Boeck.

Cassidy, T. (2013). Benefit finding through caring: The cancer caregiver experience. *Psychology & Health*, 28(3), 250–266. https://doi.org/10.1080/08870446.2012.717623

Chang, E. C. (2001). *Optimism and pessimism; Implication for theory, research, and practice*. American Psychological Association.

Chang, E. C., Maydeu-Olivares, A., & D'Zurilla, T. J. (1997). Optimism and pessimism as partially independent constructs: Relations to positive and negative affectivity and psychological well-being. *Personality and Individual Differences*, 23, 433–440.

Cheavens, J. S., Feldman, D. B., Woodward, J. T., & Snyder, C. R. (2006). Hope in cognitive psychotherapies: On working with client strength. *Journal of Cognitive Psychotherapy*, 20(2), 135–145.

Chopik, W. J. (2021). Optimism and health: Resource or delusion. *Innovation in Aging*, 5(21), 406.

Chopik, W. J., Kim, E. S., & Smith, J. (2018). An examination of dyadic changes in optimism and physical health over time. *Health Psychology*, 37, 42–50.

Chopik, W. J., Oh, J., Kim, E. S., Schwaba, T., Krämer, M. D., Richter, D., & Smith, J. (2020). Changes in optimism and pessimism in response to life events: Evidence from three large panel studies. *Journal of Research in Personality*, 88, 103985. https://doi.org/10.1016/j.jrp.2020.103985

Cornum, R., Matthews, M. D., & Seligman, M. E. P. (2011). Comprehensive soldier fitness: Building resilience in a challenging institutional context. *American Psychologist*, 66(1), 4–9. https://doi.org/10.1037/a0021420

Craig, H., Gasevic, D., Ryan, J., Owen, A., McNeil, J., Woods, R., Britt, C., Ward, S., & Freak-Poli, R. (2023). Socioeconomic, behavioural, and social health correlates of optimism and pessimism in older men and women: A cross-sectional study. *International Journal of Environmental Research and Public Health*, 20, 3259. https://doi.org/10.3390/ ijerph20043259

Diener, E., Emmons, R. A., Larsen, R. J., & Griffin, S. (1985). The satisfaction with life scale. *Journal of Personality Assessment*, 49, 71–75.

Douzenis, A., & Seretis, D. (2015). Explanatory style and health. In J. D. Wright (Ed.), *International Encyclopedia of The Social Behavioral Sciences* (pp. 598–589). Elsevier. https://doi.org/10.1016/B978-0-08-097086-8.14059-0

Eichner, K. V., Kwon, P., & Marcus, P. D. (2014). Optimists or optimistic? A taxometric study of optimism. *Psychological Assessment*, 26(3), 1056–1061.

Ey, S., Hadley, W., Nutbrock Hallen, D., Palmer, S., Klosky, J., Deptula, D., Thomas, J., & Cohen, R. (2005). A new measure of children's optimism and pessimism: The youth life orientation test. *Journal of Child Psychiatry and Psychology*, 46(5), 548–558.

Fabella, F. E. T., & Dela Paz-Aller, R. A. (2023). Optimism as a mitigator of burnout: The relationship between optimism and burnout among selected teachers. *International Research Journal of Modernization in Engineering Technology and Science*, 5(02), 414–420. https://doi.org/10.56726/IRJMETS33431

Feldman, D. B., Rand, K. L., & Kahle-Wrobleski, K. (2009). Hope and goal attainment: Testing a basic prediction of hope theory. *Journal of Social and Clinical Psychology*, 28, 479–497.

Gillham, J. E., Shatté, A. J., Reivich, K. J., & Seligman, M. E. P. (2000). Optimism, pessimism, and explanatory style. In E. C. Chang (Ed.), *Optimism & pessimism. Implications for theory, research, and practice* (pp. 53–75). APA.

Gilman, R., Schumm, J. A., & Chard, K. M. (2012). Hope as a change mechanism in the treatment of posttraumatic stress disorder. *Psychological Trauma: Theory, Research, Practice, and Policy*, 4(3), 270–277. https://doi.org/10.1037/a0024252

Han, J., Huang, K., & Shen, S. (2022). Are tourism practitioners Happy? The role of explanatory style played on tourism practitioners' psychological well-being. *Sustainability*, 14, 4881. https://doi.org/10.3390/su14094881

Hanrahan, S., Grove, J. R., & Hattie, J. A. (1989). Development of a questionnaire measure of sport-related attributional style. *International Journal of Sport Psychology*, 20, 114–134.

Ho, S., Rajandram, R. K., Chan, N., Samman, N., McGrath, C., & Zwahlen, R. A. (2011). The roles of hope and optimism on posttraumatic growth in oral cavity cancer patients. *Oral Oncology*, 47(2), 121–124. https://doi.org/10.1016/j.oraloncology.2010.11.015

Hoch, S. (1984). Conterfactual reasoning and accuracy in predicting personal events. *Journal of Experiential Psychology*, 11, 719–731.

Hood, A., Pulvers, K., Carrillo, J., Merchant, G., & Thomas, M. D. (2012). Positive traits linked to less pain through lower pain catastrophizing. *Personality and Individual Differences*, 52(3), 401–405. https://doi.org/10.1016/j.paid.2011.10.040

Irving, L. M., Snyder, C. R., Cheavens, J., Gravel, L., Hanke, J., Hilberg, P., & Nelson, N. (2004). The relationships between hope and outcomes at the pretreatment, beginning, and later phases of psychotherapy. *Journal of Psychotherapy Integration*, 14(4), 419–443. https://doi.org/10.1037/1053-0479.14.4.419

Jaycox, L. H., Reivich, K. J., Gillham, J. E., & Seligman, M. E. P. (1994). Prevention of depressive symptoms in school children. *Behaviour Research and Therapy*, 32(8), 801–816.

Jones, M., & Rakovshik, S. (2019). Inflated sense of responsibility, explanatory style and the cognitive model of social model anxiety disorder: A brief report of a case control study. *The Cognitive Behaviour Therapist*, 12, e19, 1–11. https://doi.org/10.1017/S1754470X19000047

Jose, P. E., Lim, B. T., Kim, S., & Bryant, F. B. (2018). Does savoring mediate the relationships between explanatory style and mood outcomes? *Journal of Positive Psychology and Wellbeing*, 1–19. ISSN 2587-0130

Kadlac, A. (2015). The virtue of hope. *Ethical Theory and Moral Practice*, 18(2), 337–354.

Kaslow, N. J., Tennenbaum, R. L., & Seligman, M. E. P. (1978). *The KASTAN: A children's attributional style questionnaire.* Unpublished manuscript, University of Pennsylvania.

Kavya, K., & Sannet, T. (2023). Life satisfaction: The role of happiness and optimism among young adults. *Journal of Social Sciences and Economics*, 2(1), 35–42. https://finessepublishing.com/jsse

Krafft, A. (2022). *Our hopes, our future: Insights from the Hope Barometer.* Springer.

Krafft, A., Guse, T., & Maree, D. (2021). Distinguishing perceived hope and dispositional optimism: Theoretical foundations and empirical findings beyond future expectancies and cognitions. *Journal of Well-Being Assessment.* https://doi.org/10.1007/s41543-020-00030-4

Krafft, A., Martin-Krumm, C., & Fenouillet, F. (2017). Development and validation of the perceived hope scale: Discriminant value and predictive utility vis-à-vis dispositional hope. *Assessment.* https://doi.org/10.1177/1073191117700724

Krafft, A., Perrig-Chiello, P., & Walkers, A. (2018). Hope for a good life: Results of the Hope-Barometer international research program. Springer.

Kretz, L. (2019). Hope, the environment and moral imagination. In R. Green (Hrsg.), *Theories of hope: Exploring alternative affective dimensions of human experience* (pp. 155–176). Rowman & Littlefield.

Kubzansky, L., Huffman, J., Boehm, J., et al. (2018). Positive Psychological Well-Being and Cardiovascular Disease. *Journal of the American College of Cardiology*, 72(12), 1382–1396. https://doi.org/10.1016/j.jacc.2018.07.042

Kubzansky, L. D., Boehm, J. K., Allen, A. R., Vie, L. L., Ho, T. E., Trudel-Fitzgerald, C., Koga H. K., Scheier, L. M., & Seligman, M. E. P. (2020). Optimism and risk of incident hypertension: A target for primordial prevention. *Epidemiology and Psychiatric Sciences*, 29, e157, 1–9. https://doi.org/10.1017/S2045796020000621

Lai, J. C. L. (1997). Relative predictive power of the optimism versus the pessimism index of Chinese version of the Life Orientation Test. *Psychological Record*, 47(3), 399–410.

Lopez, S. J. (2013). Making Hope happen: Create the future you want for yourself and others. Atria Books.

Martin-Krumm, C. (2012). Optimism: A synthetic analysis. *Les Cahiers Internationaux de Psychologie Sociale*, 93, 103–134.

Martin-Krumm, C., Sarrazin, P., Peterson, C., & Famose, J.-P. (2003). Explanatory style and resilience after sports failure. *Personality and Individual Differences*, 35(7), 1685–1695.

Martin-Krumm, C., Sarrazin, P., Peterson, C., & Salama-Younès, M. (2006). Optimism in sports: An explanatory style approach. In A. Delle Fave (Ed.), *Dimensions of well-being. Research and intervention* (pp. 382–399). Franco Angeli.

Martin-Krumm, C., Tarquinio, C., & Tarquinio, C. (2020). Optimism and COVID-19: A resource to support people in confinement? *Annales Médico-Psychologiques.* https://doi.org/10.1016/j.amp.2020.06.004

McAuley, E., Duncan, T. E., & Russell, D. W. (1992). Measuring causal attributions: The revised Causal Dimension Scale (CDS-II). *Personality and Social Psychology Bulletin*, 18, 566–573. https://doi.org/10.1177/01467292185006

Milona, M. (2020). *Hope and optimism.* John Templeton Foundation.

Mineka, S., Pury, C. L., & Luten, A. G. (1995). Explanatory style in anxiety and depression. In G. M. Buchanan & M. E. P. Seligman (Eds.), *Explanatory style* (pp. 135–158). Erlbaum.

Moore, M. T., Fresco, D. M., Schumm, J. A., & Dobson, K. S. (2017). Change in explanatory flexibility and explanatory style in cognitive therapy and its components. *Cognitive Therapy and Research*. https://doi.org/10.1007/s10608-016-9825-6

Moraitou, D., Kolovou, C., Papasozomenou, C., & Paschoula, C. (2006). Hope and adaptation to old age: Their relationship with individual-demographic factors. *Social Indicators Research*, 76(1), 71–93. https://doi.org/0.1007/s11205-005-4857-4

Munoz, R. T., Hanks, H., & Hellman, C. M. (2019). Hope and resilience as distinct contributors to psychological flourishing among childhood trauma survivors. *Traumatology*. Advance online publication. https://doi.org/10.1037/trm0000224

Munoz, R. T., Pearson, L. C., Hellman, C. M., McIntosh, H. C., Khojasteh, J., & Fox, M. D. (2018). Adverse childhood experiences and posttraumatic stress as an antecedent of anxiety and lower hope. *Traumatology*, 24(3), 209–218. https://doi.org/10.1037/trm0000149

Norem, J. K. (2001). Defensive pessimism, optimism, and pessimism. In E. C. Chang (Ed.), *Optimism and pessimism; Implication for theory, research, and practice* (pp. 77–100). American Psychological Association.

Norem, J. K. (1998). Why should we lower our defenses about defense mechanisms? *Journal of Personality*, 66(6), 895–917.

Norem, J. K., & Cantor, N. (1986a). Anticipatory and post hoc cushioning strategies: Optimism and defensive pessimism in "Risky" situations. *Cognitive Therapy and Research*, 10(3), 347–362.

Norem, J. K., & Cantor, N. (1986b). Defensive pessimism: Harnessing anxiety as motivation. *Journal of Personality and Social Psychology*, 51(6), 1208–1217. https://doi.org/10.1037/0022-3514.51.6.1208

Overmier, J. B., & Seligman, M. E. P. (1967). Effects of inescapable shock upon subsequent escape and avoidance learning. *Journal of Comparative and Physiological Psychology*, 63, 28–33.

Paquet, Y., Martin-Krumm, C., Junot, A., & Gilibert (2020). Attributional style and burn out at work: A cluster analysis. *L'Encéphale*. https://doi.org/10.1016/j.encep.2020.06.005

Pavani, J.-P., & Colombo, D. (2023). Appreciation and rumination, not problem solving and avoidance, mediate the effect of optimism on emotional wellbeing. *Personality and Individual Differences*, 205, https://doi.org/10.1016/j.paid.2023.112094

Peterson, C. (2000). The future of optimism. *The American Psychologist*, (55)1, 44–45.

Peterson, C., & Barrett, L. (1987). Explanatory style and academic performance among university freshmen. *Journal of Personality and Social Psychology*, 53, 603–607.

Peterson, C., Bishop, M. P., Fletcher, C. W., Kaplan, M. R., Yesko, E. S., Moon, C. H., Smith, J. S., Michaels, C. E., & Michaels, A. J. (2001). Explanatory style as a risk factor for traumatic mishaps, *Cognitive Therapy and Research*, 25(6), 633–649.

Peterson, C., & Bossio, L. M. (2000). Optimism and physical well-being. In E. C. Chang (Ed.), *Optimism & pessimism. Implications for theory, research, and practice* (pp. 127–145). APA.

Peterson, C., Schulman, P., Castellon, C., & Seligman, M. E. P. (1992). CAVE: Content Analysis of Verbatim Explanations. In C. P. Smith (Ed.), *Motivation and personality: Handbook of thematic content analysis* (pp. 383–392). Cambridge University Press.

Peterson, C., Semmel, A., Von Baeyer, C., Abramson, L. Y., Metalsky, G. I., & Seligman, M. E. P. (1982). The attributional style questionnaire. *Cognitive Therapy and Research*, 6, 3, 287–300.

Prati, G., & Pietrantoni, L. (2009). Optimism, social support, and coping strategies as factors contributing to post traumatic growth: A meta-analysis. *Journal of Loss and Trauma: International perspectives on Stress & Coping*, 14, 364–388.

Proudfoot, J. G., Corr, P. J., Guest, D. E., & Gray, J. A. (2001). The development and evaluation of a scale to measure occupational style in financial services sector. *Personality and Individual Differences*, 30, 259–270.

Reivich, K. J., & Seligman, M. E. P. (1991). *The forced-choice Attributional Style Questionnaire*. Unpublished data, University of Pennsylvania.

Rotter, J. B. (1966). Generalized expectancies for internal versus external control of reinforcement. *Psychological monographs: General and applied*, 80(1), 1.

Salama-Younes, M., Martin-Krumm, C., Hanrahan, S., & Roncin, C. (2006). Children's explanatory style in France: Psychometric properties of the Children's Attributional Style Questionnaire and reliability of a shorter version. In A. Delle Fave (Ed.), *Dimensions of well-being. Research and intervention* (pp. 191–207). Franco Angeli.

Salama-Younes, M., Martin-Krumm, C., Le Foll, D., & Roncin, C. (2009). Psychometric qualities of the Child Explanatory Mode Assessment Questionnaire. *Canadian Journal of Behavioural Science*, 40, 3, 178–184.

Scheier, M. F., & Carver, C. S. (1985). Optimism, coping, and health: Assessment and implications of generalized outcomes expectancies. *Health Psychology*, 4(3), 210–247.

Scheier, M. F., & Carver, C. S. (1987). Dispositional optimism and physical well-being: The influence of generalized outcome expectancies on health. *Journal of Personality*, 55, 169–210.

Scheier, M. F., Carver, C. S., & Bridges, M. W. (1994). Distinguishing optimism from neuroticism (and trait anxiety, self-mastery, and self-esteem): A reevaluation of the Life Orientation Test. *Journal of Personality and Social Psychology*, 67(6), 1063–1078.

Seligman, M. E. P. (1975). *Helplessness: On depression, development and death*. Freeman.

Seligman, M. E. P. (1991). *Learned optimism*. Knopf.

Seligman, M. E. P. (2011). *Flourish: A visionary new understanding of happiness and well-being*. Freeman.

Seligman, M. E. P., & Maier, S. F. (1967). Failure to escape traumatic shock. *Journal of Experimental Psychology*, 74, 1–9.

Seligman, M. E. P., Abramson, L. Y., Semmel, A., & Von Baeyer, C. (1979). Depressive attributional style. *Journal of Abnormal Psychology*, 88, 242–247.

Sharot, T. (2011). *The optimism bias: Why we're wired to look on the bright side*. Pantheon Books.

Sharot, T., Riccardi, A. M., Raio, C. M., & Phelps, E. A. (2007). Neural mechanism mediating optimism bias. *Nature*, 450 (7166), 102–105.

Showers, C., & Ruben, C. (1990). Distinguishing defensive pessimism from depression: Negative expectations and positive coping mechanism. *Personality and Social Psychology Bulletin*, 22, 193–210.

Snyder, C. R. (1994). *Psychology of hope: You can get there from here*. Free Press.

Snyder, C. R. (2002). Hope theory: Rainbows in the mind. *Psychological Inquiry*, 13(4), 249–275. https://doi.org/10.1207/S15327965PLI1304_01

Snyder, C. R., Harris, C., Anderson, J. R., Holleran, S. A., Irving, L. M., Sigmon, S. T., Yoshinobu, L., Gibb, J., Langelle, C., & Harney, P. (1991). The will and the ways: Development and validation of an individual-differences measure of hope. *Journal of Personality and Social Psychology*, 60(4), 570–585.

Snyder, C. R., Hoza, B., Pelham, W. E., Rapoff, M., Ware, L., Danovsky, M.,... & Stahl, K. J. (1997). The development and validation of the children's hope scale. *Journal of Pediatric Psychology*, 22(3), 399–421. https://doi.org/10.1093/jpepsy/22.3.399

Snyder, C. R., Irving, L. M., & Anderson, J. R. (1991). Hope and health. In C. R. Snyder & D. R. Forsyth (Eds.), *Handbook of social and clinical psychology: The health perspective* (pp. 285–305). Pergamon Press.

Snyder, C. R., Sympson, S. C., Ybasco, F. C., Borders, T. F., Babyak, M. A., & Higgins, R. L. (1996). Development and validation of the state hope scale. *Journal of Personality and Social Psychology*, 70(2), 321–335. https://doi.org/10.1037/0022–3514.70.2.321

Southwick, S. M., Vythilingam, M., & Charney, D. S. (2005). The psychobiology of depression and resilience to stress: Implications for prevention and treatment. *Annual Review of Clinical Psychology*, 1, 255–291.

Taylor, S. E., & Brown, J. D. (1988). Illusion and well-being: A social psychological perspective on mental health. *Psychological Bulletin*, 103, 193–210.

Travers, K. M., Creed, P. A., Morissey, S. (2015). The development and initial validation of a new scale to measure explanatory style. *Personality and Individual Differences*, 81, 1–6. https://doi.org/10.1016/j.paid.2015.01.045

Trudel-Fitzgerald, C., James, P., Kim, E. S., Zevon, E. S., Grodstein, F., & Kubzansky, L. D. (2019). Prospective associations of happiness and optimism with lifestyle over up to two decades. *Preventive Medicine*, 126, 105754.

Wahyuni, E., Karsih, & Cahayawulan, W. (2019). Optimism, coping skills, and life satisfaction: The implication for web-based intervention. *Advances in Social Science, Education and Humanities Research*, 464, 579–583.

Weiner, B. (1974). *Achievement motivation and attribution theory*. General Learning Press.

Weinstein, N. D. (1980). Unrealistic optimism about future life events. *Journal of Personality and Social Psychology*, 39, 806–820.

Werner, S. (2012). Subjective well-being, hope, and needs of individuals with serious mental illness. *Psychiatry Research*, 196(2–3), 214–219. https://doi.org/10.1016/j.psychres.2011.10.012

Zanchetta, M., Junker, S., & Wolf, A.-M., & Traut-Mattausch, E. (2020). "Overcoming the fear that haunts your success" - The effectiveness of interventions for reducing the impostor phenomenon. *Frontiers in Psychology*, 11, 405. https://doi.org/10.3389/fpsyg.2020.00405

Ziegler, D. J., & Hawley, J. L. (2001). Relation of irrational thinking and the pessimistic explanatory style. *Psychological Reports*, 88, 483–488.

10

PSYCHOBIOTICS, GUT HEALTH AND THE PROMISE OF POSITIVE PSYCHOLOGY

Pádraic J. Dunne

The human microbiome

The human microbiome (a collection of microbial species that co-locate in or on the human body) encompasses trillions of interactive, predominantly symbiotic microorganisms that include archaea, bacteria, viruses, yeast and fungi (Lynch & Pedersen, 2016). Human microbiome environments include the mouth (oral), genitals, skin and the gastrointestinal tract (gut) (Gilbert et al., 2018).

Our microbiomes, acquired first from our mothers, become modified over time through interaction with the surrounding environment (other humans, animals, climate, geographical location, etc.). Babies delivered by caesarean section and vaginal birth have been shown to have differing microbiomes, the former resembling their mother's skin and the latter resembling the vagina, when examined within 24 hours of birth (Dominguez-Bello et al., 2010). Emerging technologies in genetic analysis have helped establish the fact that different varieties (species) of microorganisms exist at specific anatomical sites within the same person and that these are often unique to that individual (Gilbert et al., 2018). Influences on the composition of the microbiome for each individual include the type of birth, genetic make-up, living environment, diet, lifestyle and the use of antibiotics (Fan & Pedersen, 2021; Gilbert et al., 2018).

The gut microbiome

The human gastrointestinal system (commonly referred to as the gut) is comprised of the stomach, small and large intestine (colon), rectum and anus. It contains trillions of bacterial species (among other microbes) that have co-evolved with humans over millions of years. The functional capacity of the gut microbiome reaches maturity in healthy humans around the age of 12 years

   DOI: 10.4324/9781003378426-12

and remains relatively stable for most of adult life, with a gradual decline (in function and diversity of microbial species) with advancing years (Lynch & Pedersen, 2016).

This co-evolution has meant that the gut microbiome play important roles in human health. These include: (i) the development of immunity to environmental antigens (including pathogenic organisms and food); (ii) the digestion of food (metabolism); (iii) the regulation of hormone function; (iv) the enabling of cross-talk between the gut, the nervous system and the brain; (v) the elimination of toxins (Fan & Pedersen, 2021).

The gut microbiome and the immune response

Gut-associated mucosal lymphoid tissue (GALT) is comprised of a set of anatomical areas called Peyer's Patches that are located throughout the gut. These resemble large lymph nodes that house millions of different types of immune cells from the innate (non-specific) and adaptive (specific) arms of the immune response. In addition, an array of non-specific and specific immune sentinels can be found within the tissue located just under the gut (endothelial) lining. These immune cells continuously sample the gut lining (above and below) by extending pseudopods (false feet) into the gut lumen where the microbiome and gut contents such as food reside.

Early in human infancy the co-evolved commensal (Latin for *those who share the same table*) bacteria that comprise a healthy microbiome serve to train local immune cells in recognising friend and foe. These cells become educated in what is local and helpful, in terms of food particles and commensal bacteria, and what resembles an invading disease-causing pathogen (bacterium or other microbe), as well as toxins. A specialised group of immune cells, called suppressor T cells, is subsequently cultivated to expand in the region (Travis & Romagnani, 2022). These regulatory cells dampen down (supress) would-be aggressive immune cells through chemical messengers such as Transforming Growth Factor (TGF)-β, interleukin (IL)-10 and retinoic acid (Abdelhamid & Luo, 2018; Travis & Romagnani, 2022). In addition, regional B-cells (specific antibody-producing cells) are programmed by the microbiome and suppressor T cells to produce the calming and regulatory antibody, Immunoglobulin (Ig)-A (Takeuchi & Ohno, 2022). The result is a calm, yet vigilant surveillance system, kept in check form the start by a healthy microbiome.

The gut microbiome and nutrition

B vitamins are particularly important for energy metabolism in the body. They include thiamine (B1), riboflavin (B2), niacin (B3), pantothenate (B5), pyridoxine (B6), biotin (B7), folate (B9) and cobalamin (B12) (Hossain, Amarasena, & Mayengbam, 2022). Although bacterial species in the gut microbiome can produce low amounts of B vitamins, just like humans, they require most of these important nutrients from food to function properly.

Short-Chain Fatty Acids (SCFAs)

The gut microbiota has the capacity to ferment (and digest) fibre (non-soluble carbohydrates) that we humans cannot. Fibre from the food we eat (cabbage for example), is fermented by bacteria in the gut resulting in the production of SCFAs among other metabolites (Valdes, Walter, Segal, & Spector, 2018). The most commonly produced SCFAs in the gut are butyrate, propionate and acetate. Butyrate is essential for regulating tolerogenic suppressor T cells in the gut. These cells have a role in maintaining balance in the immune system residing within gut tissue (Siddiqui & Cresci, 2021). This common SCFA also provides a primary energy source for cells lining the colon, inhibits colon cancer development and contributes to hypoxia (low oxygen environment) in the gut that prevents the growth of disease causing bacteria (dysbiosis) (Valdes et al., 2018). Finally, butyrate can also act as a neurotransmitter that signals to the vagus nerve that all is well in the gut environment (Stilling et al., 2016). This is important when it comes to the interaction between elements of the microbiome that play a role in regulating human mood and psychology, psychobiotics (Dinan, Stanton, & Cryan, 2013).

Prebiotics are usually whole foods that contain non-soluble carbohydrates (oligosaccharides) or processed oligosaccharides like inulin (taken as a supplement) that can be digested by gut bacteria to produce metabolites and functional molecules like butyrate (Pandey, Naik, & Vakil, 2015). Examples of readily available prebiotics include soybeans, Jerusalem artichoke, cabbage, garlic, onions, flax seeds, chicory, sweet potato, bananas, apples and oats (Davani-Davari et al., 2019).

The Food and Agriculture Organisation of the United Nations and the World Health Organisation (FAO/WHO) have defined probiotics as microorganisms that, when administered in adequate amounts, confer a health benefit on the host (Hill et al., 2014). Probiotic microorganisms include, *Lactobacillus rhamnosus, Lactobacillus reuteri, Bifidobacteria, Lactobacillus casei, Lactobacillus acidophilus-group* and *Bacillus coagulans,* among others (Pandey et al., 2015). Probiotic foods include fermented products such as kimchi, kombucha, sauerkraut, certain pickled vegetables, kefir and live yogurts.

The gut nervous system

The gut is wrapped in a complex web of nerves called the enteric nervous system, which helps to regulate gut function and can engage in cross talk with other parts of the nervous system, and ultimately the brain. Interestingly, gut tissue, its resident microbiome, the enteric nervous system and local immune cells all work together to manage defence, digestion and communication with local muscles and nerves, and with the brain itself. This is effected through the production of neurotransmitters (chemical messengers that allow nerves to talk to each other), hormones and immune signalling molecules (cytokines), among others (Liang, Wu, & Jin, 2018). However, unlike other organs within the body, the gut can work independently of the brain in an automatic fashion. It can regulate its own function, it plays a role in regulating human behaviour and it can even influence thinking processes and human cognition (Liang et al., 2018).

Stress and the gut

The human stress response to external or internal threats is mediated by hormones and nerves of the autonomic nervous system (ANS). The ANS is split into two arms: (1) the sympathetic nervous system (SNS), which emerges from the central spine and is largely involved with the production of adrenaline and noradrenaline; (2) the parasympathetic nervous system (PNS), which emerges from the brain stem and sacral regions of the spine. The SNS (fight or flight response), largely mediated through adrenaline, increases blood pressure, reduces appetite and libido, increases heart and breathing rates, and promotes alertness. The principle nerve in the PNS is the vagus nerve (responsible for the rest and digest response), which has a calming influence on the cardiovascular system. In fact, we now know that low vagal nerve activity is associated with inflammatory bowel disease (IBD) and irritable bowel syndrome (IBS) (Bonaz, Bazin, & Pellissier, 2018). Psychobiotics in the gut microbiome play a significant role in regulating stress through their interplay with the immune system, gut lining, enteric nervous system and the vagus nerve (Bonaz et al., 2018; Clapp et al., 2017; Siddiqui & Cresci, 2021).

SCFAs like butyrate are produced by bacteria (Psychobiotics) in the gut, by fermenting non-soluble carbohydrates form dietary fibre. The multifunctional (pleiotropic) molecule, butyrate, can stimulate specialist cells in the gut lining (enterochromaffin cells) to produce the hormone serotonin (the primary target of serotonin re-uptake inhibitor-based antidepressants). Serotonin can then activate the vagus nerve (Cryan et al., 2019). Experiments have also shown that butyrate is involved in stimulating sensory fibres of the vagus nerve, which subsequently reduces sympathetic nerve activity and lowers blood pressure (Onyszkiewicz et al., 2019). Prolonged stress and subsequent activation of the SNS can damage the gut lining by activating the local immune response, leading to leaky gut syndrome (Kelly et al., 2015). This in turn can affect the survival of psychobiotics and promote outgrowth of disease-causing, pathogenic microbes in the gut (Kelly et al., 2015). Therefore, cultivating the microbiome through diet, exercise or positive psychological interventions might have a positive impact on our mood and mental health.

Psychobiotics

Psychobiotics are defined as bacterial species found within the gut microbiome that can deliver mental health benefits to the host (Dinan et al., 2013). These bacteria have the potential to stimulate the production of neurotransmitters, immune system-related chemical messengers (cytokines), psychotropic hormones (serotonin) and SCFAs (butyrate). Common psychobiotics include members of the following bacterial families, *Lactobacilli, Streptococci, Bifidobacteria, Escherichia and Enterococci* (Dinan et al., 2013; Sharma, Gupta, Mehrotra, & Mago, 2021).

The gut and mental health

Initial experiments conducted with rodents involved the transfer of the faecal microbiomes of anxious animals to sterile (mice born to sterile mothers and raised in sterile conditions with little or no microbiome), non-stressed, identical counterparts (BALBc mice). The recipient animals displayed anxious symptoms such as increased vigilance, hyporeactivity, increased heart rates and suppressed food consumption within 24 hours (Chinna Meyyappan, Forth, Wallace, & Milev, 2020; Li et al., 2019).

A 2020 review by Chinna Meyyappan and colleagues of 21 preclinical and clinical studies in mice and humans concluded that faecal microbiome transplant (FMT) might have promise as a therapeutic procedure for psychiatric disorders (Chinna Meyyappan et al., 2020). However, more studies with greater numbers are needed. FMT was shown to mitigate psychiatric disorders (depression, anxiety, anorexia and alcoholism) in healthy donors. Conversely, psychiatric symptoms were transferable from ill donors to healthy ones (Chinna Meyyappan et al., 2020). Currently, the only Food and Drug Administration (FDA)-approved therapy using FMT is in the treatment of diarrhoea caused by the pathogen *Clostridioides Difficle* (Food and Drug Administration, 2022).

Brain–gut disorder psychotherapies

It is clear that significant crosstalk occurs between the gut and the brain in both and health disease. It is also likely that psychobiotics play a significant role in this process. Many gut-related issues can be linked to poor lifestyle practices such as the typical Western diet, excessive alcohol consumption, and lack of exercise (Appanna, 2018). It is therefore reasonable to assume that positive changes in lifestyle might mitigate these problems. However, other gut-related problems are either caused or exacerbated by chronic stress, anxiety and depression, often leading to chronic conditions like IBS (Clapp et al., 2017). The latter conditions can be targeted by psychotherapies.

In 2020, the Rome Foundation Working Team of interdisciplinary experts produced a report that recommended best practice gut–brain behaviour therapies for patients with disorders of gut–brain interaction (Laurie Keefer et al., 2022). These psychotherapies address symptoms associated with brain–gut disorders that include psychological stress, emotional distress, maladaptive cognitive processes, psychological comorbidity and somatisation, as well as abuse in early life (Laurie Keefer et al., 2022). The recommended psychotherapies include Cognitive Behavioural Therapy (CBT), mindfulness-based stress reduction (MBSR), psychodynamic interpersonal psychotherapy, gut-directed hypnotherapy and disease self-management (Farhadi, Banton, & Keefer, 2018; Laurie Keefer et al., 2022).

CBT incudes second and third wave interventions that involve cognitive techniques such as reframing, identifying automatic negative thinking, understanding that thoughts are not facts, as well as tackling avoidance behaviour, stress management and mindfulness-based approaches (MBSR; third wave CBT). Mindfulness practices cultivate enhanced, non-judgemental awareness and acceptance of thoughts, emotions, memories and sensations, including pain (Sugaya, Shirotsuki, & Nakao, 2021). Recent studies, conducted since the COVID-19 pandemic, have also shown that CBT delivered online, is just as effective for supporting individuals diagnosed with IBS, as face-to-face meetings (Sugaya et al., 2021). The online, digital approach to CBT offers patients diagnosed with gut-related disease more flexibility, choice and accessibility.

Positive psychology and the gut

Little is known about whether interventions that promote subjective wellbeing and flourishing in human beings can have a positive impact on the gut of healthy people or those diagnosed with gut-related diseases. In 2023, Madva and colleagues conducted a review of 22 research projects that studied 4,285 individuals diagnosed with IBS (Madva, Sadlonova, et al., 2023). Compared to healthy groups, individuals diagnosed with IBS had significantly lower wellbeing in terms of resilience, positive affect, self-efficacy and emotional regulation. Unsurprisingly, IBS was also associated with poorer physical and mental health, as well as lower health-related quality of life.

Existing brain–gut disorder psychotherapies for IBS generally target negative psychological factors such as negative thinking, catastrophising, frustration, avoidance behaviour, anxiety and depression. As previously mentioned, the converse relationship between positive psychological factors and IBS symptoms remains undeveloped. The same group who conducted the systematic review described above (Madva, Harnedy, et al., 2023), explored connections between positive psychological factors and IBS symptoms, in the development of a novel brain-gut behaviour therapy. Madva and colleagues recruited 23 participants diagnosed with IBS who completed self-report assessments and phone interviews to discuss the relationships between positive and negative psychological factors, IBS symptoms, health behaviour engagement, and health-related quality of life (HRQoL). Participants reported that positive psychological factors mitigated IBS symptoms, boosted health behaviour participation, and improved HRQoL. Greater positive psychological well-being was linked to managed and improved IBS symptoms, among study participants. The authors of this study suggest that interventions to cultivate greater well-being may be a novel approach to mitigating IBS symptoms, and enhancing HRQoL in individuals diagnosed with IBS (Madva, Harnedy, et al., 2023).

Dr Laurie Keefer is an academic health psychologist and Director of the Psychobehavioural Research, within the Division of Gastroenterology at Mount

Sinai Hospital, New York. Dr Keefer specialises in the psychosocial care of individuals diagnosed with gastrointestinal conditions and has written a very interesting perspective piece in Nature Reviews Gastroenterology and Hepatology (Keefer, 2018) on the potential for positive psychology interventions at mitigating gastrointestinal conditions (especially IBS). This perspective focuses on the study of positive psychology factors in the management of gastrointestinal diseases that are exacerbated by poor psychosocial health, including early-life trauma. Keefer describes the following positive psychology constructs as having a mitigating impact on GI disease symptoms:

1 **Resilience** (grit) is associated with healthy functioning of the central nervous system and can mitigate the onset and maintenance of gastrointestinal symptoms (Laurie Keefer et al., 2022).
2 **Optimism** is characterised by viewing adversity as temporary, limited, and manageable. It is associated with adaptive coping, positive healthcare interactions, and potential benefits in chronic diseases. Keefer has described a central role for cultivating optimism in promoting the reappraisal of negative events and flexible problem-solving skills, which are important for individuals coping with gastrointestinal disorders.
3 **Self-regulation**, the ability to manage thoughts, feelings, and behaviours, is essential for long-term wellness in gastrointestinal disorders, as well as other chronic conditions.
4 **Self-efficacy (mastery)** is linked to self-regulation and positive health outcomes. It reflects confidence in one's ability to succeed at disease self-management tasks.

Considering the positive psychology constructs described here can play an important role in mitigating gut-related disease, it stands to reason that they might have a protective role in otherwise healthy individuals. It makes sense that positive psychology-based interventions, which promote flourishing and wellbeing, might also stave off the development of stress, sympathetic nerve activation and associated stress hormones, thereby contributing to gut health. More quality research will provide the evidence needed to support this thesis.

Takeaways

- The human microbiome contains bacterial species called psychobiotics that can help regulate the immune system, hormone production and neurotransmitter secretion such as serotonin and butyrate.
- Poor lifestyles that include a Western diet can damage the gut and reduce the survival of psychobiotics.
- Prebiotic foods such as cabbage, onions and bananas contain non-soluble carbohydrates called oligosaccharides that psychobiotics digest for energy.
- Probiotics are fermented foods that contain bacterial species, which colonise the gut and promote health.

- Individuals diagnosed with IBS have significantly lower wellbeing in terms of resilience, positive affect, self-efficacy and emotional regulation.
- Positive psychology interventions (including mindfulness) designed to cultivate resilience (grit), optimism, self-regulation and self-efficacy (mastery) can help to mitigate symptoms related to IBS.
- It is logical to assume that the same positive psychology constructs can promote a healthy gut in thriving human beings; however, more research is needed.

Wicked questions

1 How do we reconcile conflicting scientific findings and nutritional advice related to gut health, considering that research in this field is still evolving and often subject to biases and conflicting interests?
2 What are the ethical implications of focusing on individual gut health when it may contribute to larger systemic issues such as food insecurity, environmental degradation, or animal welfare concerns?
3 What role does nutrition play in gut health and human flourishing, and how can we promote access to nutritious and gut-friendly food options for individuals of all socioeconomic backgrounds?
4 How can we integrate complementary and alternative approaches, such as mind-body therapies, probiotics, or dietary modifications, into mainstream healthcare practices to provide comprehensive care for gut health disorders?

References

Abdelhamid, L., & Luo, X. M. (2018). Retinoic acid, leaky gut, and autoimmune diseases. *Nutrients, 10*(8). https://doi.org/10.3390/nu10081016

Appanna, V. D. (2018). Dysbiosis, probiotics, and prebiotics: In diseases and health. In *Human microbes - The power within: Health, healing and beyond* (pp. 81–122). Singapore: Springer Singapore.

Bonaz, B., Bazin, T., & Pellissier, S. (2018). The vagus nerve at the interface of the microbiota-gut-brain axis. *Frontiers in Neuroscience, 12*, 49. https://doi.org/10.3389/fnins.2018.00049

Chinna Meyyappan, A., Forth, E., Wallace, C. J. K., & Milev, R. (2020). Effect of fecal microbiota transplant on symptoms of psychiatric disorders: A systematic review. *BMC Psychiatry, 20*(1), 299. https://doi.org/10.1186/s12888-020-02654-5

Clapp, M., Aurora, N., Herrera, L., Bhatia, M., Wilen, E., & Wakefield, S. (2017). Gut microbiota's effect on mental health: The gut-brain axis. *Clinics and Practice, 7*(4), 987–987. https://doi.org/10.4081/cp.2017.987

Cryan, J. F., O'Riordan, K. J., Cowan, C. S. M., Sandhu, K. V., Bastiaanssen, T. F. S., Boehme, M.,... & Dinan, T. G. (2019). The microbiota-gut-brain axis. *Physiological Reviews, 99*(4), 1877–2013. https://doi.org/10.1152/physrev.00018.2018

Davani-Davari, D., Negahdaripour, M., Karimzadeh, I., Seifan, M., Mohkam, M., Masoumi, S. J.,... & Ghasemi, Y. (2019). Prebiotics: Definition, types, sources, mechanisms, and clinical applications. *Foods, 8*(3). https://doi.org/10.3390/foods8030092

Dinan, T. G., Stanton, C., & Cryan, J. F. (2013). Psychobiotics: A novel class of psychotropic. *Biol Psychiatry, 74*(10), 720–726. https://doi.org/10.1016/j.biopsych.2013.05.001

Dominguez-Bello, M. G., Costello, E. K., Contreras, M., Magris, M., Hidalgo, G., Fierer, N., & Knight, R. (2010). Delivery mode shapes the acquisition and structure of the initial microbiota across multiple body habitats in newborns. *PNAS, 107*(26), 11971–11975. https://doi.org/10.1073/pnas.1002601107

Fan, Y., & Pedersen, O. (2021). Gut microbiota in human metabolic health and disease. *Nature Reviews Microbiology, 19*(1), 55–71. https://doi.org/10.1038/s41579-020-0433-9

Farhadi, A., Banton, D., & Keefer, L. (2018). Connecting our gut feeling and how our gut feels: The role of well-being attributes in Irritable Bowel Syndrome. *Journal of Neurogastroenterology and Motility, 24*(2), 289–298. https://doi.org/10.5056/jnm17117

Food and Drug Administration, F. (2022). *FDA approves first fecal microbiota product Rebyota approved for the prevention of recurrence of clostridioides difficile infection in adults.* Retrieved from https://www.fda.gov/news-events/press-announcements/fda-approves-first-fecal-microbiota-product

Gilbert, J. A., Blaser, M. J., Caporaso, J. G., Jansson, J. K., Lynch, S. V., & Knight, R. (2018). Current understanding of the human microbiome. *Nature Medicine, 24*(4), 392–400. https://doi.org/10.1038/nm.4517

Hill, C., Guarner, F., Reid, G., Gibson, G. R., Merenstein, D. J., Pot, B.,... & Sanders, M. E. (2014). The International Scientific Association for Probiotics and Prebiotics consensus statement on the scope and appropriate use of the term probiotic. *Nature Reviews Gastroenterology & Hepatology, 11*(8), 506–514. https://doi.org/10.1038/nrgastro.2014.66

Hossain, K. S., Amarasena, S., & Mayengbam, S. (2022). B vitamins and their roles in gut health. *Microorganisms, 10*(6). https://doi.org/10.3390/microorganisms10061168

Keefer, L. (2018). Behavioural medicine and gastrointestinal disorders: The promise of positive psychology. *Nature Reviews Gastroenterology & Hepatology, 15*(6), 378–386. https://doi.org/10.1038/s41575-018-0001-1

Keefer, L., Ballou, S. K., Drossman, D. A., Ringstrom, G., Elsenbruch, S., & Ljótsson, B. (2022). A Rome working team report on brain-gut behavior therapies for disorders of gut-brain interaction. *Gastroenterology, 162*(1), 300–315. https://doi.org/10.1053/j.gastro.2021.09.015

Keefer, L., Gorbenko, K., Siganporia, T., Manning, L., Tse, S., Biello, A.,... & Dubinsky, M. C. (2022). Resilience-based integrated IBD care is associated with reductions in health care use and opioids. *Clinical Gastroenterology and Hepatology, 20*(8), 1831–1838. https://doi.org/10.1016/j.cgh.2021.11.013

Kelly, J. R., Kennedy, P. J., Cryan, J. F., Dinan, T. G., Clarke, G., & Hyland, N. P. (2015). Breaking down the barriers: The gut microbiome, intestinal permeability and stress-related psychiatric disorders. *Frontiers in Cellular Neuroscience, 9*, 392–392. https://doi.org/10.3389/fncel.2015.00392

Li, N., Wang, Q., Wang, Y., Sun, A., Lin, Y., Jin, Y., & Li, X. (2019). Fecal microbiota transplantation from chronic unpredictable mild stress mice donors affects anxiety-like and depression-like behavior in recipient mice via the gut microbiota-inflammation-brain axis. *Stress, 22*(5), 592–602. https://doi.org/10.1080/10253890.2019.1617267

Liang, S., Wu, X., & Jin, F. (2018). Gut-brain psychology: Rethinking psychology from the microbiota-gut-brain axis. *Frontiers in Integrative Neuroscience, 12*, 33. https://doi.org/10.3389/fnint.2018.00033

Lynch, S. V., & Pedersen, O. (2016). The human intestinal microbiome in health and disease. *The New England Journal of Medicine, 375*(24), 2369–2379. https://doi.org/10.1056/NEJMra1600266

Madva, E. N., Harnedy, L. E., Longley, R. M., Rojas Amaris, A., Castillo, C., Bomm, M. D.,... & Celano, C. M. (2023). Positive psychological well-being: A novel concept for improving symptoms, quality of life, and health behaviors in irritable bowel syndrome. *Neurogastroenterology & Motility, 35*(4), e14531. https://doi.org/10.1111/nmo.14531

Madva, E. N., Sadlonova, M., Harnedy, L. E., Longley, R. M., Amonoo, H. L., Feig, E. H.,... & Celano, C. M. (2023). Positive psychological well-being and clinical characteristics in IBS: A systematic review. *General Hospital Psychiatry, 81*, 1–14. https://doi.org/10.1016/j.genhosppsych.2023.01.004

Onyszkiewicz, M., Gawrys-Kopczynska, M., Konopelski, P., Aleksandrowicz, M., Sawicka, A., Koźniewska, E.,... & Ufnal, M. (2019). Butyric acid, a gut bacteria metabolite, lowers arterial blood pressure via colon-vagus nerve signaling and GPR41/43 receptors. *Pflugers Archiv: European Journal of Physiology, 471*(11–12), 1441–1453. https://doi.org/10.1007/s00424-019-02322-y

Pandey, K. R., Naik, S. R., & Vakil, B. V. (2015). Probiotics, prebiotics and synbiotics - A review. *Journal of Food Science and Technology, 52*(12), 7577–7587. https://doi.org/10.1007/s13197-015-1921-1

Sharma, R., Gupta, D., Mehrotra, R., & Mago, P. (2021). Psychobiotics: The next-generation probiotics for the brain. *Current Microbiology, 78*(2), 449–463. https://doi.org/10.1007/s00284-020-02289-5

Siddiqui, M. T., & Cresci, G. A. M. (2021). The Immunomodulatory Functions of Butyrate. *Journal of Inflammation Research, 14*, 6025–6041. https://doi.org/10.2147/jir.S300989

Stilling, R. M., van de Wouw, M., Clarke, G., Stanton, C., Dinan, T. G., & Cryan, J. F. (2016). The neuropharmacology of butyrate: The bread and butter of the microbiota-gut-brain axis? *Neurochemistry International, 99*, 110–132. https://doi.org/10.1016/j.neuint.2016.06.011

Sugaya, N., Shirotsuki, K., & Nakao, M. (2021). Cognitive behavioral treatment for irritable bowel syndrome: A recent literature review. *BioPsychoSocial Medicine, 15*(1), 23. https://doi.org/10.1186/s13030-021-00226-x

Takeuchi, T., & Ohno, H. (2022). IgA in human health and diseases: Potential regulator of commensal microbiota. *Frontiers in Immunology, 13*. https://doi.org/10.3389/fimmu.2022.1024330

Travis, M. A., & Romagnani, C. (2022). How regulatory T cells are primed to aid tolerance of gut bacteria. *Nature, 610*(7933), 638–640. https://doi.org/10.1038/d41586-022-03368-2

Valdes, A. M., Walter, J., Segal, E., & Spector, T. D. (2018). Role of the gut microbiota in nutrition and health. *British Medical Journal, 361*, k2179. https://doi.org/10.1136/bmj.k2179

PART III

Positive health applications

Research and theory are only one aspect of Positive Health. Ultimately, the ability to apply it and make a significant difference in people's lives matters. In this section, we explore the application of Positive Health in various aspects of life.

We begin with Chapter 11, written by Prof. Beth Frates, the president of the American College of Lifestyle Medicine (USA), which discusses the application of Positive Health to self, which is particularly relevant given that healthcare professionals, coaches, and educators need to look after themselves and model the Positive Health behaviour before they encourage their clients and patients to do it. Then, Chapter 12, written by Dr Jolanta Burke, Dr Padraic Dunne, and Dr Elaine Byrne from the Centre for Positive Health, RCSI University of Medicine and Health Sciences (Ireland), will explore the concept of Positive Health Interventions. In the " Integral Theory," Ken Wilber explains that when two concepts are integrated, they evolve into something different, a step-up from the previous components, becoming a unique contribution to knowledge. As such, this chapter explores the defining features of Positive Health Interventions, how they differ from Positive Psychology and Lifestyle Medicine Interventions and what unique contribution they offer to the current psychological and medical research and practice.

In the next part of the application of Positive Health, Dr Svala Sigurðardóttir from the University of Iceland and Dr Dóra Guðrún Guðmundsdóttir from the Directorate of Health Iceland (Iceland) explores ways in which Positive Health can be applied in healthcare, specifically, in General Practice. Chapter 14, written by coaching expects, Prof. Christian van Nieuwerburg from the Centre for Positive Health Sciences, RCSI University of Medicine and Health Sciences (Ireland), and Prof. Jim Knight from the University of Kansas (USA) guide readers through a newly created model of Positive Health Coaching that will help coaches apply the amalgamation of Positive Psychology and Lifestyle Medicine

     10.4324/9781003378426-13

theory and research in their practice. Then, in Chapter 15, Dr Annalisa Setti from the University College Cork (Ireland) and Dr Tadhg Mac Intyre from Maynooth University (Ireland) explore the embodied perspectives of natural evironments and their impact on health and wellbeing.

Chapter 16, written by Dr Andrea Giraldez-Hayes from the University of East London (University of East London), examines the importance of art in decreasing the symptoms of illness and improving health and psychological flourishing. In this chapter, art is the vehicle for making a positive health change happen. This theme continues in the next Chapter 17, written by a team of Jennifer Donnelly, Dr Pádraic J. Dunne, Justin Laiti, Croía Loughnane, Dr Róisín O'Donovan from the Centre for Positive Health Sciences, RCSI University of Medicine and Health Sciences (Ireland), who explore how artificial intelligence can be used to introduce positive health changes in the population. Chapter 18, written by Dr Ciara Scott from the Centre for Positive Health Sciences, RCSI University of Medicine and Health Sciences (Ireland) and Prof. Karen Morgan, President of the RCSI and UCD Malaysia University (Malaysia), explores how motivational theories and models support Positive Health practice and ways in which they can be maximised. Chapter 19, written by, delves into health equity and how Positive Health can support it. Finally, Chapter 20, written by one of the editors, Dr Liana Lianov from the Global Positive Health Institute, summarises the research and application of Positive Psychology and the pillars of Lifestyle Medicine and its potential future contribution to making the world healthier.

11

APPLICATIONS TO SELF/SELF-CARE/ SELF-COACHING, ROLE-MODELLING

Beth Frates, MD

Definitions

Self-care has many different definitions. When someone says this word, it conjures up a variety of images and phrases in people's minds. A day at a spa, exercising, eating well, taking vacation, a massage, playing with a dog, laughing during a comedy show, yoga, sleeping 7–9 hours a night, spending time with family and friends: all of these can be considered types of self-care. The word self-care has received more and more attention in the medical literature since COVID-19. In a concept analysis of the term, 31 articles on the subject spanning from 1975 to 2020 were reviewed. Their analysis of the literature led the authors to define self-care as "The ability to care for oneself through awareness, self-control, and self-reliance in order to achieve, maintain, or promote optimal health and well-being" (Martinez et al., 2021).

The next term that requires defining is well-being. Merriam Webster Dictionary defines well-being as "the state of being happy, healthy, or prosperous" (Merriam Webster, 2022). Wellness is another term often used when discussing self-care and health. Compared to well-being, wellness is defined as "the quality or state of being in good health, especially as an actively sought goal," by the Merriam Webster Dictionary (Merriam Webster, 2022). Well-being and wellness are similar, but wellness has the added component of "an actively sought goal." There is more action implied with the word wellness. The goal is good health.

This introduces another important word, health. The World Health Organization defines health as "Health is a state of complete physical, mental and social well-being and not merely the absence of disease or infirmity" (Simons et al., 2021). This definition uses the word well-being and emphasizes the multidimensionality of the term health by identifying the physical, mental, and social components. Another definition of wellness is working towards a healthy body,

 DOI: 10.4324/9781003378426-14

peaceful mind, and joyful heart (Frates et al., 2022). This definition includes the idea of setting a goal as well as honoring the fact that health, well-being and wellness include a physical, mental, and spiritual component. Putting it all together; self-care involves awareness, self-control, and self-reliance to work toward the goal of enjoying a state of well-being with a healthy body, peaceful mind, and nourished spirit.

The last definition to be considered here is spirit. According to the Britannica Dictionary spirit is defined as "the force within a person that is believed to give the body life, energy, and power" (Britannica Dictionary, 2023). This life, energy, and power may be expressed through many different channels such as creativity and compassion. In traditional medicine, the spirit is often missing from the calculation of health. The WHO includes physical, mental, and social well-being. Social well-being includes positive social connections that feed the spirit. Barbara Frederickson and colleagues describe positivity resonance as "...a type of interpersonal connection characterized by shared positivity, mutual care and concern, and behavioral and biological synchrony" (Major et al., 2018). There is an energy force that occurs between two people and enriches their experience when they are fully engaged and connecting on a deep level. This force leads to a greater sense of well-being by nourishing the spirit. Self-care nurtures the whole person: body, mind, and spirit.

Wellness and hierarchy of needs

Maslow's hierarchy of needs emphasizes the importance of physiological and psychological human needs. At the base of the pyramid is physiological needs including water, food, warmth and rest. The next level of the pyramid is the need for safety including shelter and security. After that are love and belonging needs including intimate relationships and friends. Then comes esteem needs involving a sense of pride and accomplishment. The top of the pyramid is self-actualization meaning achieving one's full potential given their unique strengths and using their creativity. The way to the top of the pyramid or self-actualization is self-care, nurturing your whole person, body, mind, and spirit.

Maslow's hierarchy of needs created in 1954 still informs our plans and programs for well-being and self-care to this day (Maslow, 1954). In addition, there are modifications to the hierarchy that are updated. For example, Shapiro and colleagues created a physician wellness hierarchy that is similar to Maslow's original hierarchy, but this one is more detailed and specific to the current times (Shapiro et al., 2019). The journal article by Shapiro and colleagues describes the situation for physicians, but it is applicable to other healthcare professionals and other employees as well. Reviewing the levels individually makes this point and provides tips for healthcare systems and all work environments to help people enhance their sense of well-being and prioritize self-care.

The levels in the physician wellness hierarchy (Shapiro et al., 2019) are as follows. The base level is "Basics." Above the basics level is "Safety," and next is "Respect." After the respect level, there is "Appreciation." Finally, at the top is

"Heal Patients and Contribute." Looking at each level individually, for the base level and bottom of the pyramid, also known as the foundation on which all else is built, there are the "Basics." In the physician hierarchy of wellness, "Basics" involve having access to water and food as well as time to consume each. Time to sleep is part of this basics level. Being free from anxiety, depression, suicidal thoughts, and substance use are also included in this level of physician wellness needs. This "Basics" level includes three of the six pillars of lifestyle medicine: nutrition, sleep, and avoidance of risky substances.

The next level above "Basics" is "Safety." In the safety level, safety of the physician and patients as well as job security are included. These are critical and COVID-19 taught everyone that this type of safety is not something to take for granted. Having the proper personal protection equipment (PPE) was a real issue during COVID-19. After safety comes "Respect," and this level involves mutual respect and inclusion among colleagues and patients with any cultural violations being addressed. Respecting family time is specifically highlighted in this level of the physician wellness hierarchy. Also, in this level, the electronic medical record (EMR) is identified as a hassle, and in this third level of the pyramid it states, "I am not hassled by IT, EMR or bureaucracy. Objects and processes work." This is an important level and beckons the system into the wellness equation.

After the third level of "Respect" comes "Appreciation," which is such an essential level to consider, especially if one understands the power of positive psychology. Everyone wants to be known and understood in this world for the unique human being they are. This is reflected in the "Appreciation" level of the pyramid where it states, "I am noticed and appreciated. I am connected. My compensation reflects my appreciation." Connection which is another of the six pillars of lifestyle medicine, allows for the experience of positivity resonance, and helps enhance a sense of well-being. It is emphasized in this second to last level of the pyramid.

The top level of the pyramid is "Heal Patients and Contribute." This is where the all important concept of time enters the pyramid. One needs time to think, brainstorm, and use creativity to be able to make significant contributions. This top level identifies the importance of autonomy and resources for physicians to heal patients and contribute. When physicians lose a sense of autonomy, they often lose motivation and hope. This is the case with most employees. Autonomy is key. As is outlined in the self-determination theory by Ryan and Deci (Ryan and Deci, 2017), people need autonomy, connection, and competence to stay motivated. Physicians are no different than patients in many regards. They have similar basic needs. Honoring these needs will help create a culture of wellness.

Creating a culture of wellness in the hospital, academic institution, clinical practice or other work environments is often overlooked, underfunded, and over-complicated.

A culture of wellness helps open up opportunities to practice self-care and sustain this practice. A culture of wellness is one of the three domains for overall physician and healthcare professional wellness. The other two domains are personal resilience and efficiency of practice (Bohman et al., 2017). In the domain of personal resilience, the six pillars of lifestyle medicine (routine physical activity, whole food plant predominant eating pattern, restorative sleep, stress management, positive social connection, and avoidance of risky substances) and the use of positive psychology are the critical components. For the domain of efficiency of practice, areas such as administrative burden, IT hassles, work schedules, workflow, and collaboration between colleagues as well as departments and divisions are the main focus. These can also be addressed through a group coaching process during which each division meets as a group with a coach. These group coaching sessions identify pain points that are preventing the division from performing optimally. After identifying the area of focus for the division, the individuals in the division take on concrete tasks to tackle the issues. They are held to a time-frame and meet regularly for check ins over the course of the six month coaching intervention. Taking the time to hold listening sessions for each department or division and discovering what is working well, what is not working well, and what are possible solutions to problems is an excellent starting point when working on the domain of efficiency of practice. This domain heavily influences the ability of physicians and healthcare professionals to practice self-care. If people are constantly hassled and feeling time pressure, they are not likely to be able to embrace self-care with the same excitement and enthusiasm as they would if they had time. That aspect of time is the top of the physician wellness hierarchy.

The American Medical Association has acknowledged the hassles of current medical practice in the United States and offers options to mitigate these hassles with a program titled "Stop the Stupid Stuff" (Ashton, 2019). They even have a list of "Stop This, Start That" on their website to encourage physicians to take steps to change their work environment to make it more efficient and save time (American Medical Association, 2022). One of the suggestions is to turn off notifications of emails into the inbox, as this is a constant distraction and requires the physician to refocus every few minutes if they respond to each and every dinging sound of the notification system. Focus is essential for productivity and efficiency. Time is a critical resource that is often a rate limiting factor. Finding ways to take back time helps physicians, healthcare professionals, and others feel autonomy and practice self-care.

Work life harmony is also essential for well-being. Thus, working to have email free weekends and evenings can help people enjoy their time away from work and really be away from their projects physically and mentally. Many email systems allow for schedule send. People who are working on the weekend and get great ideas at that time can craft emails but delay sending them until Monday morning at 8 or 9 am. If everyone in the group or division agrees to forgo sending emails after 5 pm on weekdays and not to send any emails during the weekend, this will allow for uninterrupted family and home time. When this policy is adopted from the top (Division Chief, CEO, manager or other leaders), it is more likely to be enforced. This is why having a wellness committee encouraged by leaders with wellness ambassadors from each area of the office or department is helpful. This allows for progress in creating a culture of wellness. These types of policies give permission for employees to enjoy their time away from the office and do with it what they choose. This is another aspect of autonomy, feeling free to use your time as you wish. Having more autonomy and more time will empower individuals to prioritize self-care.

With time, people can think about their purpose and how self-care aligns with their overall purpose. Having a sense of purpose is associated with healthy lifestyle patterns. A prospective study of 13,770 US adults over age 50 followed for eight years demonstrated that a higher sense of purpose at baseline was associated with a lower likelihood of developing an unhealthy BMI, sleep problems, or physical inactivity (Kim et al., 2020). Specifically, increasing "meaning salience" has been associated with physical activity levels (Hooker et al., 2018). Meaning salience refers to identifying a sense of purpose as important and relating it to what is happening in the moment through actions or discussions. When people connect their day-to-day activities with their sense of purpose they are experiencing meaning salience. Asking individuals to identify how their day-to-day activities connect with their own sense of meaning in life may help increase well-being and even impact their self-care, especially with respect to physical activity engagement.

Self-coaching

Knowing the key ingredients of the physician wellness hierarchy including the basics, safety, respect, appreciation, time to heal patients and contribute, knowing the six pillars of lifestyle medicine, understanding the importance of purpose, and the need for time management is one part of the self-care process, but this knowing or knowledge needs to be powered by doing. The doing of self-care requires a COACH Approach™. Just as healthcare professionals use a COACH Approach™ to help empower patients to adopt and sustain healthy lifestyles, they need to use the same approach with themselves and with others when addressing self-care. The COACH Approach™ is a mnemonic in which the C stands for Curiosity, the O stands for Openness, the A stands for Appreciation, the second C stands for Compassion, and the H stands for Honesty (Frates et al., 2021).

C = Curiosity
O = Openness
A = Appreciation
C = Compassion
H = Honesty

This approach and way of being invites healthcare professionals to treat themselves with the same honor, respect and empathy that they would use with a patient. For non-healthcare professionals, this way of being invites them to treat themselves the way they would treat a family member or friend looking to enhance their well-being. The COACH Approach™ excludes shame, blame, and guilt from the process. Oftentimes, healthcare professionals are perfectionists and use a fixed mindset. The COACH Approach™ with an emphasis on curiosity encourages people to use a growth mindset whenever there is a mishap. They need to be curious about what happened in that particular situation, how can they fix it, how can they prevent it from happening again, and how can they be better and stronger as a result of the mishap. With a growth mindset, any mistake is an opportunity to learn and grow (Dweck, 2016).

The doing of coaching can be described in a five-step cycle (Frates et al., 2011) (Figure 11.1).

This five-step cycle is a roadmap to help healthcare professionals to coach patients. It can also be used to help healthcare providers help themselves. In fact, this cycle has helped all kinds of people to coach themselves. The first step in this Five Step Cycle for Collaboration is to be empathetic. The healthcare professional needs to give themselves the same empathy and compassion they would give a patient. People need to treat themselves the way they would treat a friend or family member.

Empathy is described as feeling with the other person, walking in their shoes. Taking the time to fully understand their situation. Compassion adds an element of action. Feeling the feelings and then doing something about it. Using the five-step cycle of collaboration is taking an action step.

Expressing empathy and self-compassion is difficult for many people, especially clinicians. This first step may even feel foreign to people. Dr. Kristen Neff describes self-compassion as having three components (Neff, 2023). First, self-compassion involves self-kindness and not self-judgment. Not saying things to yourself that you would not say to a friend, a family member, or even a stranger who is struggling. People tend to speak to others with kindness and respect. With self-compassion, shame, blame and guilt are excluded from the internal

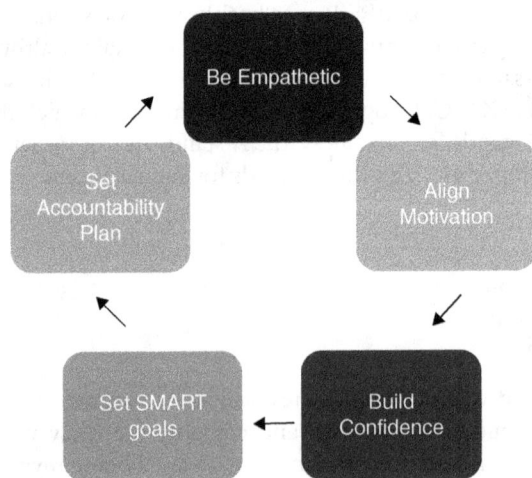

Figure 11.1 Five step cycle of coaching.[1]

dialogues. Looking for the positive and finding ways to make progress are the keys to handling mishaps. During challenging times, especially when people have made mistakes, it is often difficult to move forward. In fact, it is shame, blame and guilt that often holds people back. Knowing this is important. Speaking to oneself with compassion will help clear the way for growth and learning.

The next step after empathy is aligning motivation. What's the reason the person wants to focus on self-care? What's the motivation? For some it will be to improve attention, focus, and increase energy. Many people feel tired and fatigued. For others it will be to lose weight so they do not have to buy a whole new wardrobe and waste money. Understanding motivators is essential to making progress with self-care. Sometimes people need to think about their priorities during this step. What is most important to them right now and why? Knowing motivators and priorities paves the way for finding or reconnecting with one's purpose in life. One's reason for being or one's ikigai as the Japanese say. When one connects their motivations with their purpose, they can often more clearly see and appreciate the importance of self-care practices.

After aligning motivators, the next step is building confidence. The best way to build confidence is to list one's strengths. One option is to take the Values in Action (VIA) character strengths assessment (VIA Institute on Character, 2020). Another option is to speak with friends and family and ask them to share their opinions of the person's strengths. An exercise that can help identify a person's gifts and talents is to consider a time when the person reached a goal. Describing the process and identifying the strengths the person used to reach the goal helps to bring these strengths to life. Making a list of strengths and posting it in a place that is visible can serve as inspiration as well. Healthcare professionals and others can increase their sense of well-being by finding ways to use their strengths while they are at work and at home. Pride is a positive emotion, and positive emotions can help with creativity. In this way building confidence by pointing out strengths can help a person brainstorm around obstacles and create concrete plans for moving forward. That leads to the fourth step of setting goals.

Setting SMART goals is key to the success of the coaching process. When self-coaching, one must set goals too. Healthcare professionals and most employees set goals for their work, but they often need to learn how to set goals for their own health and self-care. SMART goals are goals that are specific, measurable, action-oriented, realistic and time sensitive. So, saying "I will exercise more" is a healthy idea, but it is not a SMART goal because it is not specific. It is not time sensitive, and it's unknown whether it is realistic. A SMART goal for exercise would include details such as "I will walk for twenty minutes after dinner on Monday, Wednesday, and Friday with my partner." It is clear that this suits the requirements for a SMART goal, if the person is free on these days at this time and has comfortable walking shoes which are all conditions that need to be in place for this to be a realistic goal.

After setting goals, the next step is to set accountability. Tracking devices, friends, apps, pen and paper, and calendars can all help with accountability. Often telling someone about self-care plans helps to solidify them and make them concrete because it is likely that the other person will check in to see how things are going. Even posting plans on social media can serve as motivation as there is a certain pressure to follow through with the plan. When people put self-care appointments in their phone calendar, computer calendar or paper calendar, they are more likely to engage in the activity or event that was planned. These self-care activities need to be taken as seriously as a doctor's appointment. The accountability with a doctor's appointment is set because the office calls the patient and often charges a fee for a missed appointment. Using this technique with other activities may help. For example, if an individual signs up for a yoga class and prepays, then they are more likely to make it to the class because they will not want to lose the money. If someone commits to meeting a friend for a hike, they are more likely to go for the hike because they do not want to let the friend down. These types of accountability measures help people stay on track and stay motivated.

After going through the five steps of expressing empathy and self-compassion, followed by aligning motivation, then building confidence, setting SMART goals, and finally setting accountability, it is back to step one with empathy and self-compassion. No matter how it went with the goal, the person needs to talk to themselves like a friend and go through the five steps again. Making sure to identify the motivators and connect with them each step of the way.

Assessments are helpful for keeping individuals on track. They provide a baseline and a starting point. Assessments that can work for self-care purposes include the 36 Item Short Form Survey (SF 36), or 12 Item Short Form Survey (SF 12), Maslach Burnout Inventory™, Satisfaction with Life Scale, Psychological Well-Being Scales (PGWB), or the Human Flourishing Scale, to name a few.

Self-care is nurturing the body, mind and spirit. An assessment tool that evaluates these three areas with evidence-based questions is the PAVING the Path to Wellness Questionnaire. Filling out the questionnaire allows people to reflect on the guidelines for healthy living and lifestyle medicine. Finding the area that is most interesting to that specific person at that particular time in their life is the key to getting started. Committing to reassessing and retaking the questionnaire is a form of accountability. If people can take the questionnaire together they can form a team and create a community small or large that can serve as motivation and inspiration.

PAVING the Path to Wellness is a program developed for patients and providers to help them thrive with a healthy body, peaceful mind and joyful heart. The book titled PAVING the Path to Wellness Workbook: A Guide to Thriving with a Healthy Body, Peaceful Mind, and Joyful Heart reviews the twelve steps recommended to prioritize self-care and to thrive at any age or stage in life (Frates et al., 2022). Harvard Health partnered with Dr. Beth Frates to create an assessment tool that helps individuals to identify strengths and areas of growth in their own self-care, lifestyles, and well-being. It is printed in the PAVING the Path to Wellness Workbook (Frates et al., 2022) and all proceeds for the book go to the non-profit www.pavingwellness.org.

In Figure 11.2 which is an image of the PAVING the Path to Wellness Wheel, all twelve steps are spelled out and separated into their respective areas: body, mind, and spirit (joyful heart). The PAVING program follows PAVING STEPSS which is a mnemonic.

P = Physical Activity
A = Attitude
V = Variety
I = Investigations
N = Nutrition
G = Goals
S = Stress Resilience
T = Time-outs
E = Energy
P = Purpose
S = Sleep
S = Social Connection

PAVING STEPSS Wheel

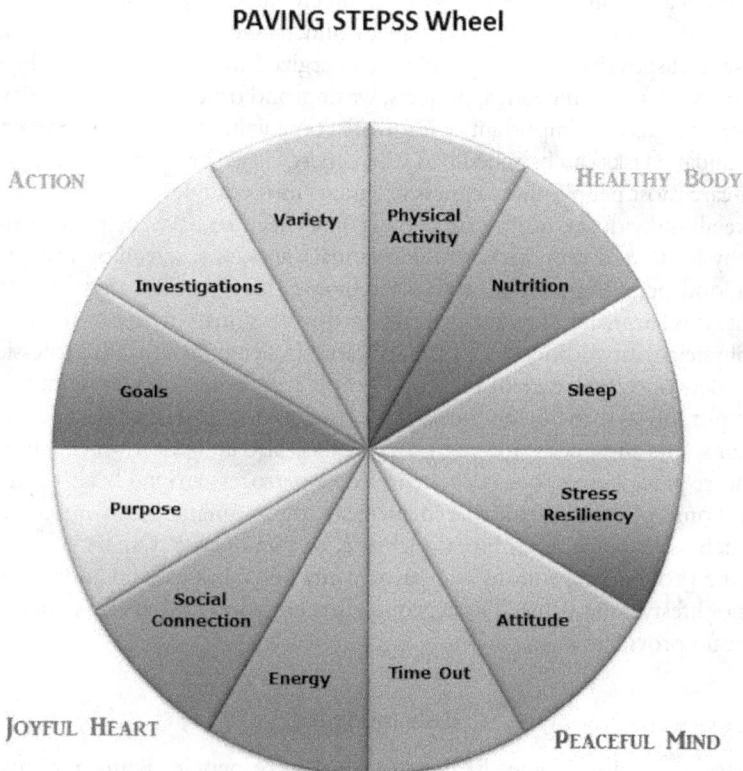

Figure 11.2 The PAVING the path to wellness wheel.

181

For a healthy body, there is a focus on the well-accepted medical areas which are also three of the lifestyle medicine pillars: physical activity, nutrition, and sleep. For a peaceful mind, one lifestyle medicine pillar is included which is stress management. Two other steps include attitude and time outs. The attitudes which are discussed and highlighted in the program include: growth mindset, positivity, gratitude and optimism. Time-outs are essential for a peaceful mind as they allow for a pause between stimulus and response. Time-outs are a form of empowerment moments. The break or pause allows the person to regroup, refocus, and strategize the best way forward, much like a sports team taking a time-out. For a joyful heart or spirit, the program focuses on two of the pillars of lifestyle medicine: social connection and avoidance of risky substances. The risks of loneliness are real and were exemplified during the COVID-19 pandemic. The health benefits of positive social connections are documented in the medical literature (Holt-Lunstad, 2022; Martino et al., 2015). Energy management involves assessing and addressing the use of substances. This includes tobacco, alcohol and caffeine, as well as other substances they may be consuming. But, energy management is more than that. People know about managing their time. Self-care involves more than time management. For example, one may have time to do four 1-hour presentations in a day but not the energy to complete these. Life involves energy management too. This requires individuals to understand their own natural energy cycles and dispositions. Some people are energized in the morning. Others are night owls. Planning meetings, projects, writing, and other important work when you are energized is important. Busy work, organizing, catching up on emails, and mundane tasks can be scheduled when energy is generally low. This is an area of self-care most people and wellness programs miss entirely.

Like all individuals, healthcare professionals need to have their own primary care physicians and keep up with their annual check-ups, screening tests, blood labs, blood pressure, weight, and other biometrics to ensure they are staying healthy. It is surprising how many healthcare professionals do not have a primary care physician. In addition to a primary care physician, healthcare professionals need a dentist to take care of their oral health and could consider working with a therapist, lifestyle medicine specialist or health and wellness coach, depending on their wants and needs. Joining group visits is also an option which allows the healthcare professional to participate in a group process around health and well-being. Some physicians run shared medical appointments based on condition type such as diabetes, high blood pressure, or menopause. Others run lifestyle medicine group interventions and participants join to assess and address all the pillars of lifestyle medicine. These group visits are good options for patients and healthcare providers alike.

Role modeling

Real stories inspire people. Real struggles inspire people. Being real inspires people. When someone sees another person walking the talk, they believe in the importance of the talk, whatever it might be. The rationale is that if someone is taking the time to walk the talk then the talk must be valuable. Two decades ago, in a survey study of primary care physicians investigating whether the physicians exercised and whether they counseled on exercise, there were interesting findings (Abramson et al., 2000). The results of the study revealed that physicians who exercised counseled on exercise. Physicians who did not exercise did not counsel on exercise. In addition, if physicians did strength training, they counseled on it, but if they did not do it, they did not counsel on it. The same finding was true for aerobic activity. So, if more physicians understood the importance and benefits of exercise, found the time to do it for themselves, and enjoyed the many benefits of exercise, they would be more likely to counsel on exercise to their entire patient panel which could impact thousands of patients. More recent studies have confirmed the finding that physicians who are physically active are more likely to counsel patients on exercise (Lobelo et al., 2009; Selvaraj and Abdullah, 2022). Thus, working on getting physicians moving could help move thousands of people closer to improved health and well-being.

Another study on this topic, which was also published two decades ago, looked at people's response to two different physician-patient interactions about exercise and nutrition (Frank, 2000). In this study, patients who were waiting to see their physician were shown two different videos: one showed a physician telling a patient all the benefits of exercise and why they should do it, and another video showed a physician disclosing their own efforts to exercise by biking to work and efforts to eat healthy by bringing an apple to work as a snack. In both scenarios, the physician spoke for a half a minute. The subjects were asked which physician in the videos was more motivating and who was more believable. The physician in the videos with the disclosure was noted to be more motivating and believable. Practicing what one preaches is powerful in the clinical setting (Oberg & Frank, 2009)

When one practices lifestyle medicine and positive health, one may serve as a role model. A role model is defined as "a person whose behavior in a particular role is imitated by others" (Merriam Webster, 2022). This could be a physician, health coach, nurse, therapist or other healthcare professional. In many cases, parents are powerful role models for children. Individuals select their role models. It is difficult to demand that a person follow a particular role model. One is often inspired to follow in the footsteps of a role model based on the connection one feels to the role model and the behaviors a particular person is looking to embody. When people are thinking about their own health, they are often looking to feel energized. People long for a sense of vitality, thriving, and flourishing. When people exude this type of energy, others want to emulate them. In fact, they often ask details such as "What do you eat? What do you do for exercise? Do you drink?" and other details so they can figure out the formula for this sense of well-being they are witnessing. Nothing is quite as powerful as a real person in front of someone walking the talk.

Does this mean that to practice lifestyle medicine and positive health, one must be perfectly healthy, happy and fit? The answer is no. First of all, there is no perfection. The focus is on progress. It is important that the healthcare professional is working on their own health and lifestyle, but no one is perfect. One of the perks of working in lifestyle medicine and positive health is that it is instant accountability. It is difficult to talk about exercise, nutrition, sleep, stress resilience and other healthy lifestyle behaviors when one does not practice them oneself.

Application

The following are strategies for each lifestyle medicine pillar and positive psychology

Physical activity strategies

1 Participate in walking meetings with colleagues, friends and patients or clients when possible.
2 Use an exercise ball as a desk chair.
3 Try a stand up workstation that can allow for flexibility with the way you work.
4 Use a treadmill workstation or a stationary bike work station that you employ when your work allows for this type of movement while you type, dictate, read or participate in meetings so that you can sit less and move more.
5 Take five to ten minute exercise breaks from sitting every hour as often as possible.
6 Use variety with your exercise and try new activities including but not limited to hiking, biking, swimming, paddleboarding, pickleball, tennis, basketball, soccer, cross-country skiing, snowshoeing, yoga, Tai Chi, Qigong, pilates, kickboxing, or rowing.
7 Have fun–hula hoop, jump rope or do something else that brings you joy and try to reach the guidelines of accumulating 150–300 minutes of moderate intensity exercise each week.

Nutritious and delicious eating patterns

1 Add vegetables to every meal and each snack when you can.
2 Add nuts and seeds into meals and snacks when you can, if you can. Pay attention to allergies.
3 Add beans and quinoa to salads to get the benefit of added plant protein.
4 Bring a snack of mixed nuts and dark chocolate (over 80% cacao).
5 Batch cook and bring left-overs to work.
6 Take cooking lessons online or in person with family and friends.
7 Follow a healthy eating plate or template like the one offered by Harvard Healthy Plate or American College of Lifestyle Medicine Healthy Plate both available online.

Sleep

1 Wake up and go to sleep at the same time each day, seven days a week, as often as possible and try to enjoy 7–9 hours of restorative sleep each night.
2 Avoid caffeine intake after 3 pm and if a person is having sleep difficulty avoid caffeine altogether.
3 Avoid alcohol within 3 hours prior to bedtime and if a person is having sleep difficulty avoid alcohol altogether.
4 Avoid blue wavelength light 3 hours prior to bedtime or use a blue wavelength blocking App or blue wavelength blocking glasses.
5 Keep the bedroom like a cave: cool (60–70 degrees Fahrenheit, with a sweet spot of 67 degrees), quiet (use earplugs or white noise), and dark (use an eye mask or curtains that block the light).
6 Follow a relaxing bedtime routine that sets the stage for a quiet night such as taking a warm bath before bed, listening to calming music, reading a book, or enjoying some herbal tea like chamomile tea.
7 Reserve the bedroom for sleep and sex only.

Stress resilience

1 Practice meditation, mindfulness based stress reduction or other techniques that help quiet the mind.
2 Practice Mind-Body practices such as yoga, Tai Chi or Qigong.
3 Find a soothing activity that speaks to you such as listening to music (whatever type you enjoy), dancing, reading, walking, talking with friends, getting out in nature, listening to and watching birds, admiring art of different forms, watching plays, watching movies, laughing with friends, praying or engaging in a spiritual practice that speaks to you, working on creative writing or poetry, taking photographs, knitting, sewing, coloring, crossword puzzles, Sudoku, word searches, board games with friend or family, playing cards (solitaire if you are alone) or any other activity that interests and relaxes you.
4 Use deep breathing to turn on the parasympathetic system or rest and digest system. Take long inhalations and extended exhalations. It is felt that the exhalation is associated with turning on the parasympathetic system.
5 Never worry alone. Reach out to a friend, colleague, religious or spiritual leader, or an anonymous hotline if you need to talk.
6 Focus on the things that you can control. There will continue to be things out of our control like pandemics, hurricanes, floods, and other disasters that we will need to respond to in the moments of these crises. It will be important to find things within our control that we can do to add value and to help ourselves and others day to day as well as in the midst of crisis.
7 If stress seems excessive to you, reach out for help from a professional.

Positive social connectedness

1. It is important to identify someone who is a "charismatic adult" meaning someone who gives you strength when you are with them. We all need at least one friend or family member who we can call in tough times as well as in good times of celebration.
2. Work to prioritize your social connections and enjoy at least one positive social connection a day or seven a week.
3. The importance of quality over quantity is important for social connectedness. High-quality connections require time and energy. Dedicating time and energy to your friends and family is time well spent. Ignoring these relationships can bring pain, misunderstandings, and heart-break.
4. Allocate time for family and friends that is uninterrupted and intentional. Make sure to put the to-do list away, the phone away, the laptop away, work of all kinds in all forms away, and put your entire focus on the person in front of you. Mindfully connecting is a gift to you and the person in your presence.
5. Spontaneous connections and gatherings are exciting but are unreliable for fostering high quality connections. Scheduled and deliberate activities are essential.
6. Phone calls, texts, FaceTime, Zoom meetings, and face-to-face gatherings can all help cultivate high quality connections.
7. Getting through tough times with loved ones and life partners is important and equally important is celebrating good times, achievements, milestones, and the simple but powerful joy of friendship.

Avoiding risky substances or harm reduction

1. Quitting smoking by any means or methodology will enhance health markedly, immediately and long term.
2. The American Heart Association and Center for Disease Control recommends that people do not start drinking. If people do drink, they recommend limiting intake to one drink of alcohol a day for women and two drinks a day for men. For example, one drink is a 12 ounce can of beer or 5 ounces of wine.
3. People are in different stages of change around the use of substances. Using the transtheoretical model of change along with motivational interviewing is the recommended approach for counseling people on substance use.
4. Healthcare professionals are human beings who can struggle with substances. No one is immune from substance use disorders. Getting help is the key, and that takes admitting there's a problem.
5. There are addiction medicine experts who can help people to reduce harm and work toward eliminating the substance depending on the specific situation.
6. Alcohol is considered a carcinogen by the National Cancer Institute. It is associated with esophageal cancer, breast cancer, colon cancer, cancer of the head and neck, and liver cancer (National Cancer Institute, 2021).
7. Instead of a glass of wine before bed, one can try a glass of tart cherry juice or herbal tea like Chamomile.

Positive psychology

1 Gratitude is a powerful positive emotion that can be used at work and at home. Start a meeting with everyone expressing one thing for which they are grateful. Start a meal by inviting people to share one thing for which they are grateful in that moment.
2 Sharing the highlights of the day can be informational and inspiring. When returning home, people can start the conversation by telling a story of the highlights of the day and asking others to share their highlights.
3 Working with strengths is an excellent way to create powerful teams at work and at home. Finding out everyone's strengths and then identifying tasks or jobs that suit those strengths will help people feel flow and joy day to day. When people are using their skills and talents and are fully engaged in a project that has the right amount of challenge to keep them mindfully present and involved, they find flow and lose track of time. This feeling of flow helps add joy and enhance well-being.
4 Asking people about their strengths helps to build their confidence.
5 Ask people about a time when they were successful or reached a goal. This helps them feel a sense of pride which is a powerful positive emotion.
6 Set goals that are achievable and realistic. Reaching goals is rewarding. Success leads to more engagement.
7 Adopt a growth mindset so that people feel comfortable going out of their comfort zones. With a growth mindset, a mishap is an opportunity to learn and grow.

Conclusion

People often view self-care as selfish. Healthcare professionals often feel their identity is wrapped up in healing others and neglecting themselves. This view is detrimental to the physical health and mental health of the healthcare professional and will not lead to positive health. As a society, it is time to give healthcare professionals the time and space to be taken care of, to see their own primary care physicians, to see their dentists, and to see any specialists they need to in order to manage their health and any medical conditions they may have themselves. Healthcare professionals are not superhuman. They are patients too. And, all patients need to prioritize self-care in order to enjoy positive health.

Individuals need time for self-care. They need space for self-care. They need tools for self-care. They should not require permission for self-care. The sooner people appreciate that self-care is synonymous with living, the better the world will be. The sooner people acknowledge that self-care involves nurturing the body, mind, and spirit, the more satisfied people will all be. Taking the time and putting energy into self-care is the best way to keep a person's batteries charged. If a car battery wears out, is overused or is malfunctioning, it may need a jump start which is much more disruptive and complicated than maintaining it with the appropriate time and attention it requires. The same is true for human beings. We need maintenance therapy and attention to our self-care, and at times, we may need a jump start for self-care.

When people are practicing and enjoying healthy living including the six pillars of lifestyle medicine as well as positive health, they often serve as role models to others, whether they know it or not. People watch other people with great interest. One important part of being a healthcare professional who works in the area of lifestyle medicine and positive health is that they are surrounded all day by the research, practices, principles, and play that accompanies these fields. It is inspiring to be among colleagues who walk the talk. Role models abound in lifestyle medicine and positive health. Patients serve as role models too. We can all learn from each other no matter who we are and what role we play.

Takeaways

General

- Self-care involves awareness, self-control, and self-reliance to work toward the goal of enjoying a state of well-being with a healthy body, peaceful mind, and nourished spirit.
- Self-care is "not exercise more and eat less." It involves all parts of a human being.
- Self-care is not a nicety. It is a necessity.
- Assessing one's well-being and self-care practices helps to get a baseline and can serve as a tracking tool.
- The COACH Approach™ involves curiosity, openness, appreciation, compassion, and honesty. Using a COACH Approach™ in self-care can be transformational.

Practical

- Make appointments for physical activity, meditation or other lifestyle medicine pillars.
- Make sure people have a primary care provider and are following up with annual visits.
- A focus on what is in a person's control helps keep people setting goals and making progress.
- Setting SMART goals is important for work and self-care.

  1 Having an accountability buddy for self-care can help.

Wicked questions

1 What policies can healthcare systems and employers put into place to acknowledge the importance of self-care?
2 What will it take to help healthcare providers take self-care seriously?
3 Will a focus on energy management help people to take care of themselves?

Note

1 From the Lifestyle Medicine Handbook, used with permission.

References

Abramson, Scott, Joel Stein, Michael Schaufele, Elizabeth Frates, and Shannon Rogan. 2000. "Personal Exercise Habits and Counseling Practices of Primary Care Physicians: A National Survey." *Clinical Journal of Sport Medicine* 10(1): 40–48. https://doi.org/10.1097/00042752-200001000-00008

American Medical Association. 2022. "STOP This, START That Checklist." https://www.ama-assn.org/system/files/ama-steps-forward-stop-this-start-that-checklist.pdf

Ashton, Melinda. 2019. "Getting Rid of Stupid Stuff." Edhub.ama-Assn.org. 2019. https://edhub.ama-assn.org/steps-forward/module/2757858

Bohman, Bryan, Liselotte N. Dyrbye, Christine A. Sinsky, Mark Linzer, Kristine C. Olson, Stewart F. Babbott, Mary Murphy, Patty Purpur deVries, Maryam S. Hamidi, and Mickey Trockel. 2017. "Physician Well-Being: The Reciprocity of Practice Efficiency, Culture of Wellness, and Personal Resilience." *NEJM Catalyst* August 7.

Dweck, Carol S. 2016. *Carol Dweck's Mindset: The New Psychology of Success: Summary.* Ant Hive Media.

Frank, E. 2000. "Physician Disclosure of Healthy Personal Behaviors Improves Credibility and Ability to Motivate." *Archives of Family Medicine* 9(3): 287–290. https://doi.org/10.1001/archfami.9.3.287

Frates, Beth, Jonathan P. Bonnet, Richard Joseph, and James A. Peterson. 2021. *Lifestyle Medicine Handbook: An Introduction to the Power of Healthy Habits.* Monterey, CA: Healthy Learning.

Frates, Beth, Michelle Tollefson, and Amy Comander. 2022. *Paving the Path to Wellness Workbook: A Guide to Thriving with a Healthy Body, Peaceful Mind, and Joyful Heart.* Monterey, CA: Healthy Learning.

Frates, Elizabeth Pegg, Margaret A. Moore, Celeste Nicole Lopez, and Graham T. McMahon. 2011. "Coaching for Behavior Change in Physiatry." *American Journal of Physical Medicine & Rehabilitation* 90(12): 1074–1082. https://doi.org/10.1097/phm.0b013e31822dea9a

Holt-Lunstad, Julianne. 2022. "Social Connection as a Public Health Issue: The Evidence and a Systemic Framework for Prioritizing the 'Social' in Social Determinants of Health." *Annual Review of Public Health* 43(1). https://doi.org/10.1146/annurev-publhealth-052020-110732

Hooker, Stephanie A., and Kevin S. Masters. 2018. "Daily Meaning Salience and Physical Activity in Previously Inactive Exercise Initiates." *Health Psychology* 37(4): 344–354. https://doi.org/10.1037/hea0000599

Kim, Eric S., Koichiro Shiba, Julia K. Boehm, and Laura D. Kubzansky. 2020. "Sense of Purpose in Life and Five Health Behaviors in Older Adults." *Preventive Medicine* 139(October): 106172. https://doi.org/10.1016/j.ypmed.2020.106172

Lobelo, F., Duperly J., and Frank E. 2009. "Physical Activity Habits of Doctors and Medical Students Influence Their Counselling Practices." *British Journal of Sports Medicine* 43(2): 89–92. https://doi.org/10.1136/bjsm.2008.055426

Major, Brett C., Khoa D. Le Nguyen, Kristjen B. Lundberg, and Barbara L. Fredrickson. 2018. "Well-Being Correlates of Perceived Positivity Resonance: Evidence from Trait and Episode-Level Assessments." *Personality and Social Psychology Bulletin* 44(12): 1631–1647. https://doi.org/10.1177/0146167218771324

Martinez, Nicole, Cynthia Connelly, Alexa Perez, and Patricia Calero. 2021. "Self-Care: A Concept Analysis." *International Journal of Nursing Sciences* 8(4): 418–425. https://doi.org/10.1016/j.ijnss.2021.08.007

Martino, Jessica, Jennifer Pegg, and Elizabeth Pegg Frates. 2015. "The Connection Prescription: Using the Power of Social Interactions and the Deep Desire for Connectedness to Empower Health and Wellness." *American Journal of Lifestyle Medicine* 11(6): 466–475. https://doi.org/10.1177/1559827615608788

Maslow, Abraham H. 1954. *Motivation and Personality.* 3rd ed. New York, NY: Addison Wesley Longman.

Merriam-Webster. 2022. "Merriam-Webster Dictionary." Merriam-Webster.com. 2022. https://www.merriam-webster.com

National Cancer Institute. 2021. "Alcohol and Cancer Risk." National Cancer Institute. Cancer.gov. July 14, 2021. https://www.cancer.gov/about-cancer/causes-prevention/risk/alcohol/alcohol-fact-sheet

Neff, Kristen. 2023. "Self-Compassion." Self-Compassion. https://self-compassion.org. Accessed September 25.

Oberg, E. B., and Frank, E. 2009. "Physicians' Health Practices Strongly Influence Patient Health Practices." *The Journal of the Royal College of Physicians of Edinburgh* 39(4): 290–291. https://doi.org/10.4997/jrcpe.2009.422

Ryan, Richard M., and Edward L. Deci. 2017. *Self-Determination Theory: Basic Psychological Needs in Motivation, Development, and Wellness.* New York, NY: Guilford Press.

Selvaraj, Christine Shamala, and Nurdiana Abdullah. 2022. "Physically Active Primary Care Doctors Are More Likely to Offer Exercise Counselling to Patients with Cardiovascular Diseases: A Cross-Sectional Study." *BMC Primary Care* 23(1). https://doi.org/10.1186/s12875-022-01657-3

Shapiro, Daniel E., Cathy Duquette, Lisa M. Abbott, Timothy Babineau, Amanda Pearl, and Paul Haidet. 2019. "Beyond Burnout: A Physician Wellness Hierarchy Designed to Prioritize Interventions at the Systems Level." *The American Journal of Medicine* 132(5): 556–563. https://doi.org/10.1016/j.amjmed.2018.11.028

Simons, Gemma, and David S. Baldwin. 2021. "A Critical Review of the Definition of 'Wellbeing' for Doctors and Their Patients in a Post Covid-19 Era." *International Journal of Social Psychiatry* 67(8): 002076402110322. https://doi.org/10.1177/00207640211032259

"Spirit Definition & Meaning | Britannica Dictionary." n.d. www.britannica.com. Accessed June 25, 2023. https://www.britannica.com/dictionary/spirit

VIA Institute on Character. 2020. "VIA Character Strengths Survey & Character Profile Reports | via Institute." Viacharacter.org. 2020. https://www.viacharacter.org

12

POSITIVE HEALTH INTERVENTIONS

An emerging concept

Jolanta Burke, Pádraic J. Dunne and Elaine Byrne

Positive Health Sciences (PHS) is an emerging field that combines Positive Psychology, Lifestyle Medicine and selected elements of health psychology. The objective of positive psychology research is to explore the factors that make life worth living (Peterson, 2006). Positive psychology recognises that not experiencing mental health problems is not, in itself, sufficient to ensure wellbeing. Aiming to help individuals flourish is a valuable societal goal that can improve the population's health not only by reducing the symptoms of mental illness but by shifting the normal distribution towards optimal health (Huppert et al., 2005).

The main objective of lifestyle medicine is to prevent non-communicable diseases (NCDs) by increasing behaviours related to six pillars (1) daily physical activity, (2) adequate sleep, (3) a diet rich in predominantly plant-based whole foods, (4) avoidance of risky substances (alcohol and tobacco), (5) stress management and (6) cultivating healthy relationships (ACLM, 2022; Frates, 2021). Thus, while lifestyle medicine focuses on preventing NCDs and helping individuals manage chronic diseases such as Type 1 diabetes or rheumatoid arthritis, positive psychology recognises that prevention is insufficient and explores ways in which individuals can go beyond wellness and experience higher levels of psychological and emotional functioning (flourishing).

Both research fields contribute significantly to developing a range of evidence-based interventions that aim to improve health and wellbeing. Positive Psychology Interventions (PPIs) are defined as psychological tools that fulfil the following criteria: (1) aim to create and enhance positive states (e.g. subjective wellbeing or meaning), (2) there is empirical evidence that they can change the state; (3) there is empirical evidence that manipulating the state will result in positive outcomes for the population (Parks & Biswas-Diener, 2013). PPIs

 DOI: 10.4324/9781003378426-15

include such interventions as practising gratitude (e.g., write about three good things), identifying one's best possible self (e.g., write about you in 10 years when everything went exactly as you hoped for), or performing random acts of kindness (Burke & Arslan, 2021; Parks & Schueller, 2014). The criteria for PPIs emphasise positive outcomes (e.g., improvements in self-esteem, experiences of positive emotions) rather than (merely) the reduction of adverse outcomes. Nevertheless, PPIs lack the non-psychological parameters for assessing high levels of physiological functioning, which the science of Lifestyle Medicine (LM) can offer.

Conversely, the LM Interventions (LMIs) aim to prevent NCDs by supporting individuals to change at least one of the pillars of lifestyle medicine. An example of a successful LM intervention comes from the Ornish Lifestyle Heart Trial (Ornish et al., 1998). Forty-eight patients with coronary artery disease were divided into control (treatment as usual) and intervention groups and monitored for five years. The intervention group were asked to engage in an intensive intervention involving a 10%-fat, vegetarian diet, moderate aerobic exercise, stress management training, smoking cessation and group psychological support. Seventy-one percent of intervention and 75% of control group participants completed a five-year follow-up assessment. Those who had adhered to the intervention programme experienced the most remarkable improvement, with regression of coronary atherosclerosis (blockage of arteries feeding the heart). Conversely, the control group experienced progressive coronary artery disease and was reported to have twice as many heart attacks.

The Diabetes Prevention Program Research Group examined the impact of a lifestyle intervention versus standard medication in preventing the development of type 2 diabetes (Group, 2002). Researchers followed 3,234 patients who initially had elevated fasting and post-load plasma glucose concentrations (pre-diabetes) over an average of three years. Participants were assigned to placebo-control, metformin (medication used to prevent Type 2 diabetes) and a lifestyle intervention consisting of a low fat, healthy balanced diet (Ernst, Cleeman, Mullis, Sooter-Bochenek, & Horn, 1988) and weekly physical activity of moderate intensity, for 150 minutes. Fifty eight percent of the intervention group experienced a reduced incidence of Type 2 diabetes, whereas 31% of the medication group demonstrated a reduction. This is one of many examples of the positive impact of lifestyle-based interventions on health and wellbeing (Bodai et al., 2018). Lifestyle medicine is still evolving and is currently focused almost exclusively on preventing disease rather than optimising health, defined more broadly. The positive health model incorporates this focus on disease prevention and attenuation but also has an added focus on optimising health and wellbeing (Keyes, 2002; O'Boyle et al., this volume) over and above ensuring the absence of disease.

Emerging evidence suggests that flourishing can support many of the pillars of lifestyle medicine. For example, tool enhancing flourishing have shown to help patients with diabetes to eat healthily, maintain their weight, engage in physical activity, take medication and monitor blood glucose (Greenberg & Bertsch, 2016). In the same vein, adherence to the Mediterranean diet or eating more fruit and vegetables is associated with higher levels of wellbeing (Conner et al., 2015; Moreno-Agostino et al., 2019; Mujcic & Oswald, 2016). In addition, researchers link physical literacy with flourishing (Durden-Myers et al., 2018) and growing evidence shows the association between engaging in physical activity and psychological flourishing (e.g., McCoy & Rupp, 2021). Increasing flourishing may also help protect individuals from substance abuse (Whiteford et al., 2013). Thus, LMIs can support PPIs and vice versa. However, further research is required to confirm this (Schotanus-Dijkstra et al., 2017).

Within positive psychology, the concept of flourishing is often limited exclusively to psychological processes such as positive affect, optimism, engagement, self-acceptance or meaning in life (e.g., Diener, 2010; Huppert & So, 2013; Ryff & Singer, 2008; Seligman, 2011). Factors such as social support, stable income, social determinants of health (economic and social conditions) and family membership impact on flourishing (Willen et al., 2022). In a survey of 2,370 participants, physical health was ranked as one of the most important contributors to psychological flourishing (Lee et al., 2021). Furthermore, we recently identified a link between the pillars of lifestyle medicine and flourishing (Burke & Dunne, 2022). In a study of 1,112 participants, all six pillars predicted psychological functioning, meaning that those who practise positive lifestyle behaviours are more likely to experience the highest level of psychological flourishing. Moreover, those who flourished were three times more likely to use 3–6 of the pillars of lifestyle medicine than those who were moderately well, and nine times more likely than languishers, whose functioning was the lowest. These studies suggest that flourishing and its associated interventions go beyond psychological outcomes and can affect physical processes. Positive Health Interventions (PHIs) aim to integrate and capitalise on the potential synergies between LMIs and PPIs.

Recently, academics at the Centre for Positive Health Sciences, RCSI University of Medicine and Health Sciences reviewed PPIs and LMIs and compiled a compendium of over 100 tools that incorporate the application of both approaches (Burke et al., 2023). They proposed two key components of PHIs, (1) the presence of positive outcomes, which extends to both psychological outcomes (such as flourishing, self-esteem, optimism, or positive affect) and physiological outcomes (such as heart-rate variability, cortisol, or intestinal permeability) and (2) the reduction of symptoms of illness, or disease measured in the context of mental and physical health. As such, PHIs aim to reflect the WHO definition of health, which refers to the absence of disease and the presence of health and wellbeing. Tools that aim to build psychological, emotional, intellectual, physiological and social resources that not only demonstrate the evidence of improving health and wellbeing, but also reduce the burden of disease.

The following are examples of PHIs suggested by Burke et al. (2022), across six categories:[1]

Calming tools

Three good things in nature (adapted from Keenan et al., 2021)

If you live in a rural area, go for a walk to a forest, park, beach, mountain, lakeside, or bog area for half an hour every day for five consecutive days. If you live in an urban area, go through a housing estate, town centre, town park or main road. Try to vary your walk each day. You can go on your own or with another person, or a group of people. It is up to you; however, this tool was assessed as a group activity. As you walk each day, try to notice three good things in nature. Then, when you are in the company of others, share the three things you noticed with each other.

Energising tools

Cook and eat mindfully (Dunn et al., 2018)

Pay attention to the food you eat. Take time before each meal to cultivate gratitude for those who grew, cultivated, harvested, processed, delivered, and cooked this food. Be grateful for the fact that you have food to eat. Savour the texture, smell, taste, and temperature of each bite. This approach will slow down the time it takes to eat a meal and assist digestion. It might also contribute to managing healthy body weight.

Coping tools

Self-compassion for binge eating (adapted from Kelly & Carter, 2015)

Over the next three weeks, follow a new routine comprising two simultaneous components:

1 Regular eating
   Avoid junk food; eat three meals a day and three snacks. Develop a healthy eating plan and each evening, make sure you have the next day's eating plan ready. Follow your plan closely, and each day write down any urges you have to binge eat.
2 Self-compassion
   It is common for people to be self-critical when experiencing a struggle, such as binge-eating. Self-blame, however, increases our anxiety and gets in the way of our motivation to eat healthily. This is why self-compassion is a more helpful approach to prevent binge-eating. In addition, when we feel cared for because we care for ourselves, we are more likely to tolerate challenges associated with the distress.

During the next three weeks, while you are completing your daily plan, practice self-compassion as frequently as you can. You can do it through imagery, self-talk or letter writing. The self-compassionate mindset you are trying to adopt may include the following:

– Encourage yourself with kindness to engage in behaviours that will help you prevent binge-eating
– Show yourself empathy and understanding about the struggle you are experiencing
– If you binge-eat through this process, forgive yourself for it. Or if you are beating yourself up for overdoing it in the past, forgive yourself for it.

Whenever you feel like binging:

– Bring back an image you associate with self-compassion or practice self-compassionate self-talk that guides you away from the food
– Talk to yourself as you would talk to a friend who struggles, with an abundance of compassionate mindset
– Accept that you feel distressed and that you struggle
– Commit to taking action that is most in line with self-compassion at this point.

Feeling-good tools

Intensely positive experiences (adapted from Burton & King, 2004)

Consider some of the happiest moments in your life. Moments that have given you an ecstatic feeling. This could include falling in love, your baby being born, being moved by music, or another memorable time of your life. Select one memory and over the next 15–20 minutes, write about it in as much detail as you can. Don't worry about any mistakes, spelling, or grammar. Instead, focus on your thoughts, feelings, emotions, circumstances, people around you, etc. Then, try to re-experience the positive emotions this happy moment gave you.

Meaning-making tools

Benefit finding or reminding (adapted from King & Miner, 2000; Tennen & Afflect, 2005)

This tool may be helpful to anyone experiencing a traumatic or adverse event. Think back to an adverse or traumatic life event you've experienced, perhaps a loss of some sort that felt devastating to you. Consider the circumstances associated with this event. Now, refocus your attention on the positive aspects of this experience. Take a piece of paper and for the next 20 minutes, write down the following:

- How has this experience benefitted you as a person?
- How has this event made you better equipped to cope with challenges in the future?

Don't worry about your spelling or grammar. Nobody is going to read this apart from you. So just let go and go deep as you write about the benefits of the bad experience.

Alternatively, take time and remind yourself daily about the benefits of your chronic illness. This tool is useful for anyone going through chronic illness, alcoholism, or experiencing ongoing pain.

Relationship tools

Letter of forgiveness (adapted from Worthington et al., 2000)

Over the next 30 minutes write a letter to someone who did you harm. In the letter (a) describe the event briefly; (b) describe your understanding of the motives of the offender; (c) describe the reasons for wanting to forgive them; and (d) state that you forgive the person who hurt or offended you.

Prospecting tools

Best possible health (Gibson et al., 2021)

Think about your best possible self. Imagine you have taken good care of your body, eating well, exercising regularly, sleeping well. You are now in excellent health as you have worked hard at accomplishing your health goals. Now consider what steps you have taken to help you get there. For the next 10 min, write down continuously what you have imagined.

These activities provide some examples of how existing LMIs and PPIs can enhance both psychological flourishing and physiological functioning. However, in addition to existing interventions, over the last few years, several researchers have proposed combining PPIs with LMIs to allow them to maximise their impact on an individual's mental and physical health (e.g., Burke & Arslan, 2021; Dunne & Schubert, 2021; Lianov et al., 2020; Morton, 2018). For example, a programme that alternated PPIs (e.g., offer a genuine compliment or write a letter of gratitude to someone and share it) and LMIs (e.g., spend 30 min of moderate exercise or 10,000 steps, or prepare a high-fibre, plant-based meal with one or more friends) over ten weeks resulted in a significant improvement in flourishing. Another programme that integrated PPIs into LMIs (e.g., at the end of the day, write down three good things you ate that day that are good for your body or engage your character strengths while doing moderate exercise in nature for at least 10 min a day) over four weeks also showed an improvement in wellbeing (Burke et al., forthcoming). Thus, the results of both interventions suggest that combining PPIs with LMIs can produce positive psychological outcomes while also engaging individuals in changing lifestyle behaviours.

Positive Health Interventions (PHIs) in practice

In order to increase understanding of PHIs and the role they play in PHSs, we have designed a PHI practice model (Figure 12.1). According to the model, disease burden can be impacted by the physical environment (e.g., levels of pollution), psychological make-up (e.g., personal beliefs, bereavement, early adverse childhood events), social factors (e.g., connectedness, lower socio-economic status) and physical lifestyle, (e.g., unhealthy diet and inactivity). PHIs can mediate

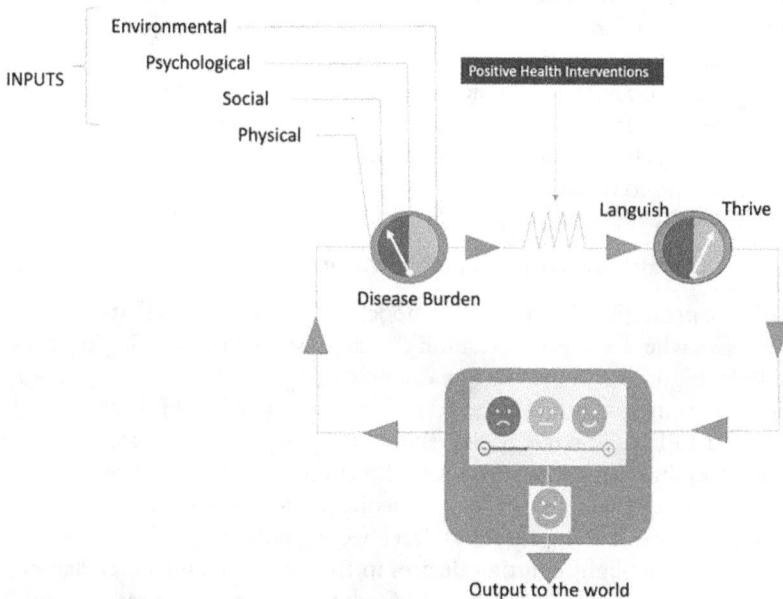

Figure 12.1 Theoretical model - impact of PHI on wellbeing with a view to improve thriving.

Wellbeing is dependent on a variety of inputs (environmental, psychological, social and physical) that when imbalanced can lead to a rise in disease burden such as a diagnosis of rheumatoid arthritis (as is the case in this example). In many cases, this diagnosis might lead to physical and psychological languishing, manifesting in specific outputs such as anxiety, depression, high inflammatory markers and swelling of joints. Conversely, PHIs might modify the mindset and perspective on this negative input, leading to a shift from languishing to thriving (as seen in this image). The resultant outputs might be positive, with improved wellbeing exemplified, for example, by a high score on the Ryff Psychological Wellbeing Scale (PWS), despite ongoing rheumatological disease.

how we live and whether we flourish or languish despite disease burden. Languishing or thriving manifests outwardly in what we do and think and how we behave in the real world (the outputs).

This model is circular, the response to disease burden existing on a languishing-to-thriving continuum. Individuals can move back and forth on this continuum throughout their lives, depending on the inputs/determinants and other factors such as age, maturity, medical treatment and the extent of the disease burden. For example, one person with multiple health conditions experiencing high disease burden and pain (despite mitigating prescribed medications) might experience languishing manifesting in outputs such as high levels of inflammatory markers, reduced subjective wellbeing, low heart rate variability (HRV) and general sickness behaviour (low appetite and libido, coupled with paradoxical anti-social tendencies). Conversely, another individual diagnosed with rheumatoid arthritis who experiences chronic pain (despite mitigating prescribed medications) might thrive despite their high disease burden. PHIs could be used to promote thriving, observed as outputs that include high subjective wellbeing, reduced blood pressure, high HRV and community engagement.

The model also allows for a bidirectional relationship between the inputs and outputs. PHIs that promote thriving and related outputs could also positively affect the physical environment and the social, physical, and psychological health of others in the community.

Health practitioners' application of the PHI circuit

Healthcare professionals can use this model to co-design PHIs that might short-circuit cases where a disease is resulting in languishing and suffering on a significant scale. Figure 12.2, provides an example of a patient, *Tony*, who was spared a life of intermittent languishing and suffering when he and his health coach co-designed a PPI-based strategy that shifted his perspective to a growth mindset by co-examining Carol Dweck's research (Dweck & Yeager, 2019). This strategy incorporates elements of lifestyle medicine such as strength training in the morning (every other day, three days each week), reduced alcohol consumption, avoidance of blue-light emitting devices in the bedroom and a diet rich in pre- and probiotics. Tony still experiences Crohn's-related symptoms, but his perspective on himself (more self-compassionate) and on his disease has changed. He thrives most days but does not despair when he feels more like languishing. Healthcare professionals can incorporate this approach into their clinics or refer their clients to qualified health coaches who can help them co-design a bespoke PHI strategy.

Mechanisms for PHI effectiveness

It is important to develop an understanding of how PHIs work in practice in order to allow us to maximise their impact and ensure the best outcomes. In positive psychology, several models exist that shed light on the intricacies of

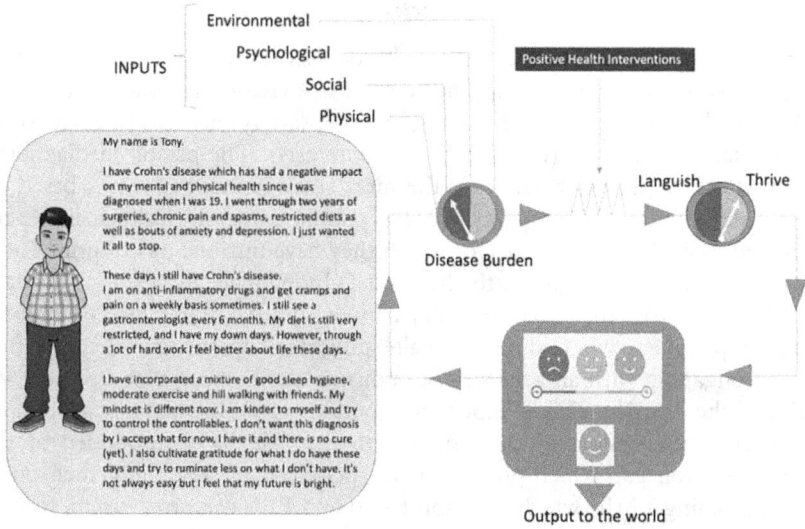

Figure 12.2   Thriving despite a high disease burden.

Healthcare practitioners can use this model to co-design PHIs that might help patients thrive despite the presence of a chronic disease.

practicing PPIs in order to evoke positive change. Some of these models can also be applied in LMI and PHI practice.

Hedonic adaptation theory

Hedonic Adaptation theory (Diener et al., 2006) proposes that individuals adapt to both positive and adverse events. Consequently, engaging in PPIs may only result in short-term effects, and individuals may need to repeat the interventions so that their wellbeing does not returns to the baseline level (Lyubomirsky & Layous, 2013). This happens because people adjust (habituate) to their affective experiences and they can also become desensitised positive life events (Armenta et al., 2014; Brickman & Campbell, 1971). Engaging in many positive activities can be tiring, particularly if an individuals' wellbeing does not change significantly over time. According to the Hedonic Adaptation model, individuals can reduce adaptation and enjoy the benefits of positive events for longer (Sheldon & Lyubomirsky, 2021). This can be achieved by taking three actions; (1) thinking and attending to a positive outcome; (2) thinking and attending to the original motivation for positive change; and (3) variety. This model suggests that in order to keep the positive change going, individuals need to actively and systematically attend to it. The challenge with daily practice of activities such as gratitude or acts of kindness is that it can become monotonous and doing the practices too often may make people more likely to disengage from them (e.g. Burke & O'Donovan, 2022; Lyubomirky & Layous, 2013).

Positive activity model

The second model is a Positive Activity Model (Lyubomirsky & Layous, 2013) which aims to explain how engaging with PPIs increases happiness. According to this model, the features of PPIs (e.g. dosage, variety) need to be matched to the features of a person (e.g. motivation, interests). The person-fit diagnostic tool that assists people in selecting the most suitable intervention is based on the self-determination theory (Ryan & Deci, 2000), whereby individuals are encouraged to engage in activities for which they have intrinsic motivation. There are a number of challenges with the model. Individuals are required to have an awareness of what dosage they may choose and, while this may be easy for some people, many will find it very challenging. Having an intrinsic motivation to start engaging with an activity, does not necessarily mean that a person will maintain the practice. This is important especially given the hedonic adaptation that occurs when engaging in positive activities. This is compounded by the intention-action gap which prevents many people from sustaining their interest. Combining LMIs, which are habit-based and PPIs can prove useful to help individuals sustain new behaviours.

Emotion-regulation theory

The third theory is the Emotion-regulation theory (Quoidbach, Mikolajczak, & Gross, 2015). This theory proposes that positive emotions can be increased in the short-term and long-term by engaging in five emotion-regulation strategies: situation selection, situation modification, attentional deployment, cognitive change, and response modulation. This theory can be extended beyond PPIs and can be used with LMIs also. For example, an individual may choose to meet with a friend or engage in physical activity. In order to amplify their positive experience, they may choose to engage in the following:

Strategies	*Meeting a friend*	*Engaging in physical activity*
Situation selection	*Make a choice of meeting them face to face*	*Make a choice to go running*
Situation modification	Choosing a restaurant, they both enjoy	Exercising in nature
Attentional deployment	While enjoying a meal, deciding to pay attention to the positive moments	Noticing trees and birds singing
Cognitive change	Counting blessings for your friendship	Thinking how grateful you are for the beauty of nature
Response modulation	Sharing your thoughts with your friend	Stopping in the middle of a meadow to admire and connect with nature

Synergistic change model

The Synergistic Change Model (Rusk, Vella-Brodrick, & Waters, 2018) challenges the reductionist approach to positive change and highlights the complexity of human beings. It explains three responses to PPIs: relapse (short-term impact of PPIs on wellbeing, returning to baseline); spill-over (positive changes in other aspects of life unrelated to PPIs); synergy (psychological processes acting in synergy).

Vantage sensitivity

The somewhat controversial "Happiness Pie" model proposes that 50% of happiness depends on genetic makeup, 10% on circumstances and 40% on planned activities such as PPIs (Lyubomirsky et al., 2005; Sheldon & Lyubomirsky, 2021). The model has been heavily criticised, especially by epigenetics researchers, as it does not consider the role of the environment in gene expression (Brown & Rohrer, 2020; Nes & Røysamb, 2017; Røysamb et al., 2014). Epigenetics is a field of research that deals with the changes in phenotype or gene expression caused by mechanisms other than changes in DNA (Keverne & Curley, 2008).

Several models exist that describe how the characteristics of individuals and their environment interact with each other. The three main models are:

1 The "Diathesis-stress" model, which proposes that individuals carry genes that put them at risk for being disproportionately susceptible to adverse events (Zubin & Spring, 1977).
2 The "Differential Susceptibility" model, according to which some individuals show more genetic plasticity in responding to positive and negative events in their lives (Belsky et al., 2007).
3 The "Vantage Sensitivity" model which proposes that some individuals benefit disproportionally from supportive conditions due to their genetic makeup (Pluess & Belsky, 2013).

The vantage sensitivity model focuses on positive activities and is, therefore, the most relevant model for discussing PPIs, LMIs and PHIs. According to the model, some individuals benefit disproportionately from supportive experiences such as wellbeing initiatives and PPIs. For example, research on children experiencing anxiety showed that those who carry the short version of the serotonin transporter gene benefit more from Cognitive Behavioural Therapy compared to those with an extended version of the gene (Eley et al., 2012). Similarly, female adolescents with higher vantage sensitivity showed longer lasting benefits from PPIs compared to those who were lower vantage sensitivity who returned to baseline within 12 months (Pluess & Boniwell, 2015; Pluess et al., 2017). Furthermore, a study of a relationship education programme for married couples showed that genome-wide genetic sensitivity was associated with the longer term benefits of the intervention (Pluess et al., 2022).

In the future, vantage sensitivity research can be extended to assess the impact of genetic predisposition when practising PHIs. It is a possible that combining PPIs and LMIs into the unique PHIs may be differentially effective depending on vantage sensitivity and some individuals may be more likely to engage with PHIs regularly or gain more significant and long-lasting outcomes. Future research needs to explore it in more depth.

PHI mechanisms

Preliminary evidence suggests that the process involved in practising PHIs may differ from PPIs in terms of impact on wellbeing (Aad et al., 2012; Burke & Dunne, 2022). Emerging experimental research shows that, when interventions are combined, the mechanisms for their effectiveness change. For example, a four-week programme that intertwined PPIs with LMIs (writing a letter of gratitude to your breath or performing three acts of kindness to your body) resulted in increased wellbeing, compared with a control group (Burke & Dunne, forthcoming). However, when the impact of the intertwined activities was assessed in relation to changes in participants' satisfaction with the use of six pillars of lifestyle medicine, there was an overall decline in satisfaction with sleep and physical activity compared to the control group. This suggests that combining PPIs and LMIs does not necessarily benefit physical and mental health equally. Further research is required to explore this and to optimise the impact and benefit of PHIs.

In summary, further research is required to explore the optimal content and application of the PHIs. Firstly, we need to identify which interventions are most effective at enhancing physical, physiological and mental health. This may involve *inter alia*: (i) combining some of the interventions from positive psychology (such as the application of character strengths) with physical activity (Hefferon, 2013); (ii) further exploring the 12 intertwined PHIs (Burke et al., forthcoming; Dunne et al., forthcoming); (iii) creating additional activities that integrate PPIs with LMIs interventions. PHIs need to be evaluated for their impact on psychological wellbeing and the extent to which their use can predict psychological flourishing. This can be done using some of the positive psychological scales, such as the PERMA profiler (Butler & Kern, 2016), the Mental Health Continuum (Keyes, 2002) or the Comprehensive Inventory of Thriving (Su et al., 2014). Furthermore, PHIs need to be assessed in the context of their impact on the lifestyle medicine pillars, using scales such as the SMILE (de Vries et al., 2008) or the RCSI Lifestyle Medicine Scale (Loughnane et al., forthcoming). Identifying the effectiveness of individual PHIs will allow comparison between them and facilitate the design of a programme that maximises the positive impact singular or combined PHIs.

In addition, conditions within which PHIs are most effective need to be explored. Whilst individual PHIs may provide positive results relating to physical, physiological and mental health improvement, combinations might prove detrimental to some aspects of individuals' health. As in the case of the PPIs, the variety, dosage of PHIs and individual preferences for them need to be explored (Lyubomirsky & Layous, 2013) in order to optimise their application.

Takeaways

- PHIs are evidence-based tools for enhancing psychological flourishing (e.g. positive affect, meaning) and improving physiological functioning.
- The mechanisms by which PHIs work may be different from those for PPIs and Lifestyle Medicine Interventions (LMIs). Therefore, future research is needed to explore their possible unique potential for maximising impact.
- PHIs can be used with clinical and non-clinical populations to improve well-being and to reduce symptoms of disease
- New interventions are required that engage body and mind to improve well-being and reduce the prevalence and impact of disease.

Wicked questions

1 Which comes first in terms of the greater impact on improving health and flourishing? PPIs or LMIs? Does it matter? Is it dependent on the circumstances for each individual?
2 What are the potential synergies between PPIs and LMIs in promoting optimal health beyond disease prevention? Is the potential impact on health greater than the sum of their parts?
3 Do different cultures place different values on PPIs versus LMIs? Should healthcare systems take cultural, age-related and gender-based differences into account when considering PHIs in total?
4 Should we include or are we including PPIs and LMIs in standard healthcare? Is the health system ready or able to integrate social prescribing of PPIs and LMIs into standard health care? What, if anything, needs to change to enable this?

Note

1 Printed with authors' permission.

References

Aad, G., Abajyan, T., Abbott, B., Abdallah, J., Abdel Khalek, S., Abdelalim, A. A., ... & Zwalinski, L. (2012). Search for magnetic monopoles in sqrt[s]=7 TeV pp collisions with the ATLAS detector. *Physical Review Letters, 109*(26), 261803.
ACLM. (2022). *What is lifestyle medicine.* Retrieved from https://www.lifestylemedicine. org/ACLM/ACLM/About/What_is_Lifestyle_Medicine_/Lifestyle_Medicine. aspx?hkey=26f3eb6b-8294-4a63-83de-35d429c3bb88

Armenta, C. Bao, K. J., Lyubomirsky, S., & Sheldon, K. M. (2014). Is lasting change possible? Lessons from the hedonic adaptation prevention model. In K. Sheldon, & R. E. Lucas (Ed.), *Stability of happiness: Theories and evidence on whether happiness can change* (pp. 57–74). Academic Press.

Belsky, J., Bakermans-Kranenburg, M. J., & van IJzendoorn, M. H. (2007). For better and for worse: Differential susceptibility to environmental influences. *Current Directions in Psychological Science*, 16(6), 300–304. https://doi-org.elib.tcd.ie/10.1111/j.1467-8721.2007.00525.x

Bodai, B. I., Nakata, T. E., Wong, W. T., Clark, D. R., Lawenda, S., Tsou, C., ... & Campbell, T. M. (2018). Lifestyle medicine: A brief review of its dramatic impact on health and survival. *The Permanente Journal*, 22, 17-025. https://doi.org/10.7812/tpp/17-025

Brickman, P., & Campbell, D. T. (1971). Hedonic relativism and planning the good society. In M. H. Appley (Ed.), *Adaptation-level theory* (pp. 287–305). Academic Press.

Brown, N. J. L., & Rohrer, J. M. (2020). Easy as (happiness) pie? A critical evaluation of a popular model of the determinants of well-being. *Journal of Happiness Studies*, 21(4), 1285–1301.

Burke, J., & Arslan, G. (2021). A new forum for sharing happiness and health research. *Journal of Happiness and Health*, 1(1), 1–3.

Burke, J., & Dunne, P. J. (2022). Lifestyle medicine pillars as predictors of psychological flourishing. *Frontiers in psychology*, 13, 963806. https://doi.org/10.3389/fpsyg.2022.963806

Burke, J., & Dunne, P. J. (forthcoming). Mind meets body: Lifestyle medicine and positive psychology interventions for school. In G. Arslan, & M. Yildrim (Eds.). *Handbook of positive school psychology interventions: Evidence-based practice for promoting youth mental health*. Springer Publishing.

Burke, J., Dunne, P. J., & Doran, A. (forthcoming). Lifestyle medicine meets positive psychology interventions: Exploring the impact of an interdisciplinary quasi-experiment in post-primary schools.

Burke, J., & O'Donovan, R. (2022). Gratitude as a protective factor against burnout in healthcare professionals: A systematic review. *British Journal of Healthcare Management*, 29(4). https://doi.org/10.12968/bjhc.2021.0163

Butler, J., & Kern, M. L. (2016). The PERMA-profiler: A brief multidimensional measure of flourishing. *International Journal of Wellbeing*, 6(3), 1–48. https://doi.org/10.5502/ijw.v6i3.526

Burton, C. M., & King, L. A. (2004). The health benefits of writing about intensely positive experiences. *Journal of Research in Personality*, 38(2), 150–163. https://doi-org.elib.tcd.ie/10.1016/S0092-6566(03)00058-8

Conner, T. S., Brookie, K. L., Richardson, A. C., & Polak, M. A. (2015). On carrots and curiosity: Eating fruit and vegetables is associated with greater flourishing in daily life. *British Journal of Health Psychology*, 20(2), 413–427. https://doi.org/10.1111/bjhp.12113

de Vries, E. N., Ramrattan, M. A., Smorenburg, S. M., Gouma, D. J., & Boermeester, M. A. (2008). The incidence and nature of in-hospital adverse events: A systematic review. *Quality & Safety in Health Care*, 17(3), 216–223. https://doi.org/10.1136/qshc.2007.023622

Diener, E. (2010). New well-being measures: Short scales to assess flourishing and positive and negative feelings. *Social Indicators Research*, 97(2), 143–156.

Diener, E., Lucas, R. E., & Scollon, C. N. (2006). Beyond the hedonic treadmill: Revising the adaptation theory of well-being. *The American Psychologist*, 61(4), 305–314. https://doi.org/10.1037/0003-066X.61.4.305

Dunn, C., Haubenreiser, M., Johnson, M., Nordby, K., Aggarwal, S., Myer, S., & Thomas, C. (2018). Mindfulness Approaches and Weight Loss, Weight Maintenance, and Weight Regain. *Current Obesity Reports*, 7(1), 37–49. doi:10.1007/s13679-018-0299-6

Dunne, P. J., & Schubert, C. (2021). Editorial: New mind-body interventions that balance human psychoneuroimmunology. *Frontiers in Psychology: Health Psychology*, 12, 706584. https://doi.org/10.3389/fpsyg.2021.706584

Durden-Myers, E. J., Whitehead, M. E., & Pot, N. (2018). Physical literacy and human flourishing. *Journal of Teaching in Physical Education*, 37(3), 308–311. https://doi-org.elib.tcd.ie/10.1123/jtpe.2018-0132

Dweck, C. S., & Yeager, D. S. (2019). Mindsets: A view from two eras. *Perspectives on Psychological Science*, 14(3), 481–496. https://doi.org/10.1177/1745691618804166

Eley, T. C., Hudson, J. L., Creswell, C., Tropeano, M., Lester, K. J., Cooper, P., Farmer, A., Lewis, C. M., Lyneham, H. J., Rapee, R. M., Uher, R., Zavos, H. M., & Collier, D. A. (2012). Therapygenetics: The 5HTTLPR and response to psychological therapy. *Molecular Psychiatry*, 17(3), 236–237. https://doi.org/10.1038/mp.2011.132

Ernst, N. D., Cleeman, J., Mullis, R., Sooter-Bochenek, J., & Horn, L. V. (1988). The National Cholesterol Education Program: Implications for dietetic practitioners from the adult treatment panel recommendations. *Journal of the American Dietetic Association*, 88(11), 1401–1409. https://doi.org/10.1016/S0002-8223(21)08024-X

Frates, B. (2021). PAVING the path to wellness: Essential aspects of helping patients improve lifestyle behaviors. *Integrative and Complementary Therapies*, 27(6), 262–264. https://doi.org/10.1089/act.2021.29359.bfr

Gibson, B., Umeh, K., Davies, I., & Newson, L. (2021). The best possible self-intervention as a viable public health tool for the prevention of type 2 diabetes: A reflexive thematic analysis of public experience and engagement. *Health expectations: an international journal of public participation in health care and health policy*, 24(5), 1713–1724. https://doi.org/10.1111/hex.13311

Greenberg, R. & Bartsch, B. (2016). The flourishing treatment approach: A strengths-based model informed by how people create health. *Diabetes Care and Education*, 37(6), 39–44.

Group, D. P. P. R. (2002). Reduction in the incidence of type 2 diabetes with lifestyle intervention or metformin. *The New England Journal of Medicine*, 346(6), 393–403. https://doi.org/10.1056/NEJMoa012512

Hefferon, K. (2013). *Positive psychology and the body: The somatopsychic side to flourishing*. Open University Press.

Huppert, F. A., & So, T. T. (2013). Flourishing across Europe: Application of a new conceptual framework for defining well-being. *Social Indicators Research*, 110(3), 837–861. https://doi.org/10.1007/s11205-011-9966-7

Huppert, F. A., Baylis, N., & Keverne, B. (2005). *The science of wellbeing*. Oxford University Press.

Keenan, R., Lumber, R., Richardson, M., & Sheffield, D. (2021). Three good things in nature: a nature-based positive psychological intervention to improve mood and well-being for depression and anxiety. *Journal of Public Mental Health*, 20(4), 243–250. https://doi-org.elib.tcd.ie/10.1108/JPMH-02-2021-0029

Kelly, A. C., & Carter, J. C. (2015). Self-compassion training for binge eating disorder: A pilot randomized controlled trial. *Psychology & Psychotherapy: Theory, Research & Practice*, 88(3), 285–303. https://doi-org.elib.tcd.ie/10.1111/papt.12044

Keverne, E. B., & Curley, J. P. (2008). Epigenetics, brain evolution and behaviour. *Frontiers in Neuroendocrinology*, 29(3), 398–412. https://doi-org.elib.tcd.ie/10.1016/j.yfrne.2008.03.001

Keyes, C. L. M. (2002). The mental health continuum: From languishing to flourishing in life. *Journal of Health and Social Behavior*, 43(2), 207–222. https://doi.org/10.2307/3090197

King, L. A., & Miner, K. N. (2000). Writing about the perceived benefits of traumatic events: Implications for physical health. Personality and Social Psychology Bulletin.

Lee, M. T., Bialowolski, P., Weziak-Bialowolska, D., Mooney, K. D., Lerner, P. J., McNeely, E., & VanderWeele, T. J. (2021). Self-assessed importance of domains of flourishing: Demographics and correlations with well-being. *The Journal of Positive Psychology*, *16*(1), 137–144. https://doi-org.elib.tcd.ie/10.1080/17439760.2020.1716050

Lianov, L. S., Barron, G. C., Fredrickson, B. L., Hashmi, S., Klemes, A., Krishnaswami, J., ... &Winter, S. J. (2020). Positive psychology in health care: Defining key stakeholders and their roles. *Translational Behavioral Medicine*, *10*(3), 637–647. https://doi.org/10.1093/tbm/ibz150

Loughnane, C., Burke, J., & Dunne, P. J. (forthcoming). *Positive lifestyle medicine scale: A validation.*

Lyubomirsky, S., King, L., & Diener, E. (2005). The benefits of frequent positive affect: Does happiness lead to success? *Psychological Bulletin*, *131*(6), 803–855.

Lyubomirsky, S., & Layous, K. (2013). How do simple positive activities increase well-being? *Current Directions in Psychological Science*, *22*(1), 57–62. https://doi.org/10.1177/0963721412469809

McCoy, S. M., & Rupp, K. (2021). Physical activity participation, flourishing and academic engagement in adolescents with obesity. *Pediatric Obesity*, *16*(10), e12796. https://doi.org/10.1111/ijpo.12796

Moreno-Agostino, D., Caballero, F. F., Martín-María, N., Tyrovolas, S., López-García, P., Rodríguez-Artalejo, F., ... & Miret, M. (2019). Mediterranean diet and wellbeing: Evidence from a nationwide survey. *Psychology & Health*, *34*(3), 321–335. https://doi.org/10.1080/08870446.2018.1525492

Morton, D. P. (2018). Combining lifestyle medicine and positive psychology to improve mental health and emotional well-being. *American Journal of Lifestyle Medicine*, *12*(5), 370–374. https://doi.org/10.1177/1559827618766482

Mujcic, R., & Oswald, A. J. (2016). Evolution of well-being and happiness after increases in consumption of fruit and vegetables. *American Journal of Public Health*, *106*(8), 1504–1510. https://doi.org/10.2105/AJPH.2016.303260

Nes, R. B., & Røysamb, E. (2017). Happiness in behaviour genetics: An update on heritability and changeability. *Journal of Happiness Studies: An Interdisciplinary Forum on Subjective Well-Being*, *18*(5), 1533–1552. https://doi-org.elib.tcd.ie/10.1007/s10902-016-9781-6

Ornish, D., Scherwitz, L. W., Billings, J. H., Brown, S. E., Gould, K. L., Merritt, T. A., ... & Brand, R. J. (1998). Intensive lifestyle changes for reversal of coronary heart disease. *JAMA*, *280*(23), 2001–2007. https://doi.org/10.1001/jama.280.23.2001

Parks, A. C., & Biswas-Diener, R. (2013). Positive interventions: Past, present, and future. In T. B. Kashdan & J. Ciarrochi (Eds.), *Mindfulness, acceptance, and positive psychology: The seven foundations of well-being* (pp. 140–165). New Harbinger Publications, Inc.

Parks, A. C., & Schueller, S. M. (Eds.). (2014). *The Wiley Blackwell handbook of positive psychological interventions*. Wiley Blackwell. https://doi.org/10.1002/9781118315927

Peterson, C. (2006). *A primer in positive psychology*. Oxford University Press.

Pluess, M., Assary, E., Lionetti, F., Lester, K. J., Krapohl, E., Aron, E. N., & Aron, A. (2018). Environmental sensitivity in children: Development of the highly sensitive child scale and identification of sensitivity groups. *Developmental Psychology*, *54*(1), 51–70. https://doi.org/10.1037/dev0000406

Pluess, M., & Belsky, J. (2013). Vantage sensitivity: Individual differences in response to positive experiences. *Psychological Bulletin*, *139*(4), 901–916. https://doi.org/10.1037/a0030196

Pluess, M., & Boniwell, I. (2015). Sensory-Processing Sensitivity predicts treatment response to a school-based depression prevention program: Evidence of Vantage Sensitivity. Personality and Individual Differences, 82, 40–45. https://doi-org.elib.tcd.ie/10.1016/j.paid.2015.03.011

Pluess, M., Boniwell, I., Hefferon, K., & Tunariu, A. (2017). Preliminary evaluation of a school-based resilience-promoting intervention in a high-risk population: Application of an exploratory two-cohort treatment/control design. *PLoS ONE*, *12*(5), 1–18. https://doi-org.elib.tcd.ie/10.1371/journal.pone.0177191

Pluess, M., Rhoades, G., Keers, R., Knopp, K., Belsky, J., Markman, H., & Stanley, S. (2022). Genetic sensitivity predicts long-term psychological benefits of a relationship education program for married couples. *Journal of Consulting and Clinical Psychology*, *90*(2), 195–207. https://doi-org.elib.tcd.ie/10.1037/ccp0000715.supp (Supplemental)

Quoidbach, J., Mikolajczak, M., & Gross, J. J. (2015). Positive interventions: An emotion regulation perspective. *Psychological Bulletin*, *141*(3), 655–693. https://doi.org/10.1037/a0038648

Røysamb, E., Nes, R. B., & Vittersø, J. (2014). Well-being: Heritable and changeable. In K. M. Sheldon & R. E. Lucas (Eds.), *Stability of happiness: Theories and evidence on whether happiness can change.* (pp. 9–36). Elsevier Academic Press. https://doi-org.elib.tcd.ie/10.1016/B978-0-12-411478-4.00002-3

Rusk, R. D., Vella-Brodrick, D. A., & Waters, L. (2018). A complex dynamic systems approach to lasting positive change: The synergistic change model. *The Journal of Positive Psychology*, *13*(4), 406–418. https://doi-org.elib.tcd.ie/10.1080/17439760.2017.1291853

Ryan, R. M., & Deci, E. L. (2000). Self-determination theory and the facilitation of intrinsic motivation, social development, and well-being. *American Psychologist*, *55*(1), 68–78. https://doi.org/10.1037/0003-066X.55.1.68

Ryff, C. D., & Singer, B. H. (2008). Know thyself and become what you are: A eudaimonic approach to psychological well-being. *Journal of Happiness Studies: An Interdisciplinary Forum on Subjective Well-Being*, *9*(1), 13–39. https://doi.org/10.1007/s10902-006-9019-0

Schotanus-Dijkstra, M., Ten Have, M., Lamers, S. M. A., de Graaf, R., & Bohlmeijer, E. T. (2017). The longitudinal relationship between flourishing mental health and incident mood, anxiety and substance use disorders. *European Journal of Public Health*, *27*(3), 563–568. https://doi-org.elib.tcd.ie/10.1093/eurpub/ckw202

Seligman, M. E. P. (2011). *Flourish: A visionary new understanding of happiness and well-being.* Free Press.

Sheldon, K. M., & Lyubomirsky, S. (2021). Revisiting the sustainable happiness model and pie chart: Can happiness be successfully pursued? *The Journal of Positive Psychology*, *16*(2), 145–154. https://doi-org.elib.tcd.ie/10.1080/17439760.2019.1689421

Su, R., Tay, L., & Diener, E. (2014). The development and validation of the Comprehensive Inventory of Thriving (CIT) and the Brief Inventory of Thriving (BIT). *Applied Psychology Health Well Being*, *6*(3), 251–79.

Whiteford, H. A., Degenhardt, L., Rehm, J., Baxter, A. J., Ferrari, A. J., Erskine, H. E., Charlson, F. J., Norman, R. E., Flaxman, A. D., Johns, N., Burstein, R., Murray, C. J. L., & Vos, T. (2013). Global burden of disease attributable to mental and substance use disorders: Findings from the global burden of disease study 2010. *The Lancet*, *382*(9904), 1575–1586. https://doi-org.elib.tcd.ie/10.1016/S0140-6736(13)61611-6

Willen, S. S., Williamson, A. F., Walsh, C. C., Hyman, M., & Tootle, W. (2022). Rethinking flourishing: Critical insights and qualitative perspectives from the U.S. Midwest. *SSM - Mental Health*, *2*, 100057. https://doi.org/10.1016/j.ssmmh.2021.100057

Worthington, E.L. Jr., Kurusu, T.A., Collins, W., Berry, J.W., Ripley, J.S., Baier, S.N. (2000). Forgiving usually takes time: A lesson learnt by studying interventions to promote forgiveness. *Journal of Psychology and Theology*, *28*(1), 3–20.

Zubin, J., & Spring, B. (1977). Vulnerability: A new view of schizophrenia. *Journal of Abnormal Psychology*, *86*(2), 103–126. https://doi.org/10.1037/0021-843X.86.2.103

13

PEOPLE MAY HAVE MANY WISHES BUT IF THEY LOSE THEIR HEALTH, THEY ONLY HAVE ONE WISH, TO BECOME HEALTHY AGAIN

Dóra Guðrún Guðmundsdóttir
and Svala Sigurðardóttir

In the Netherlands, primary care physician, Dr. Machteld Huber, at the institute for Positive Health, has proposed a new definition for health – or positive health:

"Health is broader than the absence of disease or symptoms. An increasingly central role is played by other aspects, such as resilience, sense of purpose, meaningfulness, and self-management." This definition is much more in line with the WHO definition of mental health (World Health, 2001): "Mental health is a state of mental wellbeing that enables people to cope with the stresses of life, realize their abilities, learn well and work well, and contribute to their community". WHO additionally emphasises that mental health is an integral component of health and wellbeing that underpins our individual and collective abilities to make decisions, build relationships and shape the world we live in. Mental health is a basic human right. And it is crucial to personal, community and socio-economic development.

Mental health is more than the absence of mental disorders. It exists on a complex continuum, which is experienced differently from one person to the next, with varying degrees of difficulty and distress and potentially very different social and clinical outcomes. Mental health conditions include mental disorders and psychosocial disabilities as well as other mental states associated with significant distress, impairment in functioning, or risk of self-harm. People with mental health conditions are more likely to experience lower levels of mental wellbeing, but this is not always or necessarily the case.

It is important to realise the difference between prevention and promotion. Health promotion was first defined by the World Health Organisation in

DOI: 10.4324/9781003378426-16   208

Ottawa, 1986 as "the process of enabling people to increase control over, and to improve their health" (World Health Organization. Regional Office for, 1986). Later Eriksson and Lindström (2008) demonstrated how the thoughts and the ideas behind Antonovsky's salutogenic model for health have influenced the development of health promotion.

Lifestyle change can be facilitated through a combination of efforts to enhance awareness, change behaviour, and create an environment that support good health practices (O'Donnell, 1989). The health promotion view of health is that health is created in the context of everyday life where people live, love, work and play (World Health Organization. Regional Office for, 1986). This is in line with the ideology of positive psychology.

The primary distinction between prevention and promotion lies in their focus. While prevention has its focus on the disease, promotion focuses on health. That said, the same activity can both be preventive and promoting and even treatment, like for example physical exercise. The fundamental difference lies in the focus and the aim of the activity. Is the aim to prevent or reduce symptoms, e.g. prevent weight gaining or reduce blood sugar levels (treatment) or is the aim to increase health and wellbeing which would then be health promotion and positive psychology intervention.

Unfortunately, the focus and emphasis in the healthcare systems is on treating illness instead of preventing or even better promoting health. It is well documented that resources are of much better use if spent on promoting health than treating illnesses. By enhancing health and wellbeing, there is a possibility to prevent mental health problems (Huppert, 2009) and increase flourishing. The different stages of healthcare are illustrated as a river which emphasises how important it is to work upstream in order to increase wellbeing and quality of life (Eriksson & Lindström, 2008).

Too little focus is on preventive care reflecting in extremely high numbers on the cost of care of preventable diseases (Galea & Maani, 2020). The majority of the OECD countries are spending under 1% of their GDP on preventive care (OECD, 2022). In most countries of the world, the primary care, is a part of the healthcare system, which role is to implement health promotion and prevention, but unfortunately, this is not the case. Insufficient room is made for this important aspect, instead, we are mostly putting out fires. This needs to be changed.

Although it seems relevant to apply positive psychology approaches in the healthcare system, this is not yet the case in most corners of the world. What is the obstacle? One of the main reasons why healthcare professionals are not applying positive psychology interventions is that they are not trained to use them, it is not a part of their educational curriculum. Even though interventions to increase wellbeing is not part of the training of healthcare professions, few universities, responsible for healthcare education, are opening their eyes to this field, like The Royal College of Surgeons (RCSI), and the University of Iceland to name examples. In Norway some efforts have been done, on introducing strength based focus on the patients in primary care (Jøssang et al., 2022). Nevertheless, this is new to the medical practitioner and needs further development in order to make some real changes in this field.

The *RCSI offers courses like The Science of Health and Happiness (link to course website) for health care providers and the University of Iceland, covers an introduction to the basics of positive psychology both for 6th-year medical students and 4th-year nursing students too (link to course website) and most recently, a special course for health care providers on practical basic positive psychology for health care providers fall 2022 (link to course website).*

Most HCPs do not get adequate education about the importance (and physiology) of sleep, stress, exercise, nutrition, or even health promotion. Unfortunately, most traditional schools of healthcare professionals training doctors, nurses, and psychologists still place largest focus on the disease model and therefore miss a lot of opportunities for health promotion and prevention. The guidelines provided in this chapter can be applied both as 1:1 approach, in a group setting or as a collaborate care (possibly including medical doctors, nurses, sociologist, and psychologists – some or all of those – depends). This is important to have in mind, since collaborate care is often considered a more cost beneficial model to work by.

The current and future healthcare models

As this book has covered, substantial research has been done in the field of positive psychology, more and more so in the Healthcare field over the past decade or so. With the focus on the pathology of their patients/clients, healthcare providers are not taught to be aware of the person's strength, and how that could eventually be something that could help the person deal better with what is "wrong" with them. This focus on the disease model gives rise to total ignorance of the extremely important factors influencing health, which should be the main focus.

Let's take a look at some basic theories, that can be applied in the healthcare setting, and what has been done in the field of positive psychology there. This examination of the existing research in the medical field, both in outpatient clinics and primary care, aims to be an introduction only – not a full cover of existing research – that is beyond the scope of this chapter.

As traditional psychological approaches aim to reduce symptoms and psychopathology, the person can be left without symptoms but still feeling that they are dissatisfied with their life. Positive interventions can be useful. Their goal is to enhance wellbeing and can be applied in many settings in the healthcare system. By enhancing wellbeing, there is a possibility to hinder mental health problems (Huppert, 2009) and increase flourishing.

Substantial research has been done on the application of positive psychology interventions and they have shown to be effective in both clinical and non-clinical settings (Carr et al., 2021; van Agteren et al., 2021), and optimal to apply in primary care. Research is being conducted in various corners of the world. In Spain, they have developed a group therapy called Positive psychology group therapy for patients with depression, and preliminary results show it to be as effective as CBT (Chaves et al., 2017). Positive psychotherapy (PPT) with a strength based approach, has been developed by Rashid (Rashid, 2015) is also promising (Furchtlehner et al., 2020).

In the USA, there has been a wave of positive psychology approaches and research, mostly connected to cardiology and mental health. There are ongoing research programs in cardiology, cancer (Gudmundsson et al., 2022) and atopic dermatitis (Gudmundsdóttir et al., 2022), in Iceland, that also bear elements from the field of positive psychology, like self- efficacy, mindfulness, self-determination, values and meaning.

If we take cardiovascular diseases (CVDs) as an example, it makes sense to apply positive psychology and mindfulness approaches. Studies have for example demonstrated that gratitude and optimism can increase adherence to treatment (Millstein et al., 2016) and mindfulness practice can reduce stress (Khoury et al., 2013; Levine et al., 2017) and have good effects on sleep (Thimmapuram et al., 2020) – but both lack of sleep and stress are of course well known to have detrimental effects on mental and physical health.

Further studies have exhibited effectiveness of positive interventions for people with acute coronary syndrome (Brown et al., 2019; Huffman et al., 2019) and how training optimism can be useful for these patients (Mohammadi et al., 2018) and even reduce risk of CVD's (Loucks et al., 2015). The American heart association is aware of this, and has recently published a statement, recommending that clinicians use both positive psychology and mindfulness approaches in their treatment of people with CVD (Levine et al., 2021) recognising the important connection of the mind and the body.

In the primary healthcare setting, the Dutch general physician, Dr. Machteld Huber and her team have developed a "dialogue tool" currently being used in the Netherlands and other countries, for example in the Primary Care in Iceland. This tool has shown to be a helpful and practical tool in clinical work, with patients in primary care especially. Physicians have reported that it is helpful to use this dialogue tool, in order to help their patients get to the roots of their problems. Amelioration in one area like increased score of mental wellbeing status often leads to improvement in other areas of the persons health, like quality of life.

It is a good idea to combine the application of positive interventions and this dialogue tool, sometimes called "the wheel of health", that is normally used in sessions with a patient. The practitioner and the patient discuss a problem and score the persons state in each aspect of their positive health. As homework, the person sets a goal to focus on increasing their score in one are until next time. In order to do that, the physician could suggest positive interventions known to help with this problem, to practice until they meet again. Ideally, they'd let them choose from a list of activities, or even connect them to another person like a social worker, at the primary care centre, that could further assist the person to work on this goal. For example, a person that is suffering from loneliness, might want to increase their social activities, and could be connected to a group of people that meet regularly to do things that they have in common, like gardening or visiting museums. Applying this dialogue tool with positive interventions, gives the practitioner both a concrete measurement tool, to use for goalsetting and health promotion, and enables the person to take their health in their own hands.

Application

Basic necessary knowledge that can be applied.

The following theories and applications are valuable to the HCPs work in the healthcare setting and can be applied by the therapist or the clinic, in a broader approach. Deeper introduction to each theory or model, has been covered earlier in this book.

The Salutogenetic model

The Salutgenetic model, which emphasis empowering the patient in taking an active role and responsibility when it comes to their health, is especially relevant for the health practitioner working in primary care. Being a part of the first line of healthcare, they have direct contact with their patients, and a golden opportunity to make them aware of the fact that you are not either healthy or sick, and you most certainly are not your disease. It is important to make the client aware of the factors influencing health, and how they can take their health in their own hands.

How to apply it?

The clinician, working with a patient on lifestyle change, such as exercising more and eating more healthy food. It is important to explain WHY exercise and healthy food are important, and make the client aware of how they can improve this, best if they could provide basic small steps to take to gain this and/OR even refer the client to another HCP in the clinic (e.g. the lifestyle nurse for a health-promoting interview in the clinic).

The dialogue tool (Figure11.1) could be applied, and it is essential to set a goal and give homework for next session.

Applying the broaden and build theory

The Broaden and Build theory of positive emotions (Fredrickson, 2004) is important to explain to the client, as well as clarifying that their negativity bias is normal and most of us have it. Mention that most of our negative thoughts are no longer helpful and we need to give the positive aspects in live more focus without ignoring important negative emotions which are normal and often useful. They need to understand that if we are feeling blue our negative emotions are dominating and then it can be helpful to do some exercises in noticing or savouring the positive things around, to increase the odds of "entering" the upward spiral of positive emotions.

How to apply it?

When treating a person with depression or someone going through difficulties who is ruminating and even spiralling down, it is helpful to explain this theory, and how it works. Then give them homework for next session to help them out of this negative spiral. The "3 good things" exercise or "gratitude diary" are good to train people in noticing the good things in life, but bear in mind that no one exercise is fitting for everyone. Give the person autonomy to choose from a list of activities, is a good idea, or even use Dr. Lyubomirskys person – activity – fit diagnosis tool to find the best exercise.

Self-determination theory

The self-determination approach can also be applied in clinical settings, and perfect to use with the Positive health dialogue tool in a health-promoting interview, when the client is working towards a positive lifestyle change.

How to apply it?

It is important for the person working with the client to use autonomy supportive interactions to enhance their intrinsic motivation. Here are examples:

Point out what they can do to improve their health and wellbeing.

- Encourage their knowledge – provide explanations, like why doing something, like exercising, is important for their situation.
- Recommend that they start working on something, they are likely to be able to "master" – help them chop it down to small parts.
- Try to put yourself in the persons shoes.
- Discuss the situation with them, get their input and ideas.
- Offer meaningful options.
- Show empathy and understanding – let them know that you are aware that lifestyle changes are hard.
- Try not to "order or demand" anything from the person, rather "sell the idea" of why this step is good for them.
- Complement on the effort, not the outcome or compare to others.
- Give informal feedback.

With this approach the clients are asked what outcomes really matter to them and what they would like to improve. When medical practitioners support the patient's autonomy, this enhances the patient's intrinsic motivation and perceived competence for making changes in health-compromising behaviours and taking prescribed medications.

Mindfulness and self-compassion

These are also very important factors to train, as they have shown to be essential for people working on lifestyle changes. Being mindful and self-compassionate, helps people enhance their intrinsic motivation and not to give up when they have a setback (Donald et al., 2020; Schuman-Olivier et al., 2020).

Mindfulness therapies have demonstrated multiple health benefit. They have been shown to increase mental wellbeing, decrease stress, depression and anxiety (Goldberg et al., 2018; Kuyken et al., 2008), and to be useful when going through lifestyle changes and tough times and help with weight loss (Carrière et al., 2018) to name a few examples. It is a good idea for the HPCs self and caregivers (Hansen et al., 2021; Spinelli et al., 2019) to practice mindfulness too.

How to apply it?

You could encourage your workplace to offer MBSR/MBCT ACT or CCT group therapies for your clients. You could even just recommend your clients try the free "Health minds app" or some other meditation app (e.g. CALM; HEADSPACE) to see if they like the mindfulness approach.

Character strengths

It is essential to be aware of your strengths, both for the client and you as a HCP. To be able to spot your patients strengths can get you a long way, and open people's eyes to what they CAN do, shifting the focus from what they (feel they) can't.

How to apply it?

Encourage your patient to explore their strengths and to use them for their benefits when dealing with a problem they are facing. If you know your patient well, it is powerful to point out what strengths you think they possess.

Optimism

Has been shown to increase adherence to treatment, optimistic people have numerous health benefits. For the HCP, it is much more giving to work with optimistic view of the world, to help people see what is "right" with them, not only what is "wrong" and needs fixing – (Broaden and Build theory (Fredrickson, 2004; Garland et al., 2010))

How to apply it?

Just by mentioning this theory and tell your client about it, can get them going. To help them be more aware of the good things in live, and SAVOURING, really taking in good experiences like compliments, good night with your family, etc., is very powerful and can get them "on the track" of the upward spiral of positive emotions.

Below are more general examples of how you could apply positive psychology as a health practitioner.

As a medical doctor/psychologist

When supporting a patient through rough times like a period of depression, that could need medical treatment or not, it is common in many healthcare settings, to follow–up on the patient, regularly, and sometimes the GP is the only possible therapist for the patient (waiting lists for CBT, mindfulness, psychologists are often long) so the GP could give their patients "homework" to work on between sessions, incorporating general health promoting advice with positive psychology.

An example would be to ask them to simple tasks until next time, such as, 30 minutes of physical activity (could even prescribe motion, that is possible in some countries). Give basic sleep hygiene guidance (like recommend that they go to sleep same time every night, and wake up the same time, stay away from screens 2 hours before bed, keep the bedroom cool, no meals or exercises at least 2 hours before sleep and try to make themselves a good sleep routine)

And lastly, encourage the patient to do positive interventions – either have a list with short explanations for them/link to a website, OR start with a simple "3 good things" daily after first session, moving to other simple PPI's like gratitude diary, kindness diary, strength testing, etc… there are endless options. Some research indicate that the best way to go about this is to match the person (Nelson & Lyubomirsky, 2014) but you can also start simple, with the PPIs mentioned above.

A social worker

Some primary care clinics are so lucky to have a social worker working in the same building, others must rely on social workers in the area. One good example on how they could be using positive psychology is via social prescription of various activities for example for the patient that is feeling lonely, and depressed. The GP could refer them to the social worker, that would help them find groups to join.

A nurse

Example of someone trying to quit smoking it is relevant to encourage self-compassion, mindfulness and SDT and the stages of change, plus (if possible) a prescription for motion. Teach your client to show themselves self-compassion, acknowledge that lifestyle changes are hard, recommend mindfulness and /or self-compassion exercises, and small to take small steps, don't give up if they "fail", explain how the stages of change work.

The primary healthcare sector is probably the best place to start implementing positive psychology approaches. It is highly likely that there will be a bigger need for interventions that can increase wellbeing and mental health in the light of higher depression symptoms after Covid-19 (Magnúsdóttir et al., 2022).

There is also increased demand on the healthcare system to be able to prevent diseases, by supporting healthy lifestyle choices, especially with the increased burden of obesity (Afshin et al., 2017) and related chronic diseases in the world today.

If you see this approach as something that could be beneficial for your clients, go ahead! None of the above would be considered to "cause harm" and therefore a good fit for the primary care personnel to apply.

Takeaways

- Try the PPIs out yourself, see how they make you feel? Try mindfulness meditation (or even a full MBSR seminar) and/or self-compassion and reflect on your own experience.
- Read up on the basic theories, and see if you find other relevant situations to apply in your work- you could check out the free online course at edx.org, taught at Berkeley University https://greatergood.berkeley.edu/podcasts/series/the_science_of_happiness%C2%A0
- or the science of wellbeing from Yale, taught at coursera.org, see here: https://www.coursera.org/learn/the-science-of-wellbeing
- Introduce these approaches to your staff/co-workers and make a "how to apply" brochure/guidelines for your clinic, and start applying, small steps at the time, and see how it works for you and your clinic

Wicked questions

1 What type of clients would benefit most from positive psychology approaches?
2 How can I let my client know about these approaches, I have so little time already!
3 How can I implement more health promotion in my clinic?

References

Afshin, A., Forouzanfar, M. H., Reitsma, M. B., Sur, P., Estep, K., Lee, A., Marczak, L., Mokdad, A. H., Moradi-Lakeh, M., Naghavi, M., Salama, J. S., Vos, T., Abate, K. H., Abbafati, C., Ahmed, M. B., Al-Aly, Z., Alkerwi, A., Al-Raddadi, R., Amare, A. T.,... & Murray, C. J. L. (2017). Health effects of overweight and obesity in 195 countries over 25 years. *The New England Journal of Medicine*, 377(1), 13–27. https://doi.org/10.1056/NEJMoa1614362
Brown, L., Ospina, J. P., Celano, C. M., & Huffman, J. C. (2019). The effects of positive psychological interventions on medical patients' anxiety: A meta-analysis. *Psychosomatic Medicine*, 81(7), 595–602. https://doi.org/10.1097/psy.0000000000000722
Carr, A., Cullen, K., Keeney, C., Canning, C., Mooney, O., Chinseallaigh, E., & O'Dowd, A. (2021). Effectiveness of positive psychology interventions: A systematic review and meta-analysis. *The Journal of Positive Psychology*, 16(6), 749–769. https://doi.org/10.1080/17439760.2020.1818807
Carrière, K., Khoury, B., Günak, M. M., & Knäuper, B. (2018). Mindfulness-based interventions for weight loss: A systematic review and meta-analysis. *Obesity Reviews*, 19(2), 164–177. https://doi.org/10.1111/obr.12623

Chaves, C., Lopez-Gomez, I., Hervas, G., & Vazquez, C. (2017). A comparative study on the efficacy of a positive psychology intervention and a cognitive behavioral therapy for clinical depression. *Cognitive Therapy and Research*, 41(3), 417–433. https://doi. org/10.1007/s10608-016-9778-9

Donald, J. N., Bradshaw, E. L., Ryan, R. M., Basarkod, G., Ciarrochi, J., Duineveld, J. J., Guo, J., & Sahdra, B. K. (2020). Mindfulness and its association with varied types of motivation: A systematic review and meta-analysis using self-determination theory. *Personality and Social Psychology Bulletin*, 46(7), 1121–1138. https://doi. org/10.1177/0146167219896136

Eriksson, M., & Lindström, B. (2008). A salutogenic interpretation of the Ottawa Charter. *Health Promotion International*, 23(2), 190–199. https://doi.org/10.1093/ heapro/dan014

Fredrickson, B. L. (2004). The broaden–and–build theory of positive emotions. Philosophical transactions of the Royal Society of London. *Series B: Biological Sciences*, 359(1449), 1367–1377.

Furchtlehner, L. M., Schuster, R., & Laireiter, A.-R. (2020). A comparative study of the efficacy of group positive psychotherapy and group cognitive behavioral therapy in the treatment of depressive disorders: A randomized controlled trial. *The Journal of Positive Psychology*, 15(6), 832–845. https://doi.org/10.1080/17439760.2019. 1663250

Galea, S., & Maani, N. (2020). The cost of preventable disease in the USA. *The Lancet Public Health*, 5(10), e513–e514. https://doi.org/10.1016/S2468-2667(20)30204-8

Garland, E. L., Fredrickson, B., Kring, A. M., Johnson, D. P., Meyer, P. S., & Penn, D. L. (2010). Upward spirals of positive emotions counter downward spirals of negativity: Insights from the broaden-and-build theory and affective neuroscience on the treatment of emotion dysfunctions and deficits in psychopathology. *Clinical Psychology Review*, 30(7), 849–864. https://doi.org/10.1016/j.cpr.2010.03.002

Goldberg, S. B., Tucker, R. P., Greene, P. A., Davidson, R. J., Wampold, B. E., Kearney, D. J., & Simpson, T. L. (2018). Mindfulness-based interventions for psychiatric disorders: A systematic review and meta-analysis. *Clinical Psychology Review*, 59, 52–60.

Gudmundsdóttir, S. L., Ballarini, T., Ámundadóttir, M. L., Mészáros, J., Eysteinsdóttir, J. H., Thorleifsdóttir, R. H., Hrafnkelsdóttir, S. K., Bragadóttir, H. B., Oddsson, S., & Silverberg, J. I. (2022). Clinical efficacy of a digital intervention for patients with atopic dermatitis: A prospective single-center study. *Dermatology and Therapy*, 12(11), 2601–2611. https://doi.org/10.1007/s13555-022-00821-y

Gudmundsson, G. H., Mészáros, J., Björnsdóttir, Á. E., Ámundadóttir, M. L., Thorvardardottir, G. E., Magnusdottir, E., Helgadottir, H., & Oddsson, S. (2022). Evaluating the feasibility of a digital therapeutic program for patients with cancer during active treatment: Pre-post interventional study. *JMIR Formative Research*, 6(10), e39764. https://doi.org/10.2196/39764

Hansen, N. H., Juul, L., Pallesen, K. J., & Fjorback, L. O. (2021). Effect of a compassion cultivation training program for caregivers of people with mental illness in Denmark: A randomized clinical trial. *JAMA Network Open*, 4(3), e211020. https://doi. org/10.1001/jamanetworkopen.2021.1020

Huffman, J. C., Feig, E. H., Millstein, R. A., Freedman, M., Healy, B. C., Chung, W. J., Amonoo, H. L., Malloy, L., Slawsby, E., Januzzi, J. L., & Celano, C. M. (2019). Usefulness of a positive psychology-motivational interviewing intervention to promote positive affect and physical activity after an acute coronary syndrome. *The American Journal of Cardiology*, 123(12), 1906–1914. https://doi.org/10.1016/j. amjcard.2019.03.023

Huppert, F. A. (2009). Psychological well-being: Evidence regarding its causes and consequences†. *Applied Psychology: Health and Well-Being*, 1(2), 137–164. https://doi. org/10.1111/j.1758-0854.2009.01008.x

Jøssang, I. H., Aamland, A., & Hjörleifsson, S. (2022). Discovering strengths in patients with medically unexplained symptoms–a focus group study with general practitioners. *Scandinavian Journal of Primary Health Care, 40*(3), 405–413. https://doi.org/10 .1080/02813432.2022.2139345.

Khoury, B., Lecomte, T., Fortin, G., Masse, M., Therien, P., Bouchard, V., Chapleau, M.-A., Paquin, K., & Hofmann, S. G. (2013). Mindfulness-based therapy: A comprehensive meta-analysis. *Clinical Psychology Review,* 33(6), 763–771.

Kuyken, W., Byford, S., Taylor, R. S., Watkins, E., Holden, E., White, K., Barrett, B., Byng, R., Evans, A., Mullan, E., & Teasdale, J. D. (2008). Mindfulness-based cognitive therapy to prevent relapse in recurrent depression. *Journal of Consulting and Clinical Psychology,* 76(6), 966–978. https://doi.org/10.1037/a0013786

Levine, G. N., Cohen, B. E., Commodore-Mensah, Y., Fleury, J., Huffman, J. C., Khalid, U., Labarthe, D. R., Lavretsky, H., Michos, E. D., Spatz, E. S., & Kubzansky, L. D. (2021). Psychological health, well-being, and the mind-heart-body connection: A scientific statement from the American Heart Association. *Circulation,* 143(10), e763-e783. https://doi.org/10.1161/CIR.0000000000000947

Levine, G. N., Lange, R. A., Bairey-Merz, C. N., Davidson, R. J., Jamerson, K., Mehta, P. K., Michos, E. D., Norris, K., Ray, I. B., & Saban, K. L. (2017). Meditation and cardiovascular risk reduction: A scientific statement from the American Heart Association. *Journal of the American Heart Association,* 6(10), e002218. https://www. ahajournals.org/doi/pdf/10.1161/JAHA.117.002218?download=true

Loucks, E. B., Schuman-Olivier, Z., Britton, W. B., Fresco, D. M., Desbordes, G., Brewer, J. A., & Fulwiler, C. (2015). Mindfulness and cardiovascular disease risk: State of the evidence, plausible mechanisms, and theoretical framework. *Current Cardiology Reports,* 17(12), 112. https://doi.org/10.1007/s11886-015-0668-7

Magnúsdóttir, I., Lovik, A., Unnarsdóttir, A. B., McCartney, D., Ask, H., Kõiv, K., Christoffersen, L. A. N., Johnson, S. U., Hauksdóttir, A., & Fawns-Ritchie, C. (2022). Acute COVID-19 severity and mental health morbidity trajectories in patient populations of six nations: An observational study. *The Lancet Public Health,* 7(5), e406-e416.

Millstein, R. A., Celano, C. M., Beale, E. E., Beach, S. R., Suarez, L., Belcher, A. M., Januzzi, J. L., & Huffman, J. C. (2016). The effects of optimism and gratitude on adherence, functioning and mental health following an acute coronary syndrome. *General Hospital Psychiatry,* 43, 17–22. https://doi.org/10.1016/j. genhosppsych.2016.08.006

Mohammadi, N., Aghayousefi, A., Nikrahan, G. R., Adams, C. N., Alipour, A., Sadeghi, M., Roohafza, H., Celano, C. M., & Huffman, J. C. (2018). A randomized trial of an optimism training intervention in patients with heart disease. *General Hospital Psychiatry,* 51, 46–53.

Nelson, S. K., & Lyubomirsky, S. (2014). *Finding happiness: Tailoring positive activities for optimal well-being benefits.* The Guilford Press.

O'Donnell, M. P. (1989). Definition of health promotion: Part III: Expanding the definition. *American Journal of Health Promotion,* 3(3), 5. https://doi. org/10.4278/0890-1171-3.3.5

OECD. (2022). Health expenditure and financing - preventive care share of GDP. https://stats.oecd.org/Index.aspx?DataSetCode=SHA

Rashid, T. (2015). Positive psychotherapy: A strength-based approach. *The Journal of Positive Psychology,* 10(1), 25–40. https://doi.org/10.1080/17439760.2014.920411

Schuman-Olivier, Z., Trombka, M., Lovas, D. A., Brewer, J. A., Vago, D. R., Gawande, R., Dunne, J. P., Lazar, S. W., Loucks, E. B., & Fulwiler, C. (2020). Mindfulness and behavior change. *Harvard Review of Psychiatry,* 28(6), 371–394. https://doi. org/10.1097/hrp.0000000000000277

Spinelli, C., Wisener, M., & Khoury, B. (2019). Mindfulness training for healthcare professionals and trainees: A meta-analysis of randomized controlled trials. *Journal of Psychosomatic Research,* 120, 29–38.

Thimmapuram, J., Yommer, D., Tudor, L., Bell, T., Dumitrescu, C., & Davis, R. (2020). Heartfulness meditation improves sleep in chronic insomnia. *Journal of Community Hospital Internal Medicine Perspectives*, 10(1), 10–15. https://doi.org/10.1080/20009666.2019.1710948

van Agteren, J., Iasiello, M., Lo, L., Bartholomaeus, J., Kopsaftis, Z., Carey, M., & Kyrios, M. (2021). A systematic review and meta-analysis of psychological interventions to improve mental wellbeing. *Nature Human Behaviour*, 5(5), 631–652. https://doi.org/10.1038/s41562-021-01093-w

World Health, O. (2001). The World health report: 2001: Mental health: New understanding, new hope. In. Geneva: World Health Organization.

World Health Organization. Regional Office for, E. (1986). Ottawa Charter for Health Promotion, 1986. Copenhagen: World Health Organization. Regional Office for Europe Retrieved from https://apps.who.int/iris/handle/10665/349652

14

POSITIVE HEALTH COACHING

Adopting a dialogical approach to health and wellbeing

Christian van Nieuwerburgh and Jim Knight

Interest in the use of coaching to support health and wellbeing has surged in recent years with the National Health Service in England promoting "health and wellbeing coaches" (https://www.england.nhs.uk/personalisedcare/workforce-and-training/health-and-wellbeing-coaches/) and the US setting up a National Board for Health and Wellness Coaching (https://nbhwc.org) that offers certification for health coaches. Coaching is well suited to supporting people to make behavioural changes to enhance their health and wellbeing. A large-scale meta-analysis on the effectiveness of executive, leadership and business coaching (Grover & Furnham, 2016) found links between coaching interventions and increases in wellbeing, alongside more commonly expected outcomes such as goal attainment and career satisfaction. Research specifically into the use of coaching in health settings suggests that the intervention is well suited to support people to make behavioural changes to enhance their health and wellbeing (e.g. Meng, Jiang, Yu, Song, Zhou, Xu, & Zhou, 2023; Olsen & Nesbitt, 2010). A systemic review of 12 randomized control trials of health coaching including 2,497 participants concluded that coaching improves the management of chronic diseases (Kivelä, Elo, Kyngäs, & Kääriäinen, 2014). It is further argued that it may be a cost effective intervention, reducing health service expenditure (Jonk, Lawson, O'Connor, Riise, Eisenberg, Dowd, & Kreitzer, 2015). Currently, there is growing global interest in the use of coaching in the health sector according to the Forbes Business Council (2022). In this chapter, we will be considering a change theory and current strategies before presenting "Positive Health Coaching", a new approach and framework for use in health contexts. This new approach will be presented in detail with a visual representation and an explanation of its four key components: the partnership principles; coaching skills; conversational framework and strategic knowledge.

DOI: 10.4324/9781003378426-17   220

Strategies for bringing about change

Essentially, health coaching is increasingly being seen as an effective methodology for bringing about desired behavioural change. The impact cycle (Knight, 2018) is considered as a universal framework for change. Originally designed and validated for use with educators, the cycle involves three deceptively simple stages: Identify, Learn, Improve (Figure 14.1).

Identify: During the identify stage, coaches partner with clients to identify (a) a clear picture of their current reality, (b) a motivational goal, and (c) a strategy the client will implement in an attempt to achieve their goal. Simply put, during the identify stage, clients determine where they are, where they want to go, and how they will get there.

Motivational goals have several characteristics, which we have organized around the acronym PEER. PEER goals are Powerful (they will have a lasting, significant impact on the client's health and wellbeing), Effective (the strategies are appropriate to the client's context and environment), Emotionally Compelling (clients are committed to achieving the goal), and Reachable (clients can identify pathways to their achievable goals).

Learn: During the learn stage, coaches partner with clients so that the clients are prepared to implement strategies that will enable them to meet their PEER goals. This can happen in at least two ways. Sometimes clients know the strategy they want to use to reach their goal and the coach partners with them to help them prepare themselves to implement the goal. Other times the client needs support identifying the most effective strategies, so the coach draws on their expertise to share several possible strategies the client might use to achieve their goals. In both cases, the client makes the decisions about what they will do to make progress.

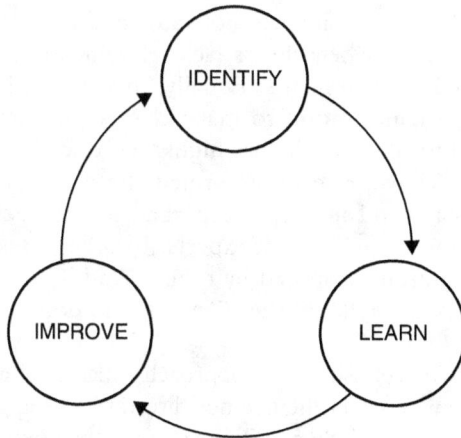

Figure 14.1 The impact cycle.[1]

Improve: During the improve stage, coaches partner with clients to make necessary adaptations to the chosen strategy so that the goal can be achieved. This can involve (a) changing how the strategy is being implemented, (b) changing the strategy, (c) reviewing the goal, or (d) changing how progress is measured.

Current context: approaches to coaching

In most situations, when people seek out coaching to support them with their health and wellbeing, there are two broad avenues available. Facilitative coaching provides clients with safe spaces to set self-identified goals, gain a better understanding of their situation and develop their own ideas for ways forward. This can be very effective when clients are well-informed, self-disciplined and highly motivated. Clients are invited to set health-related goals for themselves, and their coaches support them by asking questions, listening, summarizing and providing ongoing conversations to ensure that progress is being made. Facilitative coaches do not offer expertise or advice. Rather, they rely entirely on the resourcefulness and knowledge of their clients. The other avenue usually involves seeking support from experts in health, wellbeing or lifestyle choices. This type of coaching is more akin to sports coaching where the coach provides encouragement and expert advice. The coach's role is to motivate and instruct their clients based on their expertise. For example, a physiotherapist will provide detailed instructions about exercises that should be undertaken. The client benefits from the expertise of the coach and aims to implement recommended strategies.

Both approaches are popular and have been effective in bringing about improvements in health and wellbeing. However, they do not work for everyone and may not be the optimal intervention in many cases. The facilitative stance works for clients who are self-motivated and knowledgeable. Such an approach is not effective when clients lack relevant information about how to make the desired improvements. Equally, this approach will not work if clients lack energy or motivation to make changes. Directive interventions can be very helpful for people who are highly self-disciplined and committed to implementing effective, research-informed strategies. However, although people may understand and appreciate expert advice, many struggle while trying to implement the suggestions of experts. In other cases, people may not be motivated by solutions proposed by others. And if it feels like the expert is being judgemental or "telling" the client what to do, it can even engender resistance.

In this chapter, we propose a third approach—dialogical coaching. This approach is neither completely facilitative nor directive. The approach is based on dialogue between coach and client. The dialogical approach has been used effectively in educational settings for two decades (Knight, 2022), complementing other effective methodologies such as facilitative coaching and mentoring. This approach will be explained fully below.

A new approach: positive health coaching

Positive Health Coaching (PHC) is a form of positive psychology coaching (PPC) that adopts the dialogical approach. PPC has been defined as a "managed conversational process that supports people to achieve meaningful goals in a way that enhances their wellbeing (van Nieuwerburgh & Biswas-Diener, 2021, p. 315)". PPC is an intervention that integrates positive psychology theories (e.g. wellbeing, strengths, positive emotions, hope) with existing coaching psychology practices. PPC promotes the idea that wellbeing should be given equal weighting to goal attainment in conversations about growth and development. In a systemic literature review of PPC, Zyl et al. (2020) identified the principles of the practice. PPC

- is for relatively well-adjusted individuals
- focuses on strengths, rather than weaknesses
- takes a balanced view of strengths and areas of development
- takes a holistic approach towards development in all aspects of a client's life
- assumes that clients have an inherent capacity to grow and develop
- aims to empower the client to take ownership of their development
- works towards the client's personal vision of their ideal future self
- is facilitative, and the role of the coach is to listen supportively and empower the client

With its parallel focus on wellbeing and the achievement of goals, PPC is well-suited for use with clients who wish to improve their health and wellbeing. A number of studies suggest that clients can benefit from PPC (Fouracres & van Nieuwerburgh, 2020; Lucey & van Nieuwerburgh, 2021; Moin & van Nieuwerburgh, 2021; van Nieuwerburgh et al., 2021). Notably, study participants in all these studies reported both performance and wellbeing benefits. However, PPC is primarily a facilitative conversational intervention. In PHC, the practitioner does share information but is not directive. We propose that PHC is an intervention designed to support health and wellbeing through facilitative and dialogical approaches.

The dialogical approach

The dialogical approach to coaching lies somewhere between facilitative and directive conversational interventions (van Nieuwerburgh, Knight, & Campbell, 2019). Often, coaching is perceived to be a facilitative process, while mentoring, advising and telling are more directive ways of supporting people. When coaches take a dialogical approach to coaching, they balance asking with telling. In schools, for example, when setting goals, dialogical coaches invite teachers to describe what they would like to change and how they would like to do it. A coach might ask a teacher, for example, "You've probably thought a lot about this, what are you thinking you might do?" Then, after the teacher has shared strategies she is considering, the coach would share additional high-impact strategies that might be appropriate. The coach would then ask, "Which of these strategies gives you the most confidence?" Dialogical coaches do not "take sides," as Miller and Rollnick write (2013) by trying to talk the teacher into a particular plan. Rather, they act in ways that ensure that the client is always the person making the decisions.

The four components of positive health coaching

PHC is a form of PPC that adopts facilitative and dialogical approaches. There are four components of effective PHC. The first component is a set of partnership principles (Knight, 2011). These partnership principles underpin the type of mutually respectful, empowering relationships that are essential for PHC. The second component is having highly developed conversational skills. PHC, like all forms of coaching, is essentially an empowering conversation. Practitioners therefore need to be skilled in key conversational skills. The third component is a robust conversational framework based on the Impact Cycle (Identify-Learn-Improve) discussed earlier in this chapter. PHC is a managed conversation, so practitioners need to be familiar with a conversational framework to make best use of the time with their clients. The fourth component, which is essential for the dialogical aspect of PHC, is the ability to share strategic knowledge with confidence and clarity.

Component one: the partnership principles

Dialogical coaches interact with their clients in ways that recognize their clients' autonomy and humanity. This way of being has been articulated in a set of seven principles known as the partnership principles (Knight, 2011). These principles synthesize ideas from a wide variety of fields. In particular, the principles draw on Paulo Freire's advocacy for dialogical, mutually humanizing learning in education (1970), Peter Block's ideas about sharing knowledge in business contexts (1993), Riane Eisler's analysis of partnership and dominator social structure in communities and relationships (1987), and R. J. Bernstein's description of the role dialogue plays in overcoming incommensurability between different paradigms in scientific knowledge (1983).

The partnership principles are validated by research. In one study (Knight, 1999), participants in workshops grounded in the partnership principles reported significantly higher engagement, enjoyment, learning, and expectation to implement than those in more traditional, directive workshops. Principles provide a way for people to name and organize their behaviour, and in this case, they describe a way of being, or how coaches might act in their relationships with others. Principles help people to identify how they should act when they do what they do. The seven partnership principles, described below, provide the foundation for life-giving, mutually humanizing coaching conversations.

Equality. People want to get the status they think they deserve. Consequently, when coaches intentionally or unintentionally communicate that they think they are one-up on clients, many clients resist (Schein, 2009). People who adopt the principle of equality believe that every individual has equal dignity and value and therefore no person is more valuable than any other. When people believe in equality, they listen to others and let them speak without interruption. Importantly, they refrain from judging others moralistically.

Choice. Most people do not like to be controlled or told what to do. When people adopt the principle of choice, they recognize that autonomy is a necessary component of motivation (Deci & Ryan, 1985). Coaches who work from the principle of choice create conditions so that their clients evaluate options and choose their own plan of action.

Voice. People want to be heard, to feel like their opinions matter. Coaches who act in alignment with the principle of voice act in ways that show that they believe others' opinions matter. They ask good questions, listen effectively, and their non-verbal communication shows that they are interested in and care about what others say.

Dialogue. Dialogue is a back-and-forth conversation where all parties in a conversation share what they think, listen effectively, approaching each other with the courage to be shaped by new ideas and options. Dialogue can create thinking partnerships—dyadic learning experiences that occur between people.

Reflection. Reflection can occur when people (a) look back at past action, (b) look at their current actions, or (c) look ahead to future actions. Coaches who work from the principle of reflection encourage clients to do their own thinking by withholding advice during coaching. They ask more than they share, and they use questions to invite others to think deeper, not to try to move their clients toward a predetermined direction they have chosen for their clients.

Praxis. Praxis is the belief that real learning occurs in real life. Coaches working from this principle realize that their role involves translating research and evidence-based practice into actionable knowledge, and they partner with clients to make it as easy as possible for them to learn and apply new ideas. Then, after clients learn new strategies, they work in partnership with their clients to adapt that new knowledge so that it allows their clients to make progress.

Reciprocity. Reciprocity is the belief that learning is symbiotic, not one-directional. Coaches who work from the principle of reciprocity go into conversations expecting to learn from their clients, no matter how inexperienced their clients might be. When coaches believe in reciprocity, they see every client as a learning partner.

Component two: conversational skills

PHC is an impactful intervention because it is an empowering, respectful conversation. So it is essential for the practitioner to have highly developed conversational skills. Coaches should be good at noticing, listening, asking powerful questions and reflecting back (van Nieuwerburgh, 2020). Each of these skills is necessary for effective PHC conversations.

Listening and noticing are foundational skills in the sense that they lay the groundwork for meaningful, respectful conversations. They are practical ways that coaches can demonstrate the partnership principles. In fact, the experience of "being listened to" should be one of the consistent outcomes of any PHC conversation.

From a coaching perspective, it is helpful for practitioners to become skilled at listening actively and be aware of the various purposes of listening. The idea of "active listening" is that the coach should demonstrate that they are listening to their clients. This involves giving visual signals (nodding, tilting one's head, smiling, eye contact), making encouraging sounds ('uh huh', 'yes', 'mmm') and avoiding any distractions. By listening in this way, the practitioner can make it clear that their clients are important to them. In other words, coaches should offer their undivided attention during the conversation as a sign of respect for the other person.

Coaches will benefit from being aware of a number of different purposes of listening. Practitioners can listen to understand; listen to show empathy; listen to value; and listen to empower. In most everyday situations, people listen to understand. In this mode, one person stops talking in order to make sense of what has been said by the other person. The main purpose is to understand whatever has been said in order to respond. Practitioners can also listen in an empathetic way. By not interrupting or sharing their own experience, a practitioner can demonstrate empathy by listening compassionately as their clients talk about challenges or difficulties. It is also possible to listen in order to appreciate the other person. In this case, the primary focus is to listen for what is impressive, laudable or special about the person. In this way, the practitioner can show that they value the other person simply by listening. Finally, practitioners can listen to empower their clients. This is through fully attentive, appreciative listening and the use of silences. By listening respectfully, and not jumping in with suggestions, advice or recommendations, the coach gives time and space for the client to make their own decisions, thus building their self-esteem and self-confidence.

It is worth noting that a person cannot listen if they are talking. We advocate that practitioners should talk less in interactions with their clients. In a coaching conversation, the aim is to ensure that the coach is doing most of the listening, which means that the client should be doing most of the talking. By encouraging clients to do most of the talking, coaches are also supporting their clients to take more ownership and responsibility. In this way, the very act of listening is a way of not only valuing others, but empowering them too.

Putting it into practice

Speaking less and listening more are laudable aims for coaches. They speak less so that their clients speak more. They listen more so that their clients feel valued and respected. How can practitioners check how well they are doing in this regard? We recommend video-recording interactions that you have with your clients (of course after gaining their explicit agreement to be video recorded). Watch the video when you have a quiet moment. For the first time, watch it with the audio off. Look at the body language. Notice who is doing most of the talking. Then watch it again with the audio on. Who seems to be "in charge"? Who is making the decisions? How are you demonstrating that you are listening? Make some notes, recognize your successes and identify anything that you might work on for future conversations.

The other foundational skill is noticing. Health and wellbeing practitioners are likely to be very good at this already. In a coaching context, the practitioner should be noticing any information that is likely to be helpful for the client, the practitioner or the relationship between the client and the practitioner. Coaches can notice the body language of their clients, the words that they use or what seems to motivate them. Coaches might even notice what their clients do *not* say, what they might be avoiding or what may be causing anxiety. By noticing what may be going on for their clients, coaches are able to ask better questions, decide which avenues to pursue, guage levels of engagement, assess a client's readiness for change, and determine whether to challenge their clients or not. Coaches can also usefully notice what is happening for themselves. Are they feeling tired themselves? Do they feel frustrated as they are listening to their clients? What is their intuition telling them? Being aware of their own experiences, coaches will be better able to determine if this information relates to their client or to themselves. For example, if the coach feels a sense of frustration—is that to do with the client, or is it something personal? If it is to do with the client, then it can be brought into the conversation: "I'm picking up a sense of frustration as we talk about this—do you feel it too?". If it is not related to the client, this could be something for the coach to take to a colleague or a reflective practice session. Finally, coaches can also notice the quality of the relationship between themselves and their clients. What is the dynamic between the coach and the client? Is the client being more passive, leading the coach to take more control of the conversation? Is there a good level of trust between the coach and the client? To what extent does the relationship allow both parties to discuss topics freely? Being aware of the quality of the relationship is critically important as this influences the likelihood of positive ouctomes for the client (De Haan & Gannon, 2017).

Ready to notice

Noticing is a key skill of coaching. Take a moment to think about when you are at your best at noticing. It is likely to be when you are feeling relaxed or settled—not when you are stressed or anxious. What can you do to make sure that you are in the right state of mind to coach others? Jot down a few ideas and see if you can start implementing them in the coming weeks.

In addition to the foundational skills of listening and noticing, coaches should be good at asking questions and reflecting back. The questions that coaches ask have a significant impact on the conversation. Coaches should be adept at using a combination of closed and open questions to support their clients to commit to desired changes. Closed questions should only be asked for the purpose of clarification. For example, "so you work five days a week from your home office?", "have you tried this before?" or "do you feel confident that you will be able to make this change?" are helpful closed questions that can clarify the situation for the client or the coach. However, closed questions do not elicit much talk from the client. In general, open questions are preferable in coaching conversations. They require higher levels of engagement and thought from clients. For example, "what is your attitude to your own wellbeing?", "what is most important to you about your health?", or "how do you imagine your future if you make these changes?" are all powerful questions that are likely to elicit thoughtful answers from clients. Remember, the role of the coach is to create the ideal environment for clients to do their best thinking. Open questions often require clients to do new thinking.

Asking open questions

Most of us have been conditioned to ask closed questions on the basis that they are 'easier' to answer. "Did you have a good day?" is easier to respond to than "How was your day?" or "What was the best part of your day?". But you can see that the first question only requires a one-word answer, whereas the other two require further reflection. Start noticing your preferences in everyday conversations. Experiment with asking more open questions and see what happens!

There are two types of questions that should be avoided by coaches: leading questions and multiple questions. Leading questions are those that suggest a desired response. They are called "leading" because they lead the client in a particular direction. For example, "have you thought about walking to work rather than taking your car?" is a leading question. It suggests that walking to work may be preferable to driving. Another example is "what would happen if you started jogging every morning in the summer months?" This is simply a piece of advice disguised as a question. If the coach has specialist information that would be helpful to the client, then this should be shared explicitly at an appropriate moment in the conversation, rather than in an ambiguous way. The sharing of such information will be discussed later in the chapter.

Multiple questions are also to be avoided. This refers to a number of questions being asked consecutively without giving the client an opportunity to answer. This can cause confusion and runs counter to the aim of creating a reflective space for the client. Here is an example of multiple questions: "So what is most important to you about this? Is it more to do with your own motivation? Or are you interested in just doing something as quickly as possible?" This can often happen when the coach thinks of a follow-up question as they are talking. Multiple questions can lead to the client feeling rushed, and should be avoided. It is good practice to stop at the end of any question that has been asked, allowing the client to respond—even if the coach has thought of a "better" question. If it is still relevant, the follow-up question can be asked after the client has responded to the first one.

Reflecting back is an important and often underrated skill of coaches. This refers to the act of playing back to the client what they have said. This can be done through paraphrasing and summarizing. Clients often benefit from hearing back what have been talking about. Hearing it from someone else can often put things into perspective. Paraphrasing requires the coach to simply play back what the client has just said. For example, if the client says "sometimes I find it hard to motivate myself to get out of bed early on the weekends", the coach might respond "so, getting out of bed early can sometimes be a challenge for you, especially on weekends?". Some coaches might even repeat the words back almost verbatim: "it's hard to motivate yourself to get out of bed early on weekends". In both cases, the client has an opportunity to hear what they have just said. Importantly, this is another way in which coaches can demonstrate that they have been listening attentively to the client. Such paraphrasing supports the creation of a reflective space, and will allow the client to elaborate on the point, or to continue from there. Coaches can also summarise what clients have been saying. In this case, they would be providing a shortened version of what the client has just said. For example, if the client has spoken for about five minutes on all the reasons that they want to make a change to their work routine, the coach can say, "so it sounds like there are numerous reasons for changing your routine". Coaches should be cautious with summarizing, as it does involve making judgements about what was important in what was said. However, it again demonstrates that the coach has been listening intently, and can be a good way of capturing key points in the conversation.

This section has presented a brief description of some of the key skills of coaching. It is recommended that people wishing to become positive health coaches undertake skills training to develop and hone the conversational skills necessary to undertake coaching conversations.

Dimension three: the conversational framework

Every coaching session is essentially a conversation about change. We shared the Impact Cycle at the start of this chapter: Identify—Learn—Improve. There are numerous change theories that are relevant for positive health coaches. Essentially, most theories of change (e.g. Prochaska, Norcross and DiClemente's Transtheoretical Model (1994); Boyatzis's Intentional Change Theory (2006)) start with an identification of a desired outcome, move into reflection and then onto experimentation. The most popular coaching model, GROW, is designed to facilitate conversations that lead to change (Whitmore, 1992). The acronym sets out a conversational process that starts with Goal (G), then moves into an exploration of Reality (R). Once both the goal and current reality have been discussed, the conversation moves onto an exploration of Options (O), usually generated by the client. The final stage is a commitment from the client about what they Will (W) do before the next coaching conversation. The conversational framework of PHC builds on GROW and is an adaptation of the Coaching for Alignment model (van Nieuwerburgh & Allaho, 2018). It has been re-designed for use in health contexts. See Figure 14.2.

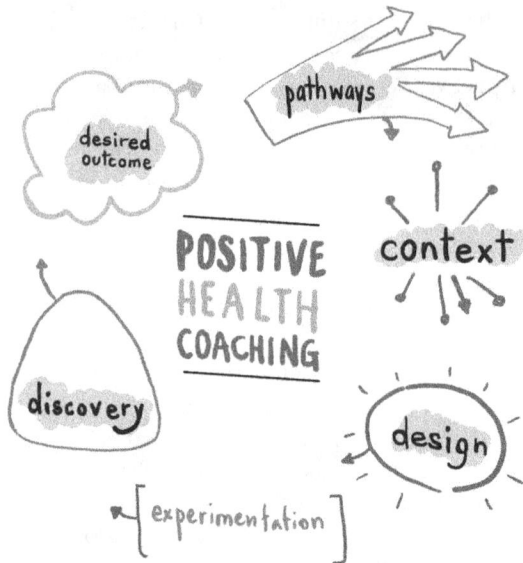

Figure 14.2 The Positive Health Coaching framework.

PHC conversations are expected to last about 30 minutes. Each conversation would cover the five phases below.

Discovery: The start of the conversation focuses on the practitioner and the client gaining a better understanding of the client's context and their attitude to health and wellbeing. In the very first conversation, this is the Discovery phase. In following conversations, this would be called the Evaluation phase, and the practitioner and the client would evaluate progress in between coaching conversations.

Desired outcome: After gaining some insight about the client's current situation and attitude, the practitioner should gain clarity about what the client seeks. Specifically, the client is asked to explain their desired outcome in relation to their health and wellbeing. In following sessions, after an evaluation of progress, the client would have an opportunity to decide whether they have achieved their desired outcome or whether further work is needed. If it has been achieved, this should be celebrated and the client can identify whether to wrap up the coaching relationship or identify a further positive step forward.

Pathways: Once the desired outcome is clear, it becomes possible for the practitioner and the client to work together to develop pathways (or possible ways forward). Both the practitioner and the client can generate pathways. The practitioner should present any pathways with clarity so that they can be easily implemented. Once a number of pathways have been identified, the client chooses one to pursue.

Context: This is a brief opportunity to check alignment and reflect on the client's context. First, does this pathway align with the positive intention that was discussed earlier? Second, how will the chosen pathway fit with the client's context? If there is good alignment, the conversation moves to the last phase. If not, another pathway that is more appropriate in the client's context might be chosen.

Design: In this final phase, the client should design the experiments that they will undertake before the next coaching conversation. The new pathway will need to be put into action. How will this be implemented? The practitioner would wrap up the conversation by checking the client's commitment to the selected experiment.

Time needs to be allowed for the client to experiment with the new behaviour or practice. Normally, there would be a gap of weeks or a couple of months before the next coaching conversation. Once the client has experimented with the new pathway, the practitioner and client meet for another coaching conversation. This time, the conversation starts with an Evaluation of the success of the pathway.

Dimension four: sharing strategic knowledge

When positive health coaches explain strategies to clients, they balance telling with asking. To accomplish this, they ensure that their explanations are precise and provisional. Of course, some personal health strategies may be so simple that detailed explanations are not needed. For example, a client who adopts Michael Pollan's diet suggestions (2019)—"eat real food, not too much, mostly plants"—likely doesn't need a checklist to understand what do to.

Other strategies, however, are more complicated. To ensure that clients use practices in ways that will have the most impact, dialogical coaches describe strategies very precisely, often using checklists to enhance their explanations (Gawande, 2009). For this reason, many coaches create information sheets with clear, simple and comprehensive checklists that they can use to describe the strategies they share with clients. To create checklists, coaches need to deeply understand, synthesize and simplify the strategies they share.

Checklists help coaches remember key components of a strategy and they keep coaches from skipping over important information that they might overlook as they run through explanations. Additionally, checklists help coaches overcome the common cognitive bias known as the curse of knowledge, the struggle many experience when explaining something they know extremely well because they forget what it is like to not know what they are explaining (Heath and Heath, 2007, p. 20).

Precise explanations are important because they increase the likelihood that clients will implement a strategy effectively. At the same time, when coaches share checklists, they should not assume that every strategy will be used in the same way by everyone. As Eric Liu has written, "teaching [or explanation] is not one-size-fits-all; it's one-size-fits-one" (2006, p. 47). During the "context" phase of the conversational framework, strategies need to be adapted so that they are most helpful for each individual in their unique setting. Additionally, since people lose motivation when they are told what to do (Deci & Ryan, 1985), dialogic coaches explain strategies provisionally—as they describe strategies, the also communicate that clients should feel free to adapt, reject, or accept any aspect of a strategy they plan to implement. Simply put, the client always decides how they will implement a strategy.

To allow for adaptation and client choices, coaches need to be provisional as well as precise. What this looks like if coaches are using checklists, for example, is that they run through the steps of the checklist, and then stop after each item and ask the client if they would like to do that aspect as it is, skip it, or change it. In the event that a client wants to adopt a strategy in ways that the coach thinks are unhealthy or dangerous, the coach is not being helpful if they do not speak up. At the same time, if a coach tells the client what to do, ironically they may decrease the likelihood that a client will adopt a strategy because most people resist being told what to do (Miller & Rollnick, 2013). Positive health coaches can offer strategies and ideas based on their expertise, perhaps by introducing their thoughts by asking, "Do you mind if I share something?" Then they can share their thoughts while also communicating that clients must choose whether or not they will integrate these ideas into their plans. Of course, the coach is simply recognizing the reality that a client will do what they choose regardless of what the coach says.

Outline of a PHC Conversation

After a brief introductory chat, the practitioner should set out the parameters of the conversation. In this part of the conversation, the practitioner explains the respective roles of the practitioner and the client, and sets out the boundaries of confidentiality.

Below, we have presented some sample questions for each of the phases. These give an indication of the types of topics that can be discussed and are not intended as a list of questions to pose to clients.

It is helpful to keep in mind that these conversations should take about 30 minutes, so it is helpful to think that there are roughly five to six minutes for each phase. The first phase of the conversation is the Discovery phase.

- In relation to your health and wellbeing, how are things going for you?
- What is working particularly well?

- What is your personal attitude to your own wellbeing?
- What would you like to talk about today?

The second phase is to identify the Desired Outcome.

- What is it that you are hoping to achieve?
- Specifically, how would you define your desired outcome?
- How will you know that you have achieved this?

The third phase is called Pathways and the purpose is to generate some ideas about ways forward.

- What have you already tried?
- What information do you need from me?
- Would you like me to share some effective strategies?
- Which of the pathways we have identified sounds most promising to you?

The fourth phase requires an exploration of the client's Context to assess the likelihood of success of the chosen pathway.

- When you think about your personal and professional contexts, what are the chances of success?
- What obstacles or challenges do you need to be aware of?
- Who can support you to ensure that you are successful?

The final phase is called Design. This is where the client designs, with the support of the practitioner, some experiments to see if the pathways will move them forward.

- How will you put this pathway into action?
- What experiments can you try over the next few weeks?
- How will you know if the pathway is successful?
- How committed are you to invest time and effort into this pathway?

Conclusion

While the indications are encouraging, the practice of PHC is still in its infancy. It builds on existing health coaching practice and draws together theories and research-informed practices from coaching, positive psychology and health psychology. PHC is essentially an intervention designed to support people to set health and wellbeing-related goals and then work towards them. At its heart are a conversational framework and coaching skills, but success of this intervention may lie in the way of being of the coach, demonstrated through the application of the partnership principles we have shared in this chapter. The intention of PHC is to treat clients with respect, empowering them and encouraging them to take more responsibility for their own health and wellbeing.

A shift in thinking may be required in situations where clients come to health professionals expecting to be given answers. The model of health practitioners prescribing medicines and behaviours is deeply engrained in many of our health systems. In this chapter, we advocate for new ways of interacting. We are not advocating a wholesale change in approach. However, we propose that adding a dialogical intervention will be helpful in certain circumstances. Ultimately, we hope that PHC will be widely adopted a respectful, effective and sustainable way of supporting people to take greater responsibility for their own health and wellbeing.

Takeaways

- Investing time listening to your clients is a powerful way of showing that you value their opinions
- Dialogical coaches take a facilitative stance but share information with their clients when it is helpful
- PHC is a respectful, empowering way of supporting clients to take responsibility for their own health and wellbeing

Wicked questions

1 How can you demonstrate that you respect the autonomy of your clients and patients?
2 How can you be at your best so that you can support others most effectively?
3 What is your own attitude to your own health and wellbeing—and how does that attitude influence your conversations with others?

Note

1 From Knight, 2018; used with permission.

References

Bernstein, R. J. (1983). *Beyond objectivism and relativism: Science, hermeneutics, and praxis.* Philadelphia: University of Pennsylvania Press.
Block, P. (1993). *Stewardship: Choosing service over self-interest.* San Francisco, CA: Berrett-Koehler.
Boyatzis, R. (2006). An overview of intentional change from a complexity perspective. *Journal of Management Development* 25: 607–623. 10.1108/02621710610678445

Deci, E. L., & Ryan, R. M. (1985). *Intrinsic motivation and self-determination in human behavior.* New York, NY: Plenum.

de Haan, E., & Gannon, J. (2017). The coaching relationship. In T. Bachkirova, G. Spence, & D. Drake (Eds.), *The SAGE handbook of coaching* (pp. 195–217). London: Sage.

Eisler, R. (1987). *The chalice and the blade: Our history, our future.* New York, NY: Harper & Row.

Forbes Business Council (2022). https://www.forbes.com/sites/forbesbusinesscouncil/2022/05/13/how-to-run-in-the-bullish-market-for-health-coaching/?sh=4459c5ae794d (accessed 12 June 2023).

Fouracres, A., & van Nieuwerburgh, C. (2020). The lived experience of self-identifying character strengths through coaching: An interpretative phenomenological analysis. *International Journal of Evidence Based Coaching and Mentoring*, 18(1): 43–56. https://doi.org/10.24384/e0jp-9m61

Freire, P. (1970). *Pedagogy of the oppressed.* New York, NY: Seabury Press.

Gawande, A. (2009). *The checklist manifesto: How to get things right.* New York, NY: Metropolitan Books.

Grover, S. & Furnham, A. (2016). Coaching as a developmental intervention in organisations: A systemic review of its effectiveness and the mechanisms underlying it. *Public Library of Science*, 11(7): 1–41.

Heath, C. & Heath, D. (2007). Made to stick: Why some ideas survive and others die. New York: Random House.

Jonk, Y., Lawson, K., O'Connor, H., Riise, K. S., Eisenberg, D., Dowd, B., & Kreitzer, M. J. (2015). How effective is health coaching in reducing health services expenditures? *Medical Care*, 53(2): 133–140. https://www.jstor.org/stable/26417909

Kivelä, K., Elo, S., Kyngäs, H., & Kääriäinen, M. (2014). The effects of health coaching on adult patients with chronic diseases: A systematic review. *Patient Education and Counseling*, 97(2): 147–157. https://doi.org/10.1016/j.pec.2014.07.026

Knight, J. (1999). *Partnership learning: Putting conversation at the heart of professional development.* Paper presented at the annual meeting of the American Educational Research Association, San Diego, California.

Knight, J. (2011). *Unmistakable impact: A partnership approach for dramatically improving instruction.* Thousand Oaks, CA: Corwin.

Knight, J. (2018). *The impact cycle: What instructional coaches should do to foster powerful improvements in teaching.* Thousand Oaks, CA: Corwin.

Knight, J. (2022). *The definitive guide to Instructional Coaching: Seven factors for success.* Alexandria, VA: ASCD.

Liu, E. (2006). Guiding lights: How to mentor—And find life's purpose. New York, NY: Ballantine.

Lucey, C. & van Nieuwerburgh, C. (2021). 'More willing to carry on in the face of adversity': How beginner teachers facing challenging circumstances experience positive psychology coaching. An interpretative phenomenological analysis. *Coaching: An International Journal of Theory, Research and Practice*, 14:1,62–77, https://doi.org/10.1080/17521882.2020.1753791

Meng, F., Jiang, Y., Yu, P., Song, Y., Zhou, L., Xu, Y., Zhou, Y. (2023). Effect of health coaching on blood pressure control and behavioral modification among patients with hypertension: A systematic review and meta-analysis of randomized controlled trials. *International Journal of Nursing Studies*, 138: 104406. https://doi.org/10.1016/j.ijnurstu.2022.104406

Miller, W. R., & Rollnick, S. (2013). *Motivational interviewing: Preparing people for change* (3rd ed.). New York, NY: Guildford Press.

Moin, F., & van Nieuwerburgh, C. (2021). 'The experience of positive psychology coaching following unconscious bias training: An interpretative phenomenological analysis'.

International Journal of Evidence Based Coaching and Mentoring, 19(1), pp. 74–89. https://doi.org/10.24384/n4hw-vz57

National Board for Health and Wellness Coaching (2023). https://nbhwc.org (accessed 12 June 2023).

National Health Service in England (2023). https://www.england.nhs.uk/personalisedcare/workforce-and-training/health-and-wellbeing-coaches/ (accessed 12 June 2023).

Olsen, J., & Nesbitt, B. (2010). Health coaching to improve healthy lifestyle behaviors: An integrative review. *American Journal of Health Promotion*, 25(1): e1–e12. https://doi.org/10.4278/ajhp.090313-LIT-101

Pollan, M. (2019). *Food rules: An Eater's manual*. New York, NY: Penguin.

Prochaska, J. O., Norcross, J. C., & DiClemente, C. C. (1994). *Changing for good*. New York, NY: Morrow.

Schein, 2009. *Helping: How to offer, receive and give help*. San Francisco, CA: Berrett-Koehler.

van Nieuwerburgh, C. (2020). *An introduction to coaching skills: A practical guide* (3rd ed.). London: Sage.

van Nieuwerburgh, C., & Allaho, R. (2018). *Coaching in Islamic culture: The principles and practice of Ershad*. London: Routledge.

van Nieuwerburgh, C., Barr, M., Fouracres, A., Moin, T., Brown, C., Holden, C., Lucey, C., & Thomas, P. (2021). Experience of positive psychology coaching while working from home during the COVID-19 pandemic: An interpretative phenomenological analysis. *Coaching: An International Journal of Theory, Research and Practice*, 15(2): 148–165. https://doi.org/10.1080/17521882.2021.1897637

van Nieuwerburgh, C., & Biswas-Diener, R. (2021). Positive psychology approach. In J. Passmore (Ed.), *The coaches' handbook: The complete practitioner guide for professional coaches* (pp. 314–321). London: Routledge.

van Nieuwerburgh, C., Knight, J., Campbell, J. (2019). 'Coaching in education'. In *Professional coaching: Principles and practice* (pp. 411–426). New York: Springer.

van Zyl, L. E., Roll, L. C., Stander, M. W., & Richter, S. (2020). Positive psychological coaching definitions and models: A systematic literature review. *Frontiers in Psychology*, 11, 793. https://doi.org/10.3389/fpsyg.2020.00793

Whitmore, J. (1992). *Coaching for Performance*. London: Brealey.

15

PERSON–NATURE FIT

Fostering well-being through nature

Annalisa Setti and Tadhg Mac Intyre

Theoretical background: people, nature and well-being

Models of nature-individual relationship for positive mental (and physical) health outcomes

In this chapter, we focus on the psychological and cognitive processes we use to interact with our environment, assuming that the physical environment itself is liveable, e.g. we do not specifically consider the effects of polluted air and water.

Definition of nature

In accordance with Frumkin et al. (2017), we define nature as an area containing plants and animals, the area can be of different size and with different levels of human intervention (e.g. an urban park and a forest) and characterized by physical features (e.g. mountains, blue spaces). We refer to 'green environment' in a comprehensive and inclusive way, considering that they may include blue features such as rivers, seaside and lakes.

Nature benefits

While we, as humans, are enjoying the advantages of a highly urbanized society, we are becoming more disconnected with nature (Beery et al., 2023). Nature exposure offers a multiplicity of positive health outcomes, ultimately reducing mortality. A recent study on 31 European countries utilized the normalized difference vegetation index and compared it with the WHO recommendations for access to green spaces (0.5 hectares accessible within 300 m of distance from one's residence) showed that meeting those could save almost 43,000 lives annually (Barboza et al., 2021). Research shows that those who are close to nature, both physically and psychologically, have positive physical and mental health outcomes, including reduced stress, anxiety, rumination, better cognitive function, and cardiovascular health (Jimenez et al., 2021). A study with 20,000 participants and over one million individual responses, showed that people report to be happier in natural environments (MacKerron & Mourato, 2013); another study with 19,806 people showed that those who had 120 min a week of nature contact reported better health and well-being than those less exposed to nature (White et al., 2019). The systematic review of nature benefits for psychological and cognitive health is beyond the scope of this chapter, we refer to different recent articles presenting more comprehensive accounts: general nature benefits (Jimenez et al., 2021), green space quality (Nguyen et al., 2021), effect of nature on attention and cognitive benefits of nature (Ohly et al., 2016; Stevenson et al., 2018); outdoor nature (Kondo et al., 2018); physical exercise in nature (Lahart et al., 2019), and lifespan perspective (Douglas et al., 2017).

Neurophysiological pathways

A classic study (Lederbogen et al., 2011) demonstrated that those living in highly populated cities (100,000+ inhabitants) showed more activation in the amygdala, i.e. the brain area related to processing of emotional stimuli, in response to social stress. On the other hand, walking in nature for 1 hour reduces activity in the amygdala, in a task where socially relevant stimuli are presented (Sudimac et al., 2022), although the effect is more reliable in women (Sudimac & Kühn, 2022). Walking in nature for 90 minutes is also associated with reduced activation in the subgenual Prefrontal Cortex (Bratman et al., 2015), a region involved in negative self-referential thought and depression, and with reduced self-reported rumination. Therefore, nature can potentially help us regulate immediate response to stressful situations, as well as reducing the aftermaths of these events such as self-referential negative thinking or what others refer to as perseverative cognition (Broschott et al., 2019). Several studies have recorded human brain activity while walking in environments with different levels of natural features showing that attentional engagement decreases when moving to green space (Aspinall et al., 2015; Neale et al., 2020). In urban settings, a dose-response effect of density of trees and self-reported stress recovery was found at behavioural level (Jiang et al., 2014). Green density related to activation of the ventral posterior cingulate cortex (Chang et al., 2021), a brain region in the limbic system also part of the Default Mode Network, conveying the effect of green environment on stress responses. Collectively, these results show nature has a role in emotions and emotion regulation both when the individual is performing a task and when they are at rest. This conclusion is supported by two recent systematic literature reviews (Bolouki, 2023; Norwood et al., 2019) on brain activity and natural versus urban environment, both concluding that natural environments are associated with higher frontal alpha band, i.e. lower stress and relaxation, less frontal activation, likely linked to lower cognitive demands and lower stress, while urban settings are associated with limbic system activation.

Conceptualizations/models of human-environment interaction

We identify five key elements of the human-environment interaction (Figure 15.1): the individual, with their access to nature (and urban environments), and their relationship with nature; the type of engagement, e.g. functional or via active participation; the type of exposure and dosage, including the quality of nature and biodiversity; the psychophysiological benefits derived from such interaction, as well as the co-benefits for the environment and the additional benefits such as increased pro-environmental behaviour; and the long term impact such as reduced healthcare burden, increased climate action and biodiversity. Our model adopts a strength-based approach, where the environment is an asset for individuals flourishing across the lifespan, provided that the individual and the environment fit each other and co-develop harmoniously. Therefore, we propose that, when applications are designed, they should consider the best person–environment fit.

This model builds on existing conceptualizations focusing on different aspects.

a Scale of the interaction. Cassarino and Setti (2016) focusing on ageing, highlighted the importance of assessing and recording benefits at different scales and their relationships. The micro scale includes perceptual information to be processed (e.g. colour, clutter), the meso scale includes the structural features of the environment and how interpretable they are for the individual (e.g. legibility, topology), the macro scale includes the type of environment (e.g. presence of nature, population density); these interact with the demographic

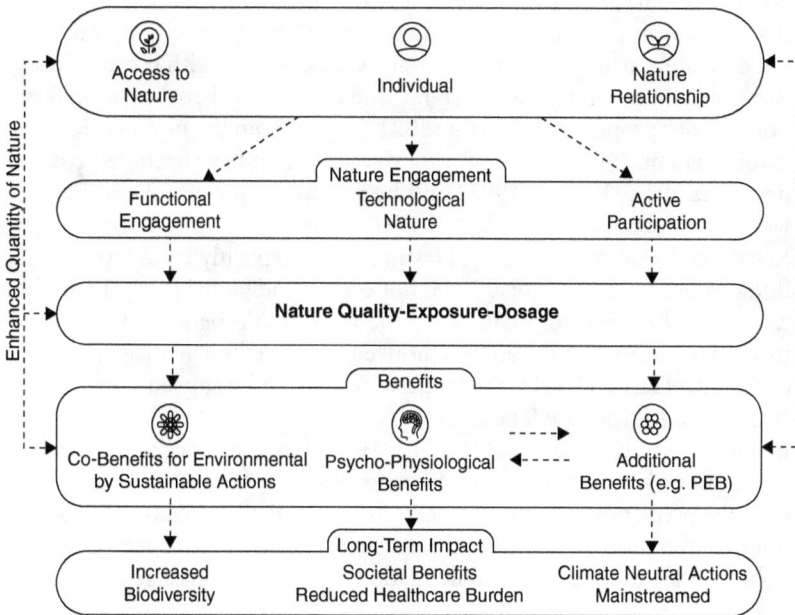

Figure 15.1 Five level model of human–nature interaction.

characteristics (e.g. socio-economic status, environment of origin), and individual response to the environment (e.g. attentional load required by the environment; perceived restorative properties; perceived usability, e.g. opportunities for social engagement) to determine behavioural outcomes (e.g. the person goes out for a nature walk frequently or not) and psychological outcomes (e.g. well-being derived from the nature walk). The person–environment fit is therefore determined by the cognitive load (or the restorative properties) of the environment (Lavie, 1995), the qualities of the environment which trigger different affective responses (Kaplan, 1995) and the affordances (e.g. perceived usability and safety) (Gibson, 1986). The importance of scale of exposure was also highlighted by Frumkin et al. (2017), who adapted a human–nature interaction model originally proposed by Shanahan et al. (2015). The spatial and temporal dimensions of nature exposure should be jointly considered when mapping nature exposure and related benefits, for example one could live in a neighbourhood rich in vegetation and therefore be exposed on an ongoing basis, while exposure to wilderness could be occasional and of shorter duration.

b Dose of exposure. Similarly to Shanahan et al. (2015) and Frumkin et al. (2017), Sumner et al. (2021) highlighted the different 'dosages' of nature exposure: 'being' in nature, where the exposure could be passive, e.g. viewing nature scenes, and of short duration, even just few minutes; 'doing' where the exposure is more prolonged as the individuals does something either with nature, e.g. gardening, or in nature, e.g. green exercise; and 'living' when the individual has prolonged exposure to nature. While more work is needed on how dissociable are these dimensions, Cox et al. (2018), for example, showed that longer durations of visits to nature were associated with lower prevalence of depression, while frequency of visits was associated with social cohesion.

c Relational dimension (with other individuals). The revised Attention Restoration Theory proposed by Hartig (2021), stems from the now classic idea that nature benefits humans by restoring resources that have been depleted (Hartig et al., 2014; Kaplan, 1995) and by replenishing psychological resources when the individual is stressed (Ulrich et al., 1991). In this framework, called Relational Restoration Theory, Hartig (2021) explicitly considers that depletion can occur at a relational level, not only at individual level, therefore one can expect benefits from nature for the relationship between individuals. In turn, social relationships can be a motive to undertake activities in nature. According to Hartig (2021), the framework can also be applied to communities (Collective Restoration Theory).

d Ecosystem services. Bratman et al. (2019) adopted an ecosystem services approach in which they define four steps to guide the understanding, and potentially the prediction, of nature benefits including the characterization of natural features, the dose of exposure, the quality of nature experience, their interactions, and the expected benefits evaluation for the individual and the ecosystem.

In our model we include elements of these previous conceptualizations, and we frame them in a multidimensional health view, where ultimately we aim to provide a pathway to foster individual well-being and health, as well as environmental and societal benefits.

First, we propose to consider the individual, with their different demographic characteristics, place of residence and mobility, co-determining the access to nature (see Barboza et al., 2021). People also differ in their relationship with nature or nature connectedness, the feeling of being part of nature. Those with higher nature connectedness, measured by different self-reported measures (e.g. Mayer & Frantz, 2004; Nisbet & Zelenski, 2013; Richardson et al., 2019) report higher levels of eudemonic well-being, in particular self-growth, as shown by a recent meta-analysis (Pritchard et al., 2020), as well as hedonic well-being (Capaldi et al., 2014). A relationship with nature can be built through different pathways (Lumber et al., 2017): positive emotions, i.e. emotions evoked by nature; contact, i.e. sensory experiences and activities like bird watching; beauty, i.e. appreciating nature aesthetic qualities; compassion, i.e. stewardship and conservation behaviours, and meaning, i.e. meaning making around nature and use of nature-related metaphors. While researchers debate what precisely nature connectedness (Murphy, MacCarthy & Petersen, 2022) emerging evidence for targeting the pathways as way to improve nature connectedness and increase well-being is accumulating (Pocock et al., 2023).

Second, we consider levels of engagement with nature. Engagement with nature can occur through our sensory modalities (e.g. multisensory or just through vision), and for different purposes (e.g. to go somewhere or to purposefully interact with nature). The vast literature on green exercise shows the benefits of activities in nature (e.g. Donnelly & MacIntyre, 2019). When exposed to nature, the more multisensory is the experience, the more memorable they are for the individual, to influence future behaviour (Thelen et al., 2014). In an Embodied Cognition perspective, mental imagery, visual and kinesthetic, could support memories of the interactions with nature and positive reinforcement for nature experiences, which constitute important ways to gain benefit from nature (Egner et al., 2020). Franco et al. (2017) reviewed the evidence for the effect of different sensory experiences on the individual (see also Myers, 2020) showing that smell, taste and touch, in addition to the more studied vision, contribute to the positive effects of nature. Nature interaction through technology also represents an interesting option for those who may be unable to access real nature due to illness or restrictions, e.g. the Covid-19 pandemic, or it could be used as a way to motivate people to experience nature, or to experience different varieties of natural environments. Based on recent conceptual accounts, digital and virtual nature are not hypothesised as being as effective as real nature interactions in terms of well-being and health benefits, possibly due to the diminished multisensory experience (Litleskare et al., 2020).

The third dimension in our model is related to the scale and dosage of the exposure, as well as the quality of the environment. Benefits on well-being have been found for 5 minutes of exposure (Barton & Pretty, 2010); for 30 minutes (Shanahan et al., 2016) during a week, and recently for spending at least 2 hours in nature a week (White et al., 2019). Experimental work utilizing digital or other virtual nature stimuli has recorded benefits on affect (e.g. O'Meara et al., 2020) and cognition (e.g. Berto, 2005, see also Neilson et al., 2021 [reads (e.g.

Berto, 2005, see also Neilson et al., 2021)]) after few minutes. Epidemiological life-course studies showed that living near nature, therefore conceivably providing consistent exposure, confers long-term benefits (Cherrie et al., 2018; Li et al., 2021). The question remains open on the durability of the effects and the best dose to obtain such benefits. As highlighted by Shanahan et al. (2016), Frumkin et al. (2017), and Sumner et al. (2021), the frequency, length and quality of the exposure are important factors, as well as the multisensory or immersive nature of the experience. Although these models propose a nature-as-medicine framework useful for potential applications, we would like to stress the importance of nature connectedness and emotions in human–nature interactions (Martin et al., 2020).

In the fourth dimension of our model, aligned to the ecosystem services perspective (Bratman et al., 2019) nature is not only of instrumental value for people, i.e. it fosters their well-being and health, but it has a relational value, whereby the individual gains fulfilment from taking care of nature (stewardship eudemonic) and perceiving such stewardship as aligned with own values (stewardship principle/virtue) (Chan et al., 2016). Indeed, nature contact and connectedness are associated with pro-environmental behaviour (Martin et al., 2020; Tzankova et al., 2023). In a recent study across seven countries, Capstick et al. (2022) showed that pro-environmental behaviour is also associated with well-being. Therefore, we propose to consider individual benefits, co-benefits for the environment and additional benefits, which include societal benefit, such as reduction of healthcare cost (Van Den Eeden et al., 2022) and social cohesion (Oh et al., 2022).

Individual differences in responding to the environment: Sensory Processing Sensitivity

Berman et al. (2021) refer to an unexplored area potentially influencing the association between well-being and natural environment: individual differences in environmental sensitivity. This difference has been conceptualized in various ways: as Differential Susceptibility (Belsky, 1997), i.e. adaptive behaviour in evolutionary perspectives based on genetic differences (Seratonin promoter gene 5-HTTLPR); as Biological Sensitivity to Context (Boyce & Ellis, 2005), emphasizing stress reactivity; as Sensory Processing Sensitivity (Aron & Aron, 1997) describing a phenotype of low sensory thresholds, enhanced responsivity, empathy, depth of processing leading to advantages or disadvantages depending on the environment the individual is in and their childhood experience. Pluess has recently integrated these approaches in a meta-framework called Environmental Sensitivity (Pluess, 2015). According to Pluess, genetic dispositions can interact with environment in a neutral, adverse, or supportive way, generating either vulnerability to poor mental and physical health, e.g. cardiovascular issues, or vantage sensitivity, e.g. flourishing in positive environments. Nature constitutes a potentially favourable environment supporting emotion regulation. Setti et al. (2022) showed that higher scores in the Highly Sensitive Person Scale are predictive of higher connectedness with nature (e.g. I often feel a sense of oneness with the natural world around me) and with animals (It is morally wrong to hunt wild animals just for sport.). The association between higher levels of sensory processing sensitivity and nature connectedness was replicated in a different study with over 800 participants, where it was found that awe is the mechanism mediating this association (Dunne et al., in press). Those who are highly sensitive have high aesthetic sensitivity and experience awe, which, in turn, supports their connectedness with the natural environment. Interestingly, in Dunne et al. (under review), high sensitivity was also predictive of higher self-reported pro-environmental behaviour, with nature connectedness as one of the mediating factors. Level of sensitivity was also a moderator of the effect of watching nature vs urban videos on positive affect in a pre-post experimental study (Cadogan et al., 2023). Those who are highly sensitive are more prone to lower subjective well-being and higher levels of perceived stress (Benham, 2006), nature could be a way for higher sensitive individuals for coping and buffer against poor well-being (Black & Kern, 2020). Nature connectedness moderated the negative association between high sensitivity and flourishing, in a study with over 900 participants (Carroll et al., submitted). This initial evidence supports that natural environments could be particularly beneficial for those who are highly sensitive.

Applications

There are multiple sectorial applications of models conceptualizing the nature–human interactions for the purpose of supporting well-being. Here we will briefly point to some of these applications (Table 15.1).

Table 15.1 Synthesis of human–nature interactions model and related examples of recommendations for applied settings

Model component	Applied recommendations (examples)
Individual, access and connectedness. There are general benefits to nature exposure, however, people differ in their: • Level of connectedness with nature (including past experiences, access to episodic memories); • Disposition to respond to positive or negative features of the environment (Environmental Sensitivity theory); • Bodily skills, demographic characteristics and cultural approaches; • Interactions with the natural environment as it presents different affordances or opportunities for engagement.	Whenever possible consider individual characteristics; for example a coach may consider whether the individual expressed connectedness with nature, and whether they indicate being sensory sensitive before introducing eco-coaching or walking coaching to obtain the best person-environment fit (which can dynamically change); a general practitioner may consider recommending an older person to join a walking group in the park, keeping in mind accessibility issues and demographic composition of the group. A teacher could consider activities that promote nature connectedness keeping in mind that pupils will have different preferred pathways to nature.

(Continued)

Table 15.1 (Continued)

Model component	Applied recommendations (examples)
Nature engagement: functional engagement, active participation, virtual nature. • Physical exercise is one of the main ways individuals engage with nature, however the actual level of engagement (e.g. 'being' or 'doing') can vary; • Active participation consists of activities involving nature contact, such as gardening, or conservation activities; mindful participation should be fostered; • When there are limited opportunities for direct engagement with nature, virtual nature offers the opportunity of access, with different levels of immersiveness and multisensory experience.	Different levels of engagement can be promoted depending on the context. For example, a business could promote active breaks in nature and promote biophilic design in the workplace; mental health practitioners could promote active engagement with nature, either real or virtual depending on the context. Health promotion officers could leverage nature benefits to promote physical activity in salutogenic places.
Nature quality, exposure, dosage. • Living near nature is a health determinant; • Benefits from nature interactions are obtained with different durations, intensities and frequencies; 120 minutes of green exposure has demonstrated benefits; • Short (few minutes) mindful exposure to nature can provide a boost to mood (and attention); • Multisensory and embodied exposure enhances the experience of nature and may help consolidate memories of nature for future recall or savoring;	A consistent exposure to nature should be encouraged, particularly the habits of engaging with nearby nature wherever available, keeping in mind the quality of the environment, which may change (e.g. peak of air pollution). Multisensory experience, where different senses are stimulated, and different actions are involved, should be fostered to provide rich experiences, memories and positive conditioning. Even a short bout of nature exposure could be helpful to improve mood and (to some extent) cognitive capacities. For example, coaches could consider a coaching session near nature if the topics to be addressed are particularly emotionally arousing; teachers could foster the use of the senses in interacting with nature.
Benefits: Psycho-physiological benefits, co-benefits (e.g. biodiversity, nature conservation), additional benefits (e.g. pro-environmental behaviour). • Appreciation of co-benefits between human health and the state of the planet is an important aspect to foster individual healthy lifestyles and climate mitigation;	Co-benefits are, for example, obtained by active transport, which increases physical activity and reduces carbon emissions; eating local or home-grown organic food, which protects the individual and the environment from chemicals. Numerous re-greening and active transport initiatives have been promoted in cities, these should be

(Continued)

Table 15.1 (Continued)

Model component	Applied recommendations (examples)
• Connectedness with nature and experiencing nature benefits are (potentially bidirectionally) associated with pro-environmental and sustainable behaviours;	grounded in the previous layers of the model and raise awareness on co-benefits. In turn, sustainable action can promote well-being by contributing to others lives.
Long-term impact: increased biodiversity, societal benefits including reduced healthcare burden, climate neutral action mainstreamed.	Communities could foster local biodiversity via grassroots movements, citizen science initiatives and education. Nature prescribing could be used as preventative strategy to promote well-being and combat depression and obesity. Teachers could promote the use of nature to foster social cohesion.
• Promoting biodiversity provides a rich environment from the ecological, aesthetic, and microbiome point of view;	
• Promoting nature exposure is associated with positive health outcomes supporting prevention of non-communicable disease;	
• Green spaces also promote positive social interactions.	

Takeaways

General

- Nature helps recovering from stress and depleted cognitive resources; it supports healthy lifestyles and fosters eudemonic and hedonic well-being;
- Studied neurophysiological benefits rest mainly on modulation of regulatory mechanisms between the Prefrontal Cortex and the Limbic system;
- Conceptualizations of nature-human interactions can help researchers and practitioners in understanding the specific determinants of such benefits and tailor interventions; different dimensions to consider are: the individual (or group) differences; type of engagement with nature; environmental quality, engagement and dosage of nature exposure; the scale of the analysis or intervention (micro-, meso- and macro-scale) the type of benefits;
- Environmental sensitivity differs in different individuals, endowing a substantial minority of the population with a particular sensitivity to positive and negative environments. Natural environments could foster flourishing in these individual, contributing to preventing mental illness, however, more evidence is needed.

Practical

- Any intervention of nature-based solutions should consider the individual as co-designer. Individuals and groups have different ways to interact with nature, they perceive the urban and natural environment in different ways and these aspects need to be considered from the outset.

- Modifying the environment to support human well-being has a series of consequences for the individual and the environment, which should be considered. One way is to start with the models presented here and adopt a systems thinking perspective.
- Our perception of the world is grounded in multisensory experiences and our body, to harness benefits of nature we need to consider the individual as a whole.

Wicked questions

- Do benefits at different levels of analysis relate to each other? Cassarino and Setti (2016) and Berman et al. (2021) highlight the necessity to establish whether and how benefits at different scales relate to each other. For example, at the micro-scale would faster/better processing of environmental scenes with a certain level of visual complexity, relate to perceived restorative potential by self-report, and how that relates to real-life behaviours such as accessing more natural vs urban environments? A notable exception is a study (Tost et al., 2019) where participants were followed for a week with Ambulatory Momentary Assessment, collecting data at different times per day on their mood and the presence of nearby green space. The same participants were then scanned with fMRI after the week, while performing an emotion processing task. Those participants who benefitted more of the presence of green during the week, also showed reduced activation in the Dorso-Lateral Prefrontal Cortex (i.e. brain area associated with self-regulation) in response to negative emotional stimuli in the task, indicating that individual reactivity to green exposure was modulating activation to negative social stimuli. This kind of approach, merging different paradigms and spatio-temporal scales, is a promising avenue to explore the impact of nature on well-being in real-life contexts, while maintaining the advantages of an experimental neuroimaging approach.
- What is the role of the quality of the natural environment? A gap in the literature exists between evidence supporting the role of nearby nature to promote health and reduce mortality and the quality of that environment. We suggest that a simple dose-response approach overlooks both the requirements for environmental quality (e.g. reduced noise and air pollution) and personal preferences for different typologies. We suggest that individuals experiencing eco-anxiety for example may not benefit from access to green space unless certain levels of biodiversity are present. Assessment of the quality of the environment using both quantitative measures and person-centred perception of quality is a next step for researchers.
- How can we ensure that benefits foster co-benefits and additional benefits? We distinguished between individual benefits, co-benefits (for the environment) and additional benefits (for society). Considering only benefits that we can derive from nature contact, while recognizing the importance of nature, means still adopting an anthropocentric perspective, where nature 'serves' the

individual. All of those who aim to harness the benefits of nature, e.g. medical professions, eco-coaches, teachers, businesses, need to be aware that those benefits should be considered an entry point to foster sustainability and adopt an ecosystem centric rather than an anthropocentric perspective.

References

Aron, E. N., & Aron, A. (1997). Sensory-processing sensitivity and its relation to introversion and emotionality. *Journal of Personality and Social Psychology*, 73(2), 345–368. https://doi.org/10.1037/0022-3514.73.2.345

Aspinall, P., Mavros, P., Coyne, R., & Roe, J. (2015). The urban brain: Analysing outdoor physical activity with mobile EEG. *British Journal of Sports Medicine*, 49(4), 272–276. https://doi.org/10.1136/bjsports-2012-091877

Barboza, E. P., Cirach, M., Khomenko, S., Iungman, T., Mueller, N., Barrera-Gómez, J., Rojas-Rueda, D., Kondo, M., & Nieuwenhuijsen, M. (2021). Green space and mortality in European cities: A health impact assessment study. *The Lancet Planetary Health*, 5(10), e718–e730. https://doi.org/10.1016/S2542-5196(21)00229-1

Barton, J., & Pretty, J. (2010). What is the best dose of nature and green exercise for improving mental health? A multi-study analysis. *Environmental Science & Technology*, 44. https://doi.org/10.1021/es903183r

Beery, T., Stahl Olafsson, A., Gentin, S., Maurer, M., Stålhammar, S., Albert, C., Bieling, C., Buijs, A., Fagerholm, N., Garcia-Martin, M., Plieninger, T., & Raymond, C. M. (2023). Disconnection from nature: Expanding our understanding of human–nature relations. *People and Nature*, 5(2), 470–488. https://doi.org/10.1002/pan3.10451

Belsky, J. (1997). Variation in susceptibility to environmental influence: An evolutionary argument. *Psychological Inquiry*, 8, 182–186. https://doi.org/10.1207/s15327965pli0803_3

Benham, G. (2006). The highly sensitive person: Stress and physical symptom reports. *Personality and Individual Differences*, 40(7), 1433–1440. https://doi.org/10.1016/j.paid.2005.11.021

Berman, M. G., Cardenas-Iniguez, C., & Meidenbauer, K. L. (2021). An environmental neuroscience perspective on the benefits of nature. In A. R. Schutte, J. C. Torquati, & J. R. Stevens (Eds.), *Nature and psychology: Biological, cognitive, developmental, and social pathways to well-being* (pp. 61–88). Springer International Publishing. https://doi.org/10.1007/978-3-030-69020-5_4

Berto, R. (2005). Exposure to restorative environments helps restore attentional capacity. *Journal of Environmental Psychology*, 25(3), 249–259. http://dx.doi.org/10.1016/j.jenvp.2005.07.001

Black, B. A., & Kern, M. L. (2020). A qualitative exploration of individual differences in wellbeing for highly sensitive individuals. *Palgrave Communications*, 6(1), 103. https://doi.org/10.1057/s41599-020-0482-8

Bolouki, A. (2023). Neurobiological effects of urban built and natural environment on mental health: Systematic review. *Reviews on Environmental Health*, 38(1), 169–179. https://doi.org/10.1515/reveh-2021-0137

Boyce, W. T., & Ellis, B. J. (2005). Biological sensitivity to context: I. An evolutionary-developmental theory of the origins and functions of stress reactivity. *Developmental and Psychopathology*, 17(2), 271–301. https://doi.org/10.1017/s0954579405050145

Bratman, G. N., Anderson, C. B., Berman, M. G., Cochran, B., de Vries, S., Flanders, J., Folke, C., Frumkin, H., Gross, J. J., Hartig, T., Kahn, P. H., Kuo, M., Lawler, J. J., Levin, P. S., Lindahl, T., Meyer-Lindenberg, A., Mitchell, R., Ouyang, Z., Roe, J., ... & Daily, G. C. (2019). Nature and mental health: An ecosystem service perspective. *Science Advances*, 5(7), eaax0903. https://doi.org/10.1126/sciadv.aax0903

Bratman, G. N., Hamilton, J. P., Hahn, K. S., Daily, G. C., & Gross, J. J. (2015). Nature experience reduces rumination and subgenual prefrontal cortex activation. *Proceedings of the National Academy of Sciences*, 112(28), 8567–8572. https://doi.org/10.1073/pnas.1510459112

Brosschot, J. F., Gerin, W., & Thayer, J. F. (2006). The perseverative cognition hypothesis: a review of worry, prolonged stress-related physiological activation, and health. *Journal of Psychosomatic Research*, 60(2), 113–124. https://doi.org/10.1016/j.jpsychores.2005.06.074

Cadogan, E., Lionetti, F., Murphy, M., & Setti, A. (2023). Watching a video of nature reduces negative affect and rumination, while positive affect is determined by the level of sensory processing sensitivity. *Journal of Environmental Psychology*, 102031. https://doi.org/https://doi.org/10.1016/j.jenvp.2023.102031

Capaldi, C. A., Dopko, R. L., & Zelenski, J. M. (2014). The relationship between nature connectedness and happiness: A meta-analysis [Original Research]. *Frontiers in Psychology*, 5(976). https://doi.org/10.3389/fpsyg.2014.00976

Capstick, S., Nash, N., Whitmarsh, L., Poortinga, W., Haggar, P., & Brügger, A. (2022). The connection between subjective wellbeing and pro-environmental behaviour: Individual and cross-national characteristics in a seven-country study. *Environmental Science & Policy*, 133, 63–73. https://doi.org/10.1016/j.envsci.2022.02.025

Carroll, S., O'Reilly, A., Lionetti, F., & Setti, A. (2023). Environmental sensitivity, nature and flourishing: A mixed method study.

Cassarino, M., & Setti, A. (2016). Complexity as key to designing cognitive-friendly environments for older people [review]. *Frontiers in Psychology*, 7. https://doi.org/10.3389/fpsyg.2016.01329

Chan, K. M. A., Balvanera, P., Benessaiah, K., Chapman, M., Díaz, S., Gómez-Baggethun, E., Gould, R., Hannahs, N., Jax, K., Klain, S., Luck, G. W., Martín-López, B., Muraca, B., Norton, B., Ott, K., Pascual, U., Satterfield, T., Tadaki, M., Taggart, J., & Turner, N. (2016). Why protect nature? Rethinking values and the environment. *Proceedings of the National Academy of Sciences*, 113(6), 1462–1465. https://doi.org/10.1073/pnas.1525002113

Chang, D. H. F., Jiang, B., Wong, N. H. L., Wong, J. J., Webster, C., & Lee, T. M. C. (2021). The human posterior cingulate and the stress-response benefits of viewing green urban landscapes. *NeuroImage*, 226, 117555. https://doi.org/10.1016/j.neuroimage.2020.117555

Cherrie, M. P. C., Shortt, N. K., Mitchell, R. J., Taylor, A. M., Redmond, P., Thompson, C. W., Starr, J. M., Deary, I. J., & Pearce, J. R. (2018). Green space and cognitive ageing: A retrospective life course analysis in the Lothian Birth Cohort 1936. *Social Science & Medicine*, 196, 56–65. https://doi.org/10.1016/j.socscimed.2017.10.038

Cox, D. T. C., Shanahan, D. F., Hudson, H. L., Fuller, R. A., & Gaston, K. J. (2018). The impact of urbanisation on nature dose and the implications for human health. *Landscape and Urban Planning*, 179, 72–80. https://doi.org/10.1016/j.landurbplan.2018.07.013

Donnelly, A. A., & MacIntyre, T. E. (2019). *Physical activity in natural settings*. Routledge. https://doi.org/10.4324/9781315180144

Douglas, O., Lennon, M., & Scott, M. (2017). Green space benefits for health and wellbeing: A life-course approach for urban planning, design and management. *Cities*, 66, 53–62. https://doi.org/10.1016/j.cities.2017.03.011

Dunne, H., Lionetti, F., Pluess, M., & Setti, A. (in press). Individual traits are associated with pro-environmental behaviour: Environmental sensitivity, nature connectedness and consideration for future consequences. *People and Nature*.

Egner, L. E., Sütterlin, S., & Calogiuri, G. (2020). Proposing a framework for the restorative effects of nature through conditioning: Conditioned restoration theory. *International Journal of Environmental Research and Public Health*, 17(18). https://doi.org/10.3390/ijerph17186792

Franco, L. S., Shanahan, D. F., & Fuller, R. A. (2017). A review of the benefits of nature experiences: More than meets the eye. *International Journal of Environmental Research and Public Health*, 14(8). https://doi.org/10.3390/ijerph14080864

Frumkin, H., Bratman, G. N., Breslow, S. J., Cochran, B., Kahn, P. H., Jr., Lawler, J. J., Levin, P. S., Tandon, P. S., Varanasi, U., Wolf, K. L., & Wood, S. A. (2017). Nature contact and human health: A research agenda. *Environ Health Perspect*, 125(7), 075001. https://doi.org/10.1289/ehp1663

Gibson, J. J. (1986). *The ecological approach to visual perception.* Psychology Press.

Hartig, T. (2021). Restoration in nature: Beyond the conventional narrative. In A. R. Schutte, J. C. Torquati, & J. R. Stevens (Eds.), *Nature and psychology: Biological, cognitive, developmental, and social pathways to well-being* (pp. 89–151). Springer International Publishing. https://doi.org/10.1007/978-3-030-69020-5_5

Hartig, T., Mitchell, R., de Vries, S., & Frumkin, H. (2014). Nature and health. *Annual Review of Public Health*, 35(1), 207–228. https://doi.org/10.1146/annurev-publhealth-032013-182443

Jiang, B., Li, D., Larsen, L., & Sullivan, W. C. (2014). A dose-response curve describing the relationship between urban tree cover density and self-reported stress recovery. *Environment and Behavior*, 48(4), 607–629. https://doi.org/10.1177/0013916514552321

Jimenez, M. P., DeVille, N. V., Elliott, E. G., Schiff, J. E., Wilt, G. E., Hart, J. E., & James, P. (2021). Associations between nature exposure and health: A review of the evidence. *International Journal of Environmental Research and Public Health*, 18(9). https://doi.org/10.3390/ijerph18094790

Kaplan, S. (1995). The restorative benefits of nature: Toward an integrative framework. *Journal of Environmental Psychology*, 15(3), 169–182. https://doi.org/10.1016/0272-4944(95)90001-2

Kondo, M. C., Jacoby, S. F., & South, E. C. (2018). Does spending time outdoors reduce stress? A review of real-time stress response to outdoor environments. *Health Place*, 51, 136–150. https://doi.org/10.1016/j.healthplace.2018.03.001

Lahart, I., Darcy, P., Gidlow, C., & Calogiuri, G. (2019). The effects of green exercise on physical and mental wellbeing: A systematic review. *International Journal of Environmental Research and Public Health*, 16(8), 1352. https://doi.org/10.3390/ijerph16081352

Lavie, N. (1995). Perceptual load as a necessary condition for selective attention. *Journal of Experimental Psychology: Human Perception and Performance*, 21(3), 451–468. https://doi.org/10.1037/0096-1523.21.3.451

Lederbogen, F., Kirsch, P., Haddad, L., Streit, F., Tost, H., Schuch, P., Wüst, S., Pruessner, J. C., Rietschel, M., Deuschle, M., & Meyer-Lindenberg, A. (2011). City living and urban upbringing affect neural social stress processing in humans. *Nature*, 474(7352), 498–501. https://doi.org/10.1038/nature10190

Li, D., Menotti, T., Ding, Y., & Wells, N. M. (2021). Life course nature exposure and mental health outcomes: A systematic review and future directions. *International Journal of Environmental Research and Public Health*, 18(10). https://doi.org/10.3390/ijerph18105146

Litleskare, S., MacIntyre, T. E., & Calogiuri, G. (2020). Enable, reconnect and augment: A new ERA of virtual nature research and application. *International Journal of Environmental Research and Public Health*, 17(5). https://doi.org/10.3390/ijerph17051738

Lumber, R., Richardson, M., & Sheffield, D. (2017). Beyond knowing nature: Contact, emotion, compassion, meaning, and beauty are pathways to nature connection. *PLoS ONE*, 12(5), e0177186. https://doi.org/10.1371/journal.pone.0177186

MacKerron, G., & Mourato, S. (2013). Happiness is greater in natural environments. *Global Environmental Change*, 23(5), 992–1000. https://doi.org/10.1016/j.gloenvcha.2013.03.010

Martin, L., White, M. P., Hunt, A., Richardson, M., Pahl, S., & Burt, J. (2020). Nature contact, nature connectedness and associations with health, wellbeing and pro-environmental behaviours. *Journal of Environmental Psychology*, 68, 101389. https://doi.org/10.1016/j.jenvp.2020.101389

Mayer, F. S., & Frantz, C. M. (2004). The connectedness to nature scale: A measure of individuals' feeling in community with nature. *Journal of Environmental Psychology*, 24(4), 503–515. https://doi.org/10.1016/j.jenvp.2004.10.001

Murphy, C., MacCarthy, D., Petersen, E. (2022). Emerging concepts exploring the role of nature for health and well-being. In *The Palgrave Encyclopedia of Urban and Regional Futures*. Cham: Palgrave Macmillan. https://doi.org/10.1007/978-3-030-51812-7_250-1

Myers, Z. (2020). Multisensory nature and mental health. In Z. Myers (Ed.), *Wildness and wellbeing: nature, neuroscience, and urban design* (pp. 71–110). Singapore: Springer. https://doi.org/10.1007/978-981-32-9923-8_3

Neale, C., Aspinall, P., Roe, J., Tilley, S., Mavros, P., Cinderby, S., Coyne, R., Thin, N., & Ward Thompson, C. (2020). The impact of walking in different urban environments on brain activity in older people. *Cities & Health*, 4(1), 94–106. https://doi.org/10.1080/23748834.2019.1619893

Neilson, B. N., Craig, C. M., Curiel, R. Y., & Klein, M. I. (2021). Restoring attentional resources with nature: A replication study of Berto's (2005) paradigm including commentary from Dr. Rita Berto. *Human Factors*, 63(6), 1046–1060. https://doi.org/10.1177/0018720820909287

Nguyen, P. Y., Astell-Burt, T., Rahimi-Ardabili, H., & Feng, X. (2021). Green space quality and health: A systematic review. *International Journal of Environmental Research and Public Health*, 18(21). https://doi.org/10.3390/ijerph182111028

Nisbet, E., & Zelenski, J. (2013). The NR-6: A new brief measure of nature relatedness [Original Research]. *Frontiers in Psychology*, 4. https://doi.org/10.3389/fpsyg.2013.00813

Norwood, M. F., Lakhani, A., Maujean, A., Zeeman, H., Creux, O., & Kendall, E. (2019). Brain activity, underlying mood and the environment: A systematic review. *Journal of Environmental Psychology*, 65, 101321. https://doi.org/10.1016/j.jenvp.2019.101321

O'Meara, A., Cassarino, M., Bolger, A., & Setti, A. (2020). Virtual reality nature exposure and test anxiety. *Multimodal Technologies and Interaction*, 4(4), 75. https://www.mdpi.com/2414-4088/4/4/75

Oh, R. R. Y., Zhang, Y., Nghiem, L. T. P., Chang, C.-c., Tan, C. L. Y., Quazi, S. A., Shanahan, D. F., Lin, B. B., Gaston, K. J., Fuller, R. A., & Carrasco, R. L. (2022). Connection to nature and time spent in gardens predicts social cohesion. *Urban Forestry & Urban Greening*, 74, 127655. https://doi.org/10.1016/j.ufug.2022.127655

Ohly, H., White, M. P., Wheeler, B. W., Bethel, A., Ukoumunne, O. C., Nikolaou, V., & Garside, R. (2016). Attention restoration theory: A systematic review of the attention restoration potential of exposure to natural environments. *Journal of Toxicology and Environmental Health, Part B*, 19(7), 305–343. https://doi.org/10.1080/10937404.2016.1196155

Pluess, M. (2015). Individual differences in environmental sensitivity. *Child Development Perspectives*, 9(3), 138–143. https://doi.org/10.1111/cdep.12120

Pocock, M. J. O., Hamlin, I., Christelow, J., Passmore, H.-A., & Richardson, M. (2023). The benefits of citizen science and nature-noticing activities for well-being, nature connectedness and pro-nature conservation behaviours. *People and Nature*, 5(2), 591–606. https://doi.org/10.1002/pan3.10432

Pritchard, A., Richardson, M., Sheffield, D., & McEwan, K. (2020). The relationship between nature connectedness and eudaimonic well-being: A meta-analysis. *Journal of Happiness Studies*, 21(3), 1145–1167. https://doi.org/10.1007/s10902-019-00118-6

Richardson, M., Hunt, A., Hinds, J., Bragg, R., Fido, D., Petronzi, D., Barbett, L., Clitherow, T., & White, M. (2019). A measure of nature connectedness for children and adults: Validation, performance, and insights. *Sustainability*, 11(12), 3250. https://www.mdpi.com/2071-1050/11/12/3250

Setti, A., Lionetti, F., Kagari, R., Motherway, L., & Pluess, M. (2022). The temperament trait of environmental sensitivity is associated with connectedness to nature and affinity to animals. *Heliyon*, 8(7). https://doi.org/10.1016/j.heliyon.2022.e09861

Shanahan, D. F., Bush, R., Gaston, K. J., Lin, B. B., Dean, J., Barber, E., & Fuller, R. A. (2016). Health benefits from nature experiences depend on dose. *Scientific Reports*, 6(1), 28551. https://doi.org/10.1038/srep28551

Shanahan, D. F., Lin, B. B., Bush, R., Gaston, K. J., Dean, J. H., Barber, E., & Fuller, R. A. (2015). Toward improved public health outcomes from urban nature. *American Journal of Public Health*, 105(3), 470–477. https://doi.org/10.2105/ajph.2014.302324

Stevenson, M. P., Schilhab, T., & Bentsen, P. (2018). Attention restoration theory II: A systematic review to clarify attention processes affected by exposure to natural environments. *Journal of Toxicology and Environmental Health. Part B, Critical Reviews*, 21(4), 227–268. https://doi.org/10.1080/10937404.2018.1505571

Sudimac, S., & Kühn, S. (2022). A one-hour walk in nature reduces amygdala activity in women, but not in men [Original Research]. *Frontiers in Psychology*, 13. https://doi.org/10.3389/fpsyg.2022.931905

Sudimac, S., Sale, V., & Kühn, S. (2022). How nature nurtures: Amygdala activity decreases as the result of a one-hour walk in nature. *Molecular Psychiatry*, 27(11), 4446–4452. https://doi.org/10.1038/s41380-022-01720-6

Sumner, R. C., Cassarino, M., Dockray, S., Setti, A., & Crone, D. M. (2021). Moving towards a multidimensional dynamic approach to nature and health: A bioavailability perspective. *People and Nature*, 4(1), 44–52. https://doi.org/10.1002/pan3.10266

Tzankova, I., O'Sullivan, C., Facciuto, A. I., Sacchetti, L., Fini, F., Cicognani, E., & Setti, A. (2023). Engagement with Nature and the Home Environment: Wellbeing and Proenvironmental Behavior among Irish and Italian University Students during the COVID-19 Emergency. *International Journal of Environmental Research and Public Health*, 20(14). https://doi.org/10.3390/ijerph20146432

Thelen, A., Matusz, P. J., & Murray, M. M. (2014). Multisensory context portends object memory. *Current Biology*, 24(16), R734–R735. https://doi.org/10.1016/j.cub.2014.06.040

Tost, H., Reichert, M., Braun, U., Reinhard, I., Peters, R., Lautenbach, S., Hoell, A., Schwarz, E., Ebner-Priemer, U., Zipf, A., & Meyer-Lindenberg, A. (2019). Neural correlates of individual differences in affective benefit of real-life urban green space exposure. *Nature Neuroscience*, 22(9), 1389–1393. https://doi.org/10.1038/s41593-019-0451-y

Ulrich, R. S., Simons, R. F., Losito, B. D., Fiorito, E., Miles, M. A., & Zelson, M. (1991). Stress recovery during exposure to natural and urban environments. *Journal of Environmental Psychology*, 11(3), 201–230. https://doi.org/10.1016/S0272-4944(05)80184-7

Van Den Eeden, S. K., Browning, M. H. E. M., Becker, D. A., Shan, J., Alexeeff, S. E., Thomas Ray, G., Quesenberry, C. P., & Kuo, M. (2022). Association between residential green cover and direct healthcare costs in Northern California: An individual level analysis of 5 million persons. *Environment International*, 163, 107174. https://doi.org/10.1016/j.envint.2022.107174

White, M. P., Alcock, I., Grellier, J., Wheeler, B. W., Hartig, T., Warber, S. L., Bone, A., Depledge, M. H., & Fleming, L. E. (2019). Spending at least 120 minutes a week in nature is associated with good health and wellbeing. *Scientific Reports*, 9(1), 7730. https://doi.org/10.1038/s41598-019-44097-3

16

ARTS AS MEDICINE

Using art interventions to promote health and wellbeing

Andrea Giraldez-Hayes

"Within the arts lies a powerful but largely untapped force for healing. The arts and science are two sides of the same coin, which is our shared humanity. Our ability to live fulfilling, healthy lives depends on bringing these two forces together." Vivek H. Murthy, MD, MBA. 19th Surgeon General of the United States

The use of arts in health and wellbeing, including shamanic healing rituals, can be traced back c. 40,000 years ago, and the therapeutic value of arts has been profusely documented throughout history (Fancourt, 2017). However, it was not until the mid-twenty century that, following medical theories and traditions, different art forms were systematically and scientifically used in health and mental health, giving rise to various modalities of art therapy and therapeutic arts (Pamelia, 2015; St. John, 1986). It can be argued that these developments were possible as medicine moved away from the biomedical model to a psychosomatic one, influenced by Freudian and other psychoanalytic theories highlighting the connection between the mind and physical illness. Later developments also paved the way for considering art as medicine and the therapeutic value of arts. Among them, it is worth mentioning the biopsychosocial model (Engel, 1977) and the shift from psychoanalytic theories to humanistic psychology with representatives such as Maslow and Rogers. Humanistic psychology recovered ancient Greeks and Renaissance ideas advocating the significance of happiness, self-actualisation, and the creative nature of human beings.

Additionally, over the past two decades, we have seen a significant increase in the number of research studies exploring the effects of music, drama, painting, creative writing, and other art forms on health and wellbeing (Fancourt & Finn, 2019), and artists have worked side by side with health and mental health professionals, psychologists, researchers, and policymakers to explore and understand the complex and varied links between arts, health, and wellbeing (Daykin,

DOI: 10.4324/9781003378426-19   252

2019). In this endeavour, a nascent but growing number of professionals have explored arts through the lenses of positive psychology; among them, Tay, Pawelski and Keith (2018) and Wilkinson and Chilton (2017).

This chapter considers these developments aiming to explore and bring together some of the theories and research findings underpinning the use of art interventions to promote health, as defined by the World Health Organisation (WHO) back in 1946: "A state of complete physical, mental and social wellbeing and not merely the absence of disease or infirmity" (World Health Organisation, 2002, p. 1), and the use of arts and arts activities as or in positive psychology interventions.

Arts, health and wellbeing: research and governmental reports

The arts, health and wellbeing field integrates practices, policies, and research on many different experiences and art forms, including visual arts, drama, music, dance, photography, creative writing, and film. These experiences happen in various settings, including communities, hospitals, prisons, art centres, care homes, schools, libraries, theatres, and museums. They may involve diverse individuals, including those considered "functioning" or "healthy" and those with presenting health or mental health conditions.

Research has been essential to support these activities, give them visibility and allow the establishment of arts, health and wellbeing as an academic field backed by publications such as the *Journal of Arts and Health*; *Arts & Health: An international Journal of Research, Policy and Practice*; the *Nordic Journal of Arts, Culture and Health*; *Music and Medicine* or the *Journal of Applied Arts and Health*. In addition, other journals, such as the *Journal of Health Psychology* (2008) or *Perspectives in Public Health* (2013) have published special issues on arts, health and wellbeing. Furthermore, several scoping and systematic reviews have identified and examined ways in which the arts have been and are used to promote or address health and wellbeing for individuals and communities. Among others, Fancourt and Finn (2019) looked at the evidence on the role of the arts in improving health and wellbeing; Curtis et al. (2018) considered the impact of art on health, wellbeing and quality of life of older people living in care homes; Jensen and Bonde (2018) concluded that participatory arts activities are effective non-medical interventions to promote mental health and wellbeing, and Pesata et al. (2022) identified and examined how the arts have been used to promote wellbeing in communities in the United States of America. These and other reviews found evidence for the crucial role the arts play in health prevention and promotion (Corbin et al., 2021) and the potential of the arts to improve individuals' and communities' wellbeing (Johnson & Stanley, 2007; Stuckey & Nobel, 2010), prevent mental health issues (Stickley & Duncan, 2007), delay age-related physical and cognitive decline (Lee et al., 2019; Noice et al., 2014), reduce stress levels (Abbott et al., 2013; Curl, 2008), decrease anxiety levels (Jakobsson, 2022), enhance mood (Henry et al., 2021; Kim et al., 2023) or assist in end-of-life care (McConnell et al., 2016).

The actions encouraged by the WHO European Region have also contributed to the understanding and support of art, health and wellbeing projects. For example, in the United Kingdom, the Arts Council England and the National Health Service's Arts and Health Working Group reviewed the role of the Department in Health in promoting arts and health. After interviewing workers in the health service, the Arts Council, Local Government, professional bodies and organisations, charities, patients and artists, they concluded "the arts are undoubtedly essential for human wellbeing" (Cayton, 2007, p. 1).

The Creative Health: The Art for Health and Wellbeing report, commissioned by the All-Party Parliamentary Group on Arts, Health and Wellbeing (2017) also identified examples and evidence of the powerful contribution of the arts to health and wellbeing and concluded that the arts help people to get well, aid their recovery and support longer lives better lived; help to face significant challenges in health and social care, such as ageing, loneliness, long-term conditions or mental health, and have the potential to save money in social care and health services. Their report includes a series of recommendations to the government and professional bodies and organisations. Similar reports have been completed in other European countries, including Norway (Theorell et al., 2015), Ireland (The Arts Council, 2010) or Finland (Liikanen, 2010). It is worth noticing that most of these projects work around a broad and inclusive concept of arts, such as the one presented below.

From high art to mass cultures

When people think about art, they usually think of artworks exhibited in galleries and museums or music, dance, or drama performances in theatres. In other words, they think about arts as the result of the activity and production of professional artists. However, that is a narrow-minded view. As human beings, we are surrounded by art and, either as public, producers or creators, we engage in art activities in our everyday lives, both for personal enjoyment and to foster human connection. These activities are opportunities for aesthetic experiences, creativity, social interaction, physical recreation, sensory activation, cognitive stimulation, imagination or emotions perceived and expressed through music, visual arts, crafts, dance, design, drama, photography, film or, increasingly, digital media (Fancourt & Finn, 2019).

The opportunities are endless and the perception of art production as restricted to professionals with formal training shifted, driven by the emergence of community art in the 1960s, which originated from the idea of cultural democracy (Mathews, 1975). Community art, also known as or related to similar practices such as participatory art, relational practice, socially engaged art, interactive art or activist art can be defined as a range of artistic activities "based in a community setting, characterised by interaction or dialogue with the community and often involving a professional artist collaborating with people who may not otherwise engage in the arts" (Tate, n.d.). The momentum for the development of arts, health and wellbeing projects has direct links to the community art movements. Because of these movements, the cultural, social and symbolic functions of arts shifted from the territories of the "high arts" to those of "mass cultures" or "popular cultures" to propose and impose an urgent review of our aesthetic assumptions (Aguirre, 2005). As a result, we can identify a contemporary function of the arts that is basically integrative and relational, which aims to connect with all the facets of reality we share, and not only as a superior manifestation of the human spirit. In short, a function sustained from the need to understand that cultural productions are not a privilege of the few who produce and distribute culture but a right of every individual. This clarification is important, as art activities related to health and wellbeing are not limited to high art (although they may play an essential role in some projects) but include a wide range of possibilities recognising, as the German artist Joseph Beuys once said, that "every human being is an artist" (Beuys, as cited in Harrison & Wood, 2003, p. 929). This is the perspective used in a variety of approaches in the field of arts, health and wellbeing, including art therapy, therapeutic art, arts-based health and mental health promotion, arts in hospitals, arts on prescription and the most recent developments of arts activities and interventions in positive psychology.

Arts and positive psychology

For the last ten years, positive psychologists and art-therapists have developed an increasing interest in the role of arts in human flourishing and examined how engagement with arts helps people to thrive individually and collectively (Darewych & Riedel Bowers, 2018; Lomas, 2016; Tay & Pawelski, 2016; Wilkinson & Chilton, 2017). According to Seligman (2021), "As positive psychology was twenty years ago, so the positive humanities are now: a new field poised to become a worldwide movement" (p. XV). A significant number of research studies and publications contribute to and increase the vast amount of research on arts, health and wellbeing already produced in different professional and academic fields, including psychology, education, health, mental health, sociology, and philosophy.

The use of arts in and as positive psychology interventions, that is evidence-based, "intentional activities aimed at cultivating positive feelings, positive behaviours, or positive cognitions" (Sin & Lyubomirsky, 2009, p. 467) and "to increase wellbeing in non-clinical populations" (Pawelski, 2011, p. 643), has been more and more frequent. Furthermore, art-based positive psychology interventions have also been used with clinical populations through new therapeutic methods influenced by positive psychology approaches to diagnosis and treatment, including positive clinical psychology (Seligman & Peterson, 2003), positive psychotherapy (Seligman et al., 2006), and positive art-therapy (Wilkinson & Chilton, 2017).

Arts have been used in positive psychology interventions for different purposes, for example, children's drawing to promote gratitude and think about their best possible selves (Owens & Patterson, 2013); taking pictures to improve emotional wellbeing, involving mood, affect and satisfaction with life (Lee et al., 2021) or to reflect on meaning in life (Steger et al., 2014); listening to uplifting music to improve wellbeing in self-critical and needy individuals (Sergeant & Mongrain, 2011); using a creative journal art-therapy to assist Latina/o teenagers to increase resilience and decrease depressive symptoms (Vela et al., 2019); activating and expressing positive emotions (Chilton et al., 2015); engaging with a self-administered online positive psychology intervention on the beauty in nature, arts and behaviours to increase levels of happiness and ameliorate depressive symptoms (Proyer et al., 2916); or using music and dance to enhance positive affect and divergent thinking (Campion & Levita, 2014).

To illustrate these and other arts-based projects and positive psychology interventions, the following ones will be described in greater detail: Seeing Happy, Singing with us, Submit your Poetry, Long COVID wellness project, People dancing and a selection of projects under the umbrella of social prescribing. We will also describe two community and participatory art projects that promote wellbeing, Before I die and The sewing rooms. Finally, we will suggest several art-based activities that can be used to increase wellbeing.

Art projects to promote health and wellbeing

The number and variety of art projects is enormous. Therefore, our intention is not to present all the options available, but a small sample of art projects that stand out for their power and, at the same time, their simplicity.

Seeing happy

https://seeinghappy.org

Research in positive psychology has highlighted the importance of experiencing positive emotions. Fredrickson (1998) broaden-and-build theory suggests that experiencing positive emotions such as joy, contentment, love or interest, broaden people's attention, expand cognition (e.g., curiosity and creative thinking) and behaviours (e.g., playfulness) and helps people to build resilience and perdurable personal, intellectual, physical and social resources which, in turn, have an impact on emotional regulation, psychological wellbeing, social connection, and physical health. Kobau et al. (2011) suggested "greater synergy between positive psychology and public health might help promote mental health in innovative ways" (p. e1) and Fredrickson (2016) suggested positive emotions stimulate human health and longevity. The power of mindful photography as a tool to increase positive emotions and appreciation has also been observed in different studies, including Kurtz and Lyubomirsky (2013) or McKee et al. (2020).

The main aim of Seeing Happy is to cultivate happiness and promote flourishing through photography and "to make the world happier by encouraging others to be mindful of the good, to focus on it (literally), share one photo at a time, and create a communal work of art" (SeeingHappy, 2022) that showcases people's positive emotions. Lead by psychologist and photographer Mandy Seligman, the project's team includes educators, artists, photographers, and psychologists. Everyone is invited to participate by taking and posting a photo representing what makes them happy. The project is organised around five elements, namely beauty, connections, gratitude, happy and hope, each one representing a psychological experience which, when paid attention, can increase happiness and wellbeing.

Singing with us

https://performancescience.ac.uk/singwithus

A compelling body of research demonstrates the power of music and it has been proved that a wide variety of activities, including individual and shared music listening, singing, and instrument playing, both formally or informally, song writing, creating (exploring, improvising, composing) or movement and dance have a positive impact on individuals' and communities' health, wellbeing and social connection (Croom, 2015; Sheppard & Broughton, 2020; Welch, 2014, 2020). Hallam and Himonides (2022) explore the evidence and observe that, among other elements, music plays an essential role and has an impact on engagement, positive relationships, positive emotions, achievement, self-esteem, optimism, meaning, vitality, stress reduction, increased relaxation and, more broadly, in psychological wellbeing and good health through the different stages of the lifespan. They also offer a review of research related to participation in choirs and identify benefits such as physical relaxation and release of tension; emotional release; positive psychobiological effects (reduced levels of cortisol and increased concentration of oxytocin); enhanced breathing and posture; a sense of greater emotional and physical wellbeing or an increased sense of self-confidence or self-esteem.

The aim of Singing with us was to explore the psychobiological and psychosocial benefits of singing in choirs on mental health, quality of life, social support and wellbeing for people affected by cancer. The results of a pilot study with 193 participants suggested that a single choir session was enough to increase the levels of immune proteins and reduce stress hormones, while the longitudinal study showed a decrease in anxiety and building resilience (Fancourt et al., 2016).

Submit your poetry!

The benefits of writing poetry have been observed in different research studies, including Rickett et al. (2011) and Soter (2016). According to Croom (2015), a number of studies on poetry therapy have suggested that poetry can be an effective therapeutic tool and contribute to people's flourishing and increasing wellbeing.

Submit your poetry!, a recent initiative promoted by a peer-reviewed journal, Health Promotion Practice, aims to create new narratives for health and wellbeing by inviting people to write and submit poems that reflect on health (in)equity and wellbeing from different perspectives. Poems can be written by

257

individuals or groups, adopting the form of collaboratively written poetry, and fostering positive relationships.

People dancing

https://www.communitydance.org.uk/creative-programmes/health-and-wellbeing

The contribution of dance and movement to health and wellbeing has also been demonstrated by different research studies. For example, Chappell et al. (2021) after conducting a systematic review, found that dance makes seven contributions, including "embodiment, identity, belonging, self-worth, aesthetics, affective responses and creativity" (p. 1) and McGonigal (2019), in her book The Joy of Movement: How exercise helps us find happiness, hope, connection and courage suggests that exercising, including dancing, are health-enhancing and life-extending.

People dancing illustrate the possibilities of developing movement and dance programmes to support people's health and wellbeing. The programme aims to support dancers, educators, and organisations to make dance and its benefits more accessible and reduce the negative impact of physical inactivity.

Long COVID wellness project

https://www.oldvictheatre.com/discover/community/long-covid-wellness-project

This programme, created collaboratively between movement and voice theatre practitioners and drama therapists, aims to use movement and breathing techniques to support patients with long COVID symptoms. The intervention has been evaluated by a group of researchers working at the University College London, who observed a decrease in depressive symptoms and anxiety, loneliness, shortness of breath, and chronic fatigue, and an increase in mental wellbeing. The eight weeks workshop was delivered online and in person and focused on the use of movement and breathing techniques.

Arts on prescription

Different art modalities play an important role in social prescribing, sometimes called community referral, that is "A mechanism for linking patients with non-medical sources of support within the community" (Centre Forum Mental Health Commission, 2014, p. 6), which is becoming a favoured resource for the NHS England and Scotland. The term refers to the practice of referring patients to social and art activities, to complement or replace other conventional modalities of medicine. Independently of their age, cultural or social background, everyone, and in particular people who have long-term conditions, are lonely or isolated, experience mild mental health issues or have social needs which affect their wellbeing, can be referred by their doctor, nurse, mental health professional, a social worker, charity staff or by themselves to engage with art activities in their communities, including singing in choirs, visiting museums, libraries, etc.). According to the All-Party Parliamentary Group on Arts, Heath and Wellbeing (2017) inquire report, Arts on Prescription Gloucestershire shown a drop in of 37% in GP consultation rates and a reduction of 27% in hospital admissions. Social prescribing is consistent with the WHO (2002) recommendations and aims to consider health from a holistic perspective, providing solutions to psychosocial problems that may have an impact on people's health. A review of community referral schemes conducted by Thomson et al. (2015) found that the most frequent effects of community referrals were a greater sense of control and empowerment, increases in self-esteem and confidence, reductions in anxiety and depression and an increased psychological wellbeing. A free life-learning course developed by the University College London for Culture, Health and Wellbeing Alliance, Culture, Health and Wellbeing: An online training course (see https://www.culturehealthandwellbeing.org.uk/culture-health-and-wellbeing-online-training-course) aims to help participants to learn about the impact of arts and culture on health and wellbeing. The course includes an evidence-based programme, Museums on Prescription, which refers lonely older people to activities in museums in London and Kent (see https://www.ucl.ac.uk/culture/projects/museums-on-prescription).

The programme described below, The line, is an example of an arts on prescription programme.

The line

The line is a public art programme in East London. It is an outdoor exhibition and a space for quiet contemplation and discovery. One of its programmes is intended to promote the health and wellbeing benefits of taking a walk and being in intimate contact with the beauty of art and nature by following the waterways and the line of the Greenwich Meridian. The line is offered as a social prescription activity in which individuals can connect with other participants, reducing isolation and creating new connections. For more information, go to https://the-line.org.

Community and participatory arts

Although there is no consensus to define community arts, participatory arts and other related approaches, "the term is being used widely to refer to art practices that encourage active participation by people who can be identified by their membership of designated communities rather than their skills and/or experience as artists" (Mills, 2006, cited by Mulligan et al., 2008). Research has also shown that community arts projects have the potential to fostering people's wellbeing and play an increasing important role in mental health promotion (Johnson & Stanley, 2007; Swindells et al., 2013).

Before I die

In an increasingly alienating world, artist Candy Chang activate public spaces around the world inviting people to think, feel and connect. One of her most famous works is Before I die, a community art project that is an invitation to "reimagine how the walls of our cities can help us grapple with mortality and meaning as a community today". Anyone walking and passing by her walls can take a piece of chalk, reflect on their lives, and share their personal aspirations in a public space. People write things such as "before I die I want to live off the grid", "before I die I want to hold her, one more time", "before I die I want to find love", "before I die I want to abandon my insecurities". The artist has also created online resources (see https://beforeidieproject.com/participate) encouraging people all over the world to create a wall. Over the time, the project has become a global movement with over 5,000 walls created in 75 countries and more than 35 languages. Before I die, as well as other projects created by Candy Chang connect with wellbeing factors such as positive relationships by knowing you are not alone and meaning by making place for reflection and contemplations and remember what really matters to us.

Artworks can be an inspiration to create community art projects. In my role as director of the Postgraduate Course of Arts Education, Culture and Citizenship for the Organisation of Ibero-American States for Education, Science and Culture (OEI) between 2007 and 2017, I promoted several community art projects inspired in artists artwork. The idea was to bring these projects to communities that will hardly have the opportunity to engage with arts and, by doing so, promote and increase their resilience, hope and wellbeing. The photograph (Figure 16.1) was taken when working on one of these projects in a landfill in Dominican Republic. With a group of postgraduate students, we invited the workers to connect to their dreams and aspirations and participate by writing and sharing them in an improvised wall.

The sewing rooms

https://www.remendandoytejiendoafectos.com/costureros

The sewing rooms ("los costureros", in Spanish) is a project promoted by the ICESI University in Colombia. The sewing rooms are conceived as spaces for dialogue, allowing the exchange of experiences between people from different contexts and backgrounds. They are scenarios of co-creation and circulation of knowledge. These meeting and creation spaces revolve around textile practices, reading and the weaving of collective memories that inhabits the "Casa de Mono", in Cali. One of these sewing rooms was "Ancestor. Conversations with a flavour of equality", a space to talk to other women about human rights and their systematic violations. This sewing kit was designed and guided by Maritza Sánchez Hernández, creator of Ancestra. Ancestra's methodological proposal has conversations and personal stories at the centre. In this sense, the aim was to elaborate a joint letter quilt that captures the stories, complaints, feelings and

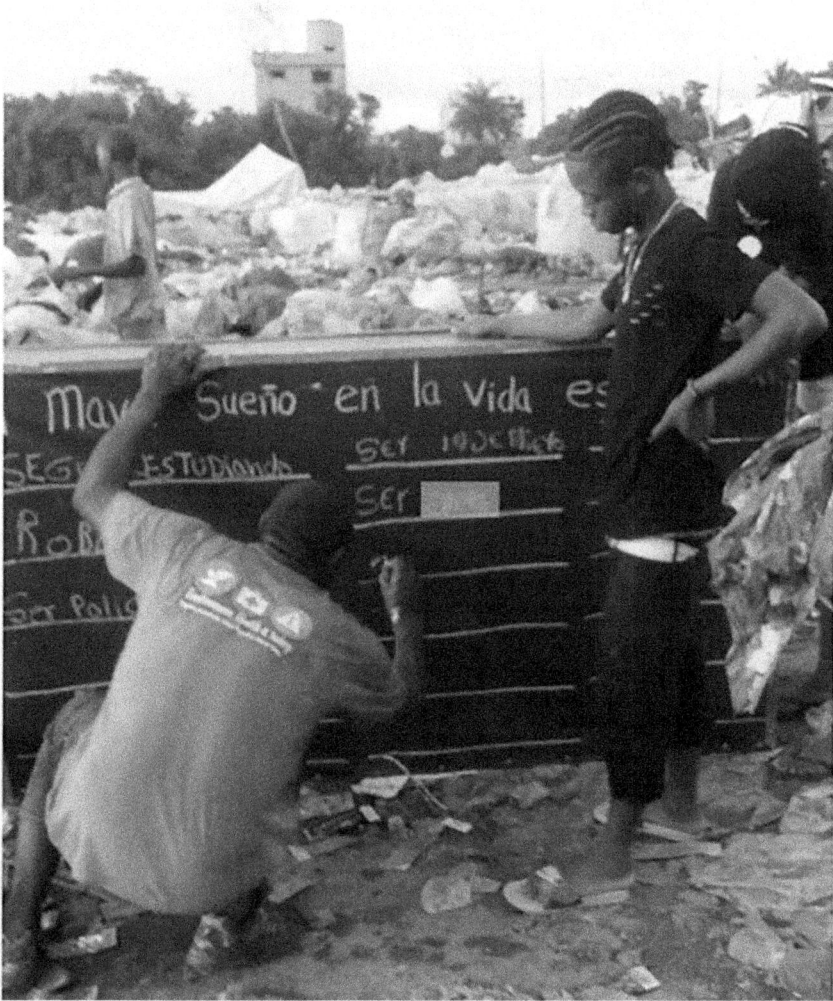

Figure 16.1 My dream in life. Dominican Republic, 2015. Picture taken as part of the
    Pos Andrea Giraldez-Hayes

experiences the participants want to share with other women as a "textile message". In addition, an epistolary exercise was encouraged on paper that answers
different open questions, which provoke personal reflection and, in turn, collective discussions.

Takeaways

• Remember that there is enough evidence that experiencing or participating
  in arts and art-based activities can have a positive impact on physical, mental,
  and emotional wellbeing, and there are several ways in which this can happen:

creative expression, community arts programmes, participating in expressive art experiences or art therapy, among others.

- Engage yourself in arts-based activities to experience and explore their impact on your health, mental health, and wellbeing.
- Become familiar with community and participatory art projects as well as other art activities (e.g., choirs, book clubs, cinema forums, museums) in your area. There will be some open to social prescribing referrals, and others accessible to public.
- Create a collection of positive arts-based activities that you can recommend to your patients and clients to enhance to experience positive emotions, identify and use their strengths, engage in the act of flow, experience gratitude, explore their creativity, engage in positive relationships, find meaning, connect with hope, increase their resilience, raise their self-awareness and, in general, cultivate their wellbeing.

Wicked questions

1 How could you revise unhelpful beliefs and myths about arts and what it takes to take part in arts-based activities?
2 Knowing what you know now, how would you integrate art-based activities in your work?
3 How can arts be used as tools in positive psychology interventions?

References

Abbott, K. A., Shanahan, M. J., & Neufeld, R. W. (2013). Artistic tasks outperform non-artistic tasks for stress reduction. *Art Therapy*, 30(2), 71–78.

Aguirre, I. (2005), *Teorías y prácticas en educación artística. Ideas para una revisión pragmática de la experiencia estética*. Octaedro.

All-Party Parliamentary Group on Arts, Health and Wellbeing (2017). *Creative health. The arts for health and wellbeing*. Retrieved from https://www.culturehealthandwellbeing.org.uk/appg-inquiry

Campion, M., & Levita, L. (2014). Enhancing positive affect and divergent thinking abilities: Play some music and dance. *The Journal of Positive Psychology*, 9(2), 137–145.

Cayton, H. (2007). *Report of the review of arts and health working group*. Leeds: Department of Health. http://www.artsandhealth.ie/wp-content/uploads/2011/09/Report-of-the-review-on-the-arts-and-health-working-group-DeptofHealth.pdf

Centre Forum for Mental Health Commission (2014). *The Pursuit of Happiness. A New Ambition for our Mental Health*. https://centreforum.org/assets/pubs/the-pursuit-of-happiness.pdf

Chappell, K. et al. (2021). The aesthetic, artistic and creative contributions of dance for health and wellbeing across the lifecourse: A systematic review. *International Journal of Qualitative Studies on Health and Well-being*, 16(1), 1950891.

Chilton, G. et al. (2015). The art of positive emotions: Expressing positive emotions within the intersubjective art making process (L'art des émotions positives: Exprimer des émotions positives à travers le processus artistique intersubjectif). *Canadian Art Therapy Association Journal*, 28(1–2), 12–25.

Corbin, J. H., Sanmartino, M., Hennessy, E. A., & Urke, H. B. (2021). *Arts and health promotion: Tools and bridges for practice, research, and social transformation.* Springer.

Croom, A. M. (2015). Music practice and participation for psychological well-being: A review of how music influences positive emotion, engagement, relationships, meaning, and accomplishment. *Musicae Scientiae,* 19(1), 44–64.

Croom, A. M. (2015). The practice of poetry and the psychology of well-being. *Journal of Poetry Therapy,* 28(1), 21–41.

Curl, K. (2008). Assessing stress reduction as a function of artistic creation and cognitive focus. *Art Therapy,* 25(4), 164–169.

Curtis, A., Gibson, L., O'Brien, M., & Roe, B. (2018). Systematic review of the impact of arts for health activities on health, wellbeing and quality of life of older people living in care homes. *Dementia,* 17(6), 645–669.

Darewych, O. H., & Riedel Bowers, N. (2018). Positive arts interventions: Creative clinical tools promoting psychological well-being. *International Journal of Art Therapy,* 23(2), 62–69.

Daykin, N. (2019). *Arts, health and well-being: A critical perspective on research, policy and practice.* Routledge.

Engel, G. L. (1977). The need for a new medical model: A challenge for biomedicine. *Science,* 8;196(4286), 129–36.

Fancourt, D. (2017). *Arts in health: Designing and researching interventions.* Oxford University Press.

Fancourt, D., & Finn, S. (2019). *What is the evidence on the role of the arts in improving health and well-being?* A scoping review. World Health Organisation. Regional Office for Europe. Health Evidence Network Synthesis Report 97. https://apps.who.int/iris/bitstream/handle/10665/329834/9789289054553-eng.pdf

Fancourt, D., Williamon, A., Carvalho, L. A., Steptoe, A., Dow, R., & Lewis, I. (2016). Singing modulates mood, stress, cortisol, cytokine and neuropeptide activity in cancer patients and carers. *Ecancermedicalscience,* 10. https://doi.org/10.3332/ecancer.2016.631

Fredrickson, B. L. (1998). What good are positive emotions? *Review of General Psychology,* 2(3), 300–319.

Fredrickson, B. L. (2016). The eudaimonics of positive emotions. In J. Vittersø (Ed.), *Handbook of Eudamonic wellbeing* (pp. 183–190). Springer.

Hallam, S., & Himonides, E. (2022). *The power of music: An exploration of the evidence.* Open Book Publishers.

Harrison, C., & Wood, P. (2003). *Art in Theory 1900–2000.* Blackwell.

Henry, N., Kayser, D., & Egermann, H. (2021). Music in mood regulation and coping orientations in response to COVID-19 lockdown measures within the United Kingdom. *Frontiers in Psychology,* 12, 647879.

Jakobsson Støre, S., & Jakobsson, N. (2022). The effect of mandala coloring on state anxiety: A systematic review and meta-analysis. *Art Therapy,* 39(4), 173–181.

Jensen, A., & Bonde, L. (2018). The use of arts interventions for mental health and well-being in health settings. *Perspectives in Public Health,* 138(4), 209–214. https://doi.org/10.1177/1757913918772602

Johnson, V., & Stanley, J. (2007). Capturing the contribution of community arts to health and well-being. *International Journal of Mental Health Promotion,* 9(2), 28–35.

Kim, K. S., Lor, M., & Rakel, B. (2023). Evaluation of art making activity as a pain management strategy for older adults and their experience using an art making intervention. *Geriatric Nursing,* 50, 109–116.

Kobau, R., Seligman, M. E., Peterson, C., Diener, E., Zack, M. M., Chapman, D., & Thompson, W. (2011). Mental health promotion in public health: Perspectives and strategies from positive psychology. *American Journal of Public Health,* 101(8), e1–e9.

Kurtz, J. L., & Lyubomirsky, S. (2013). Happiness promotion: Using mindful photography to increase positive emotion and appreciation. In J. J. Froh & A. C. Parks (Eds.), *Activities for teaching positive psychology: A guide for instructors* (pp. 133–136). American Psychological Association. https://doi.org/10.1037/14042-021

Lee, J. A., Efstratiou, C., Siriaraya, P., Sharma, D., & Ang, C. S. (2021). SnapAppy: A positive psychology intervention using smartphone photography to improve emotional well-being. *Pervasive and Mobile Computing*, 73, 101369.

Lee, R. et al. (2019). Art therapy for the prevention of cognitive decline. *The Arts in Psychotherapy*, 64, 20–25.

Liikanen, H.-L. (2010). *Art and culture for well-being: Proposal for an action programme 2010–2014*. Helsinki: Ministry of Education and Culture.

Lomas, T. (2016). Positive art: Artistic expression and appreciation as an exemplary vehicle for flourishing. *Review of General Psychology*, 20(2), 171–182.

Mathews, J. D. H. (1975). Arts and the people: The new deal quest for a cultural democracy. *The Journal of American History*, 62(2), 316–339.

McConnell, T., Scott, D., & Porter, S. (2016). Music therapy for end-of-life care: An updated systematic review. *Palliative Medicine*, 30(9), 877–883.

McGonigal, K. (2019). *The joy of movement: How exercise helps us find happiness, hope, connection, and courage*. Penguin.

McKee, L. G., Algoe, S. B., Faro, A. L. & O'Leary, J. L. (2020). What do daily reports add to the picture? Results from a photography intervention designed to increase positive emotion. *The Journal of Positive Psychology*, 15(5), 639–644.

Mulligan, M. et al. (2008). Renegotiating community life: Arts, agency, inclusion and wellbeing. *Gateways: International Journal of Community Research and Engagement*, 1, 48–72.

Noice, T., Noice, H., & Kramer, A. F. (2014). Participatory arts for older adults: A review of benefits and challenges. *The Gerontologist*, 54(5), 741–753.

Owens, R. L., & Patterson, M. M. (2013). Positive psychological interventions for children: A comparison of gratitude and best possible selves approaches. *The Journal of Genetic Psychology*, 174(4), 403–428.

Pamelia, E. (2015). *Therapeutic art-making and art therapy: Similarities and differences and a resulting framework*. [Master's Dissertation, University Graduate School, Indiana University]. Retrieved from https://core.ac.uk/download/pdf/46960356.pdf

Pawelski, J. O. (2011). Questions conceptuelles en psychologie positive. In C. Martin-Krumm, & C. Tarquinio (Eds.), *Traité de psychologie positive* (pp. 643–657). De Boeck.

Pawlski, J. O., & Tay, L. (2016). Better together. The sciences and the humanities in the quest of human flourishing. In S. J. Lopez, L. M. Edwards & S. Marques (Eds.), *The Oxford Handbook of Positive Psychology* (pp. 108–124). Oxford University Press.

Pesata, V. et al. (2022). Engaging the arts for wellbeing in the United States of America: A scoping review. *Frontiers in Psychology*, 6524. https://doi.org/10.3389/fpsyg.2021.791773

Rickett, C. et al. (2011). Something to hang my life on: The health benefits of writing poetry for people with serious illnesses. *Australasian Psychiatry*, 19(3), 265–268.

Seeing Happy (2022). *Seeing Happy*. https://seeinghappy.org

Seligman, M. E. (2021). Foreword. In L. Tay & J. O. Pawelski (Eds.), *The Oxford handbook of the positive humanities* (pp. XIII–SV). Oxford University Press.

Seligman, M. E., & Peterson, C. (2003). Positive clinical psychology. In L. G. Aspinwall & U. M. Staudinger (Eds.), *A psychology of human strengths: Fundamental questions and future directions for a positive psychology* (pp. 305–317). American Psychological Association. https://doi.org/10.1037/10566-021

Seligman, M. E., Rashid, T., & Parks, A. C. (2006). Positive psychotherapy. *American Psychologist*, 61(8), 774.

Sergeant, S., & Mongrain, M. (2011). Are positive psychology exercises helpful for people with depressive personality styles?. *The Journal of Positive Psychology*, 6(4), 260–272.

Sheppard, A., & Broughton, M. C. (2020). Promoting wellbeing and health through active participation in music and dance: A systematic review. *International Journal of Qualitative Studies on Health and Well-being*, 15(1), 1732526.

Sin, N., & Lyubomirsky, S. (2009). Enhancing well-being and alleviating depressive symptoms with positive psychology interventions: A practice-friendly meta-analysis. *Journal of Clinical Psychology*, 65, 467–487.

Soter, A. O. (2016). Reading and writing poetically for well-being: Language as a field of energy in practice. *Journal of Poetry Therapy*, 29(3), 161–174.

St. John, P. (1986). Art Education, Therapeutic Art, and Art Therapy: Some Relationships. *Art Education*, 39(1), 14–16. https://doi.org/10.1080/00043125.1986.11649719

Steger, M. F., Shim, Y., Barenz, J., & Shin, J. Y. (2014). Through the windows of the soul: A pilot study using photography to enhance meaning in life. *Journal of Contextual Behavioral Science*, 3(1), 27–30.

Stickley, T., & Duncan, K. (2007). Art in Mind: Implementation of a community arts initiative to promote mental health. *Journal of Public Mental Health*, 6(4), 24–32. https://doi.org/10.1108/17465729200700025

Stuckey, H. L., & Nobel, J. (2010). The connection between art, healing, and public health: A review of current literature. *American Journal of Public Health*, 100(2), 254–263.

Swindells, R. et al. (2013). Eudaimonic well-being and community arts participation. *Perspectives in Public Health*, 133(1), 60–65.

Tate (n.d.). *Community art*. Tate. https://www.tate.org.uk/art/art-terms/c/community-art

Tay, L., Pawelski, J. O., & Keith, M. G. (2018). The role of the arts and humanities in human flourishing: A conceptual model. *The Journal of Positive Psychology*, 13(3), 215–225.

The Arts Council (2010). *Arts and health policy and strategy*. Arts Council of Ireland.

Theorell, T. et al. (2015). Culture and public health activities in Sweden and Norway. In S. Clift & Camic P. M. (Eds.), *Oxford textbook of creative arts, health, and wellbeing: International perspectives on practice, policy and research* (pp. 171–177). Oxford University Press.

Thomson, L. et al. (2015). *Social prescribing: A review of community referral schemes*. CCCU Research Space Repository. Retrieved from https://repository.canterbury.ac.uk/download/b4200c5d0d0b31dfd441b8efedffae2865b13569e44cb4a662898a3ed20c1092/3729872/Social_Prescribing_Review_2015.pdf

Vela, J. C., Smith, W. D., Rodriguez, K., & Hinojosa, Y. (2019). Exploring the impact of a positive psychology and creative journal arts intervention with Latina/o adolescents. *Journal of Creativity in Mental Health*, 14(3), 280–291.

Welch, G. F. et al. (2014). Singing and social inclusion. *Frontiers in Psychology*, 5, 803. Retrieved from https://www.frontiersin.org/articles/10.3389/fpsyg.2014.00803/full

Welch, G. F., Biasutti, M., MacRitchie, J., McPherson, G. E., & Himonides, E. (2020). The impact of music on human development and well-being. *Frontiers in Psychology*, 11, 1246.

Wilkinson, R. A., & Chilton, G. (2017). *Positive art therapy theory and practice: Integrating positive psychology with art therapy*. Routledge.

World Health Organisation (2002). International Health Conference. Constitution of the World Health Organization. 1946. *Bulletin of the World Health Organization*, 80(12), 983–984. https://apps.who.int/iris/handle/10665/268688

17

DIGITAL POSITIVE HEALTH PLATFORMS, SUPPORTED BY ARTIFICIAL INTELLIGENCE, MEASURED USING WEARABLE DEVICES

*Jennifer Donnelly, Pádraic J. Dunne, Justin Laiti,
Croía Loughnane and Róisín O'Donovan*

The digitalisation of healthcare has increased in popularity over the last decade and has been further accelerated by the onset of the COVID-19 pandemic. The World Health Organisation (WHO) has urged that "digital health should be an integral part of health priorities" (WHO, 2021, p. 8). In order to support this, the WHO has developed a digital positive health" strategy to ensure digital literacy, equality of access to technologies and the incorporation of digital interventions into healthcare systems (WHO, 2021).

Although, as yet in its infancy, the benefits of digitalising heath interventions and education are becoming clear. Digital technology can facilitate distribution of healthcare to a wider audience, across different locations and time zones (Kanatouri, 2020) while keeping costs low (Rossett & Marino, 2005). The flexibility and scalability of Digital Positive Health (DPH) makes it an effective tool to overcome barriers to accessing healthcare and health education. This approach has been applied to a wide range of cohorts, most notably for chronic disease management, smoking cessation, stress reduction, and overall lifestyle management (Semwal et al., 2019; Seixas et al., 2021; Singh et al., 2022). As DPH is an emerging field, there is no 'gold standard' approach. Neither is there a preferred modality, communication style or technique for delivering DPH interventions. It is therefore understandable for questions to be raised about the sustainability and acceptability of DPH. In this chapter, we will first describe the relevant theoretical models that can be applied to digital technologies in positive health. We will then describe the different ways in which positive health can be utilised, and how practitioners can effectively facilitate such approaches. Finally, we will describe practical applications of the DPH theory.

Digital transformation in positive health

Digital Transformation (DT) encompasses all changes taking place in society and industries using digital technologies (Vial, 2021). DT of sciences is complex and multifaceted and requires the collaboration and buy-in of multiple stake-holders (e.g. participants, tech developers, healthcare practitioners, managers, and government agencies). For health practitioners, DT can facilitate new ways of providing positive health interventions. This can contribute to the achievement of sustainable health goals like quality, efficiency, equity, affordability, and accessibility without requiring trade-offs between goals (Ricciardi et al., 2019; WHO, 2021). In addition, the World Economic Forum (WEF) predicts that the most crucial impact of DT will be the move to person-centred healthcare, allowing for increased autonomy and responsibility of individuals in managing their own health (Ricciardi et al., 2019; WHO, 2021). Although DT in healthcare can be disruptive, technologies such as digital health platforms, wearables and artificial intelligence (AI) can help create a continuum of care between health practitioners and participants. This has been shown to improve health outcomes by promoting self-management of care, data-based treatment decisions and person-centred digital therapeutics as well as creating more evidence-based knowledge, skills and competence for practitioners (WHO, 2021).

Digital platforms

The arrival of digital platforms has resulted in a cultural shift in how people communicate, disseminate, and consume health information (Andersson & Mattsson, 2015). This was dramatically accelerated by the COVID-19 global pandemic with digital platforms becoming the new normal in education, healthcare and business settings (Alshammary & Alhalafawy, 2023). The many opportunities for digital platforms to be utilised in positive health interventions will be explored further in the following sections of this chapter.

Within a positive health context, we propose the following categories of digital platforms: Media Sharing, Social
Media, Knowledge-Based and Service-Based (Kaushal, 2022).

1 **Media Sharing Platforms** (e.g., websites and applications allowing for the sharing of videos, podcasts and blogs). Both video and audio media can be utilised to disseminate health information. Furthermore, the use of blogs, podcasts and online video can appeal to a variety of learning styles (Boulos et al, 2006). Digital media can provide more variation in sound and imagery than traditional analogue health content and this can provide a more stimulating and engaging experience (Shutikova & Beshenkov, 2020). A further

benefit of using media sharing platforms for positive health is that they can disseminate educational content on a global scale to a wide variety of individuals and groups, and they also allow for content to be accessed without the need for formal appointments and settings (Donovan et al., 2022; Liu et al., 2019)

2 **Social Media Sites** (e.g., websites and applications allowing participants to communicate with each other and share personal experiences, media and services). Social media sites are now part of everyday life, with many health practitioners using these platforms to communicate health messages (Frankish et al., 2012; Lim et al., 2022). Economically, it has become feasible to develop content and provide it to participants. Conversely, the rise in ease of access to health promotion via social media has seen a rise in "health influencers" providing free health and wellness content. Unfortunately, this ease of access has increased the prevalence of unvalidated claims and fallacious advice (Gisondi et al., 2022). Despite this, it is important to consider the potential for digital platforms to support and increase access to positive health interventions. Social media content also allows the participant to "discover" health-related information for themselves, from people they see as similar to themselves. This can increase autonomy and competence, resulting in increased self-determination concerning positive health behaviours (Gudka, Gardiner & Lomas, 2023).

3 **Knowledge-Based Platforms** (e.g., platforms that include guides, information and media related to the questions the participant may have). Knowledge-based platforms allow the user to access moderated or evidence-based health information. This form of knowledge acquisition allows for increased autonomy over a one's health and can reduce the demands on positive health coaches. The use of online chat forums can increase supportive relationships and connections for individuals experiencing illness, loss, or other negative life experiences (Griffin & Roy, 2019). Individuals can easily communicate with those who have similar experiences to themselves, and this can lead to positive psychological outcomes (Montali et al., 2021). These informal groups can however also be potentially misused (Au & Eyal, 2021). Therefore, if such groups are to be utilised, it is important to provide moderation or ground rules that can support the sharing of support, while ensuring that these spaces encourage positive emotions and provide meaning for participants.

4 **Service Based Platforms** (e.g., platforms that allow practitioners and coaches to provide interventions or support to participants). Mobile applications can allow positive health coaches and other health practitioners to communicate with participants and provide positive health interventions. Digital platforms can facilitate new forms of communication such as online video calls, voice notes and text-based chat (Nguyen et al., 2021). Furthermore, the option of text-based communication can open more opportunities for participants seeking anonymity (Weinberg & Rolnick, 2020). Digital health promotion messages can also be tailored and personalised for individuals, aligning with theories of positive health by taking a person-centred approach to digital

communication (Sequeira et al., 2021). Incorporating push notifications can act as automated reminders which can support health-related goal setting and adherence (Valdagno et al., 2014).

Wearable devices as an adjunct to support DPH

The DT of health has seen an increase in the popularity of wearable devices for health promotion and it is now common for people to track their steps, heart rate, calories and sleep quality (Iqbal et al., 2021). However, despite growing research on wearable use, the application of such devices in health science and coaching is still relatively unexplored (Tahri Sqalli & Al-Thani, 2020). Wearable devices can provide the wearer with previously unattainable objective data such as heart rate, respiration rate or calories burned during exercise. Such objective data provide for greater awareness of health-related behaviours, and this can increase autonomy and control over one's health (Kerner & Goodyear, 2017). The objective data obtained from these devices are well suited to digital platforms especially within the context of positive health. Knowledge and service-based platforms can be used to connect a coach or community with a person's wearable data thereby increasing interconnectedness and motivation (Jung & Kang, 2022). The impact of objective specific data from wearable devices is limited by their being disconnected from the broader context of health. For example, a wearable device can count steps but cannot determine whether those steps were taken while on a sociable hike with friends or a solitary walk to work. A health coach may provide valuable insights into wearable device data that can elevate a person's awareness of their health as well as the coach's knowledge of the person.

Wearable devices can be expensive, require a level of digital literacy and often need to come into contact with skin and these factors may prevent a some people from using them. There may also be some negative impacts of using such devices. For example, if a person becomes fixated on counting steps at the expense of other activities and relationships the device could have an overall negative impact on their health. The use of such devices should be approached with caution especially with individuals suffering from anxiety or obsessive-compulsive related disorders (El-gendi & Menon, 2019). Despite these downsides, wearable devices offer a unique advantage in that they provide measurable health related goals which can support positive health while instilling a sense of self-efficacy in relation to one's health.

AI in digital positive health

The increased use of both digital platforms and wearable devices leads to growing data sets which can be used by AI applications to enhance DPH. AI is the use of technology to make human-like decisions that are based on data inputs without real-time assistance from a human. The application of AI in DPH can enhance positive change by increasing the scalability and efficiency of applications and by analysing complex datasets to provide targeted insights. However, AI can also increase risks associated with privacy and bias. For example, the human inputs and even the data included in the development of AI can create biases in AI algorithms that can negatively impact the ability of AI systems to make well-informed unbiased decisions. The European Commission has compiled ethical guidelines for the development and evaluation of AI that is trustworthy and fair AI (Ala-Pietilä et al., 2019). The development of AI should reflect the principles of positive technologies and participant-centred design to ensure that this powerful tool is used to help support psychological needs of users and to account for the diverse needs of individuals and communities.

There are various approaches within AI that have their own strengths and applications. Two common approaches include machine learning which continues to learn without or with minimal human intervention and deep learning which mimics the decision-making process of the human brain. In the context of DPH, AI could be used in wellbeing management to make decisions about which wellbeing resources to provide to participants based on a combination of inputs about their thoughts, feelings and emotions. Machine learning could increase the effectiveness of such decisions by learning from participants' previous interactions with such systems. Deep learning could further enhance this learning process by generating personalised conversation-like feedback with referenced resources. The various levels of complexity of AI can be leveraged for various desired outcomes within DPH such as educational resource recommendations based on client activity (Figure 17.1). Defining the need for AI in supporting specific aspects of digital platforms can help identify what approach is most beneficial.

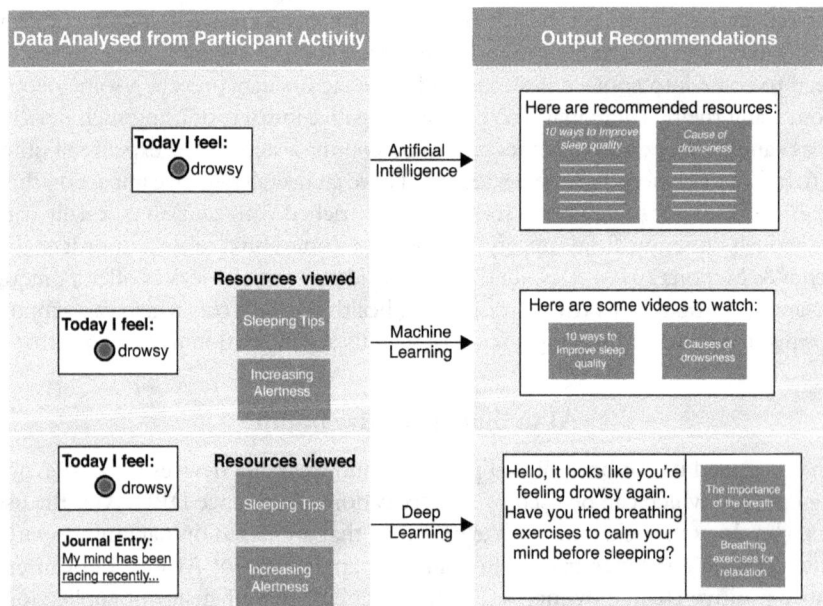

Figure 17.1 Levels of AI in Digital Positive Health.

AI can be applied within DPH sciences to enhance the functions of digital tools and effectively improve the wellbeing of participants. It is important to note that while AI is used to make "human-like" decisions, it is not intended to replace the role of humans, but rather to work alongside humans by helping utilise information that can be gathered from large datasets. For example, we discuss later the use of AI to assist health coaches working on digital platforms. The growing use of digital platforms, wearables and AI has been met with some concerns relating to privacy, bias, literacy for text-based communication and potential barriers (cost, access, lack of digital literacy) (Inkster et al., 2020). In the following sections, we explore theories that aim to incorporate positive psychology and business analysis into both the design of digital products and the use of digital platforms.

Business analysis in DPH

DT can feel daunting, especially when it involves digital platforms, wearables, and other digital technologies like AI, automation and associated application designs. These can present challenges to our sense of control. Business Analysis can mitigate these fears by providing clarity about DT, promoting collaboration between stakeholders in digital technology development and creating co-designed roadmaps that explain the DT process. Business analysis is the practice of enabling change by defining needs and recommending solutions that deliver tailored value to stakeholders (IIBA, 2015). It focuses on implementing technologies to reach business goals or rebuilding business models using technology that caters to consumers' needs and expectations (Mashhood & Senapathi, 2021). The role of the business analyst is to act as a broker between end-users and information technology (IT) practitioners who design and develop DPH solutions (Mashhood & Senapathi, 2021).

The business analyst core competencies model

Business analyst core competencies can be applied to many different sectors including the DT of healthcare. The six core competencies – changes, solutions, context, value, stakeholder, and needs – are all equal, necessary and dependent on each other (IIBA, 2015). Thus, if one competency changes (i.e., stakeholders), all other competencies must be re-evaluated for changes and impact. Core competencies help address questions as listed in Figure 17.2.

- What kinds of changes are we making?
- What are the needs we are trying to satisfy?
- What are the solutions we are creating or changing?
- Who are the stakeholders involved?
- What do stakeholders consider to be of value?
- What are the contexts that we and the solutions are in?

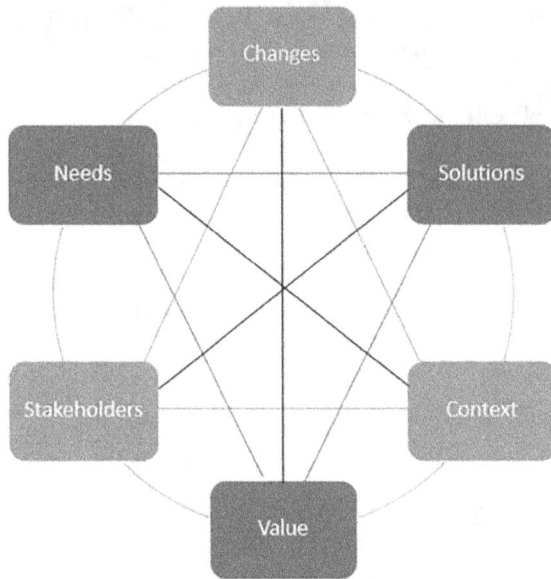

Figure 17.2 The Business Analyst Core Competencies Model (adapted from IIBA, 2015).

The role of the business analyst in this model is to engage with each of the competencies, to understand how each interacts with and impacts on the others and how each competency can contribute to overall DPH solutions. Business analysis, which is an effective strategy for creating participant-centred digital platforms and business models, can help facilitate participant and public involvement (PPI) in planning and generating inclusive positive technology applications.

Participant-centred DPH research

PPI is crucial to the design and development of effective positive health science-based interventions (Hoddinott et al., 2018). This is especially relevant for research involving digital technology. Most available health and wellbeing digital platforms are designed for a broad range of participants and do not address the unique needs of specific cohorts or individuals (Eyles et al., 2016). PPI offers an approach to addressing this issue by involving stakeholders in the development of strategies and tools that support specific cohorts.

PPI facilitates the broad involvement of stakeholders in guiding research practices. Techniques range from informal discussions to 'partnership approaches' that gather specific data to inform research and development (Hoddinott et al., 2018). The term 'partnership approaches' acknowledges the equal voices and reciprocity between the researcher and the participant. This approach encourages the on-going involvement of participants allowing them to lead the direction of the research. Co-design is one way that partnership can help in the development of research projects and applications. In the context of DPH research, this is an important phase where applications and interventions can be personalised for specific participants. This can increase the acceptability and effectiveness of digital tools and ultimately leads to better outcomes for participants (Byrne, 2019). It is beneficial to include on-going feedback throughout the development of a research project to ensure alignment between the project goals and the needs of the participants.

Whether studies include existing applications, wearable devices or are creating new technologies, it is important to optimise participant involvement in the study design and evaluation. Participant-centred research practices are important for the positive health sciences since the resulting alignment between the needs of participants and the content of the digital applications can encourage behaviour change and in turn improve health and wellbeing.

Positive technology

As digital health and wellbeing applications evolve, we must ensure that these tools are designed and used to support the psychological needs of the individual. Including a broad range of stakeholders increases the relevance of the applications. For example, the field of cyberpsychology explores ways in which relationships with technology can impact human psychology and overall wellbeing (Naz, Ilyas, & von Humboldt, 2019). When this is combined with a positive health approach, the focus is shifted from the psychological impacts of these technologies to understanding how the influencing factors can be adapted to optimally support wellbeing. This can be seen in the emerging fields of positive cyberpsychology and positive technologies in which researchers examine how technology can be created and used for better living (Gaggioli et al., 2019; Riva, 2012).

Positive Product Design is a positive psychology informed approach that seeks to limit the negative psychological impacts of technology on participants. Products designed in this way can be used to encourage participants to reach their full potential and optimise their wellbeing (Bigony, 2022). This approach is designed to inform practices in technology development that have human flourishing as their end goal. Additionally, the partnership approach provides a key component of a positive technology approach that allows developers to work closely with participants in the design of interventions. Examples of a partnership approach include gathering feedback and wellbeing assessments to understand the impact that technology has on the psychological health of participants.

DPH coaching as a vehicle for positive health

DPH coaching involves the integration of Positive Health Coaching previously defined in Chapter X with digital technology. PHC is a "managed conversational process that supports people to achieve meaningful goals in a way that enhances their wellbeing" (van Nieuwerburgh & Biswas-Diener, 2020, p. 315)". DPH Coaching is dialogical in its approach, which lies between facilitative and direction conversational interventions (van Nieuwerburgh, Knight & Campbell). More information on PHC can be found in Chapter 16. DPH coaching can be self-directed, coach directed or automated through AI and machine learning (e.g. chatbots), and/or a blend of all three forms (Hultgren et al., 2016).

Digitalisation of coaching

Using technology to facilitate coaching adds flexibility and expands reach, regardless of geography and time zone (Kanatouri, 2020). However, it is important to whether and to what extent technology as a mediator affects the coaching relationship. DPH coaching differs from traditional coaching in that there are three moving parts in the coaching conversation instead of two: the coach, the participant and the technology. With digital coaching (regardless of the platform used or the mode of communication), the technology is always present as a mediator between coach and participant. Kanatouri (2020) suggest that when the technology is seamless and easy to use, the coach and participant can embody the technology and speak through this digital space. Here, the technology fades into the background of the conversation and the connection between coach and participant is placed at the forefront. Any disruption to the technology (i.e., internet outage, platform failure, computer issues) causes the technology to suddenly become highly salient and to interrupt the connection between coach and participant. If not managed properly, disruptions in technology can create barriers between coach and participant and can have a negative impact on the relationship. In order to mitigate such disruption, it is important to (1) invest in stable and reliable technology, (2) to manage expectations about the capabilities of the technology and (3) to have technical support available for the participants.

Technology-mediated communication

The way we communicate is integral to coaching relationships. Video, audio, and text-based communication are all effective modes of communication. However, it is important to understand the respective benefits each mode of communication for DPH coaching.

Video call

Video-based conversations are almost identical to traditional face-to-face (FTF) coaching. They allow the parties to interact FTF through encrypted web-based video conferencing tools like Skype, Zoom, Microsoft Teams, and Facetime. Participants have reported enjoying the closeness provided by video call communication. Likewise, individuals have shown to build trust quicker through video

(Bos et al., 2002). However, they have also reported that the interaction is more effortful and difficult than text-based communication (Mallen, Day, & Green, 2003; McKenna & Green, 2002; Okdie et al., 2001). While video-based conversations are still the most common mode of communication for DPH coaching, there is growing research examining text and audio-based communication.

Audio call

Audio calls represent an alternative and effective form of communication. These can occur through telephone networks or online via software-based, digital platforms. Audio calls share some features of video calls but with the added advantage of allowing participants to engage in a wider range of settings (i.e., on lunch breaks or while out for a walk).

Voice messages

Voice messaging is an instant communication technology in which messages are transmitted via voice media. This form of communication is closer to text-based communication but retains some sensory cues from audio calls. Voice messages are stored and can be accessed through instant messaging chat boxes at any time, with the option to reply via text or voice message. Voice messages offer greater flexibility than audio calls and are more inclusive of people with limited literacy skills than text-based communication. Likewise, research shows that voice messages generate high levels of satisfaction, comprehension, and learning, and can help build rapport and trust more quickly than text-based communication (Crawford et al., 2014).

Text-based conversation

Text-based communications include, but are not limited to, e-mail, text messages, in-app or web-based instant messaging and online forums. Text-based communication is growing in popularity in DPH coaching because of its accessibility, effectiveness and scalability, in addition to being low cost, easy to use, and lightweight (i.e., less demanding, less effort, and easier for participants to share information) (Battestini et al., 2010; Crawford et al., 2014; Marcolino et al., 2018). Text-based communication has the added benefit of being available at the participants' convenience and can be received even if phones are turned off or during internet outages (Crawford et al., 2014). Instant messages and, to an extent, text messaging are the most effective form of text-based communication. Text-based communication naturally creates the spaces between stimulus and response that coaches work to create in face to face, video, and audio communication. Participants and coaches can take more time to think about and articulate thoughts (Walther, 2007; Okdie et al., 2011). Okdie and colleagues suggested that the lower cognitive load required for text-based communication (due to reduced visual processing and behavioural and emotional management) increases self-awareness and provides participants with more cognitive resources to direct towards their own thoughts and desires (Okdie et al., 2011).

Choosing modes of communication in DPH interventions depends on various aspects of the coaching process such as context, personality, timing, and participants' needs and preferences (Bardi & Brady, 2010; Okdie et al., 2011; Reid & Reid, 2007). Each mode has strengths and weaknesses when used to facilitate coaching interactions. For example, richer medias like video and audio can build trust quicker than text, and allows for nonverbal communication, but text communication can help encourage disclosure, increase awareness, and is more convenient and private than video or audio and (Battestini et al., 2010; Bos et al., 2002; Crawford et al., 2014; Marcolino et al., 2018). As a result, we do not recommend one mode of communication, but rather recommend incorporating and offering all types of communication.

Inclusivity

The capacity for inclusivity ranges across different modes of communication. However, each mode of communication poses its own accessibility problems for some individuals. For example, FTF is inclusive in that it can easily be adapted to the needs and limitations of participants. Conversely, the same approach can exclude citizens who live in areas lacking FTF facilities. Likewise, text-based communication is accessible for those with impaired hearing but inaccessible for those with literacy issues.

Scalability, accessibility, and flexibility

There is a trade-off between the availability of nonverbal cues and accessibility, scalability and flexibility, as communication moves from FTF to text. For example, text-based communication has the advantage of being able to facilitate multiple conversations at once but at the expense of nonverbal communication. Although voice messaging also sacrifices some nonverbal cues, while still maintaining audio cues like emotional tone, it does create reflective space between stimulus and response and between coach and participant.

AI and digital positive health coaching

AI has the potential to improve DPH coaching by automating certain human tasks at a vastly reduced cost. This has the potential to make such coaching more affordable and accessible especially for marginalised and low-income groups (Terblanche et al., 2022). However, research shows that there is still a boundary between AI automation and human support on DPH platforms. Clutterbuck (2020, p. 24) argues that, "The doing of coaching can be replicated by AI with relative ease. The 'being' of coaching requires presence, intuition and immense compassion". Understanding the boundary between AI and human coaching has several consequences. Delegating the 'doing' of PHC to AI and allowing human coaches to provide the 'being' through digital technologies allows for scalability and accessibility while maintaining motivation, accountability for change, support, and positive affect from human connection. (Clutterbuck, 2020)

Emerging evidence shows that AI can complement person based coaching (Fadhil, Wang, & Reiterer, 2019; Moreno-Blanco and colleagues, 2021). One approach has been to use an intelligent coaching assistant (ICA) which is based on the principle of intelligence augmentation: assisting human intelligence rather than replacing it (Moreno-Blanco et al., 2021). ICA uses advances in machine learning, AI, and human–computer interaction to provide human-centred AI (Islas-Cota et al., 2022). ICA technology has the potential to transform the coaching profession by supporting the online human coach to be more accessible and to reach a greater number of people. AI techniques and intelligent software agents are used to bridge the gap between remote coaches and their clients. These techniques can boost the efficacy and efficiency of coaches by automating aspects of their daily tasks (i.e., administrative tasks, booking appointments, and follow-ups), as well as improving data collection and analysis (Azvine et al., 2000; Fadhil, Wang, & Reiterer, 2019; Islas-Cota et al., 2022). Research has shown that clients using automated systems value having a human coach in the background to personalise their activities (Fadhil, Wang, & Reiterer, 2019). (ED: is there a reference to the work done in the CPHS?)

Takeaways

General

- Digitalisation of positive health interventions is needed to provide equitable, scalable, and sustainable care.
- A user-centred approach to the design and implementation of digital technologies is essential for the sustainability of DPH interventions.
- Digital platforms can be enhanced using wearable devices and AI to benefit both users and practitioners.
- DPH coaching can be used to replace traditional FTF interventions.
- Understanding the potential impact of digital technology on PHC and developing competence and confidence in digital technology will become increasingly important for all practitioners interested in DPH.

Practical

- The DT of positive health interventions is needed to create equitable, accessible, scalable, and sustainable tools that facilitate positive health for everyone.
- It is important to recognise the psychological impacts of technology throughout the design and implementation phases of a project. Adopting a positive design approach through existing frameworks such as positive product design and business analysis can contribute to enhanced outcomes for participants.

- Individuals must always be at the centre of the design, development, and implementation phases of each project. This will ensure the creation of meaningful, impactful, and sustainable DPH solutions.
- The rapid advancement of AI can be used to benefit both practitioners and participants using DPH technology. It is helpful to understand how AI can augment DPH interventions to different degrees and how it can be created and used ethically. It is important to maintain control of AI in positive health and use digital technologies for the benefit of all stakeholders.
- It can be a challenge for coaches and participants to find the best way to communicate using digital technology. The key is to be flexible with the modes of communication, engage in trial and error and attempt to meet the needs of all parties.

Wicked questions

1 How can we scale traditional FTF coaching with digital technologies without losing quality?
2 How can the development and implementation of digital platforms be guided by the participant using them?
3 How can we ensure wearable devices, designed to support mental health don't create mental health issues e.g., obsessive engagement?

References

Ala-Pietilä, P. et al. (2019). High level expert group on artificial inteligence: Ethics guidelines for trustworthy AI. Merlin.obs.coe.int. Retrieved September 25, 2023, from https://merlin.obs.coe.int/article/8608#:~:text=The%20Guidelines%20begin%20by%20noting

Alshammary, F. M., & Alhalafawy, W. S. (2023). Digital platforms and the improvement of learning outcomes: Evidence extracted from meta-analysis. *Sustainability*, 15(2), 1305. https://doi.org/10.3390/su15021305

Andersson, P., & Mattsson, L.-G. (2015). Service innovations enabled by the "internet of things." *IMP Journal*, 9(1), 85–106. https://doi.org/10.1108/imp-01-2015-0002.

Au, L., & Eyal, G. (2021). Whose advice is credible? Claiming lay expertise in a Covid-19 online community. *Qualitative Sociology*. https://doi.org/10.1007/s11133-021-09492-1

Azvine, B., Djian, D., Tsui, K. C., & Wobcke, W. (2000). The intelligent assistant: An overview. *Intelligent Systems and Soft Computing*, 215–238.

Bardi, C. A., & Brady, M. F. (2010). Why shy people use instant messaging: Loneliness and other motives. *Computers in Human Behavior*, 26(6), 1722–1726.

Battestini, A., Setlur, V., & Sohn, T. (2010, September). A large scale study of text-messaging use. In *Proceedings of the 12th international conference on Human computer interaction with mobile devices and services* (pp. 229–238).

Bigony, C. (2022). A Guide to Positive Product Design™: Building human potential technology.

Bos, N., Olson, J., Gergle, D., Olson, G., & Wright, Z. (2002, April). Effects of four computer-mediated communications channels on trust development. In *Proceedings of the SIGCHI conference on human factors in computing systems* (pp. 135–140).

Boulos, M. N. K., Maramba, I., & Wheeler, S. (2006). Wikis, blogs and podcasts: a new generation of Web-based tools for virtual collaborative clinical practice and education. *Bmc Medical Education*, 6(1), 1–8.

Byrne, M. (2019). Increasing the impact of behavior change intervention research: Is there a role for stakeholder engagement? *Health Psychology*, 38(4), 290–296. https://doi.org/10.1037/hea0000723

Clutterbuck, D. (2020). *The challenges of coaching and mentoring in a digitally connected world*. Coaching im digitalen Wandel.

Crawford, J., Larsen-Cooper, E., Jezman, Z., Cunningham, S. C., & Bancroft, E. (2014). SMS versus voice messaging to deliver MNCH communication in rural Malawi: Assessment of delivery success and user experience. *Global Health: Science and Practice*, 2(1), 35–46.

Donovan, G., Hall, N., Ling, J., Smith, F., & Wilkes, S. (2022). Influencing medication taking behaviors using automated two-way digital communication: A narrative synthesis systematic review informed by the Behavior Change Wheel. *British Journal of Health Psychology*. https://doi.org/10.1111/bjhp.12580

Elgendi, M., & Menon, C. (2019). Assessing anxiety disorders using wearable devices: Challenges and future directions. *Brain Sciences*, 9(3), 50.

Eyles, H., Jull, A., & Dobson, R. et al. (2016). Co-design of mHealth delivered interventions: A systematic review to assess key methods and processes. *Current Nutrition Reports*, 5, 160–167. https://doi.org/10.1007/s13668-016-0165-7

Fadhil, A., Wang, Y., & Reiterer, H. (2019). Assistive conversational agent for health coaching: A validation study. *Methods of Information in Medicine*, 58(01), 009–023.

Frankish, K., Ryan, C., & Harris, A. (2012). Psychiatry and online social media: Potential, pitfalls and ethical guidelines for psychiatrists and trainees. *Australasian Psychiatry*, 20(3), 181–187.

Gaggioli, A., Villani, D., Serino, S., Banos, R., & Botella, C., eds. (2019). *Positive technology: Designing E- experiences for positive change*. Lausanne: Frontiers Media. https://doi.org/10.3389/978-2-88963-023-3

Gisondi, M. A., Barber, R., Faust, J. S., Raja, A., Strehlow, M. C., Westafer, L. M., & Gottlieb, M. (2022). A deadly infodemic: Social media and the power of COVID-19 misinformation. *Journal of Medical Internet Research*, 24(2), e35552. https://doi.org/10.2196/35552

Griffin, L., & Roy, J. (2019). A great resource that should be utilised more, but also a place of anxiety: Student perspectives on using an online discussion forum. *Open Learning: The Journal of Open, Distance and E-Learning*, 1–16. https://doi.org/10.1080/02680513.2019.1644159

Gudka, M., Gardiner, K. L., & Lomas, T. (2023). Towards a framework for flourishing through social media: a systematic review of 118 research studies. *The Journal of Positive Psychology*, 18(1), 86–105.

Hoddinott, P., Pollock, A., O'Cathain, A., Boyer, I., Taylor, J., MacDonald, C., Oliver, S., Donovan, J. L. (2018, June 18). How to incorporate patient and public perspectives into the design and conduct of research. *F1000Research. 7*, 752. https://doi.org/10.12688/f1000research.15162.1. PMID: 30364075; PMCID: PMC6192439.

Hultgren, U., Palmer, S., & O'Riordan, S. (2016). Developing and evaluating a virtual coaching programme: A pilot study. *The Coaching Psychologist*, 12(2), 67–75.

IIBA, (2015). *A guide to the Business Analysis Body of Knowledge (BABOK Guide) Version 3.0*. International Institute of Business Analysis, Ontario.

Inkster, B., O'Brien, R., Selby, E., Joshi, S., Subramanian, V., Kadaba, M., Schroeder, K., Godson, S., Comley, K., Volmer, S. J., & Mateen, B. A. (2020). Digital health management during and beyond the COVID-19 pandemic: Opportunities, barriers, and recommendations (Preprint). *JMIR Mental Health*, 7(7). https://doi.org/10.2196/19246

Iqbal, S. M., Mahgoub, I., Du, E., Leavitt, M. A., & Asghar, W. (2021). Advances in healthcare wearable devices. *NPJ Flexible Electronics*, 5(1), 9.

Islas-Cota, E., Gutierrez-Garcia, J. O., Acosta, C. O., & Rodríguez, L. F. (2022). A systematic review of intelligent assistants. *Future Generation Computer Systems*, 128, 45–62.

Jung, E. H., & Kang, H. (2022). Self-determination in wearable fitness technology: The moderating effect of age. *International Journal of Human–Computer Interaction*, 38(15), 1399–1409.

Kanatouri, S. (2020). Digital coaching: A conceptually distinct form of coaching?. Coaching im digitalen Wandel.

Kaushal, D. (2022, October 31). *Digital products vs digital platforms: What's the difference*. Insights - Web and Mobile Development Services and Solutions. https://www.netsolutions.com/insights/digital-products-vs-digital-platforms/

Kerner, C., & Goodyear, V. A. (2017). The motivational impact of wearable healthy lifestyle technologies: A self-determination perspective on fitbits with adolescents. *American Journal of Health Education*, 48(5), 287–297. https://doi.org/10.1080/19325037.2017.1343161

Lim, M. S. C., Molenaar, A., Brennan, L., Reid, M., & McCaffrey, T. (2022). Young adults' use of different social media platforms for health information: Insights from web-based conversations. *Journal of Medical Internet Research*, 24(1), e23656. https://doi.org/10.2196/23656

Liu, D., Baumeister, R. F., Yang, C., & Hu, B. (2019). Digital communication media use and psychological well-being: A meta-analysis. *Journal of Computer-Mediated Communication*, 24(5), 259–273. https://doi.org/10.1093/jcmc/zmz013

Mallen, M. J., Day, S. X., & Green, M. A. (2003). Online versus face-to-face conversation: An examination of relational and discourse variables. *Psychotherapy: Theory, Research, Practice, Training*, 40(1–2), 155.

Marcolino, M. S., Oliveira, J. A. Q., D'Agostino, M., Ribeiro, A. L., Alkmim, M. B. M., & Novillo-Ortiz, D. (2018). The impact of mHealth interventions: Systematic review of systematic reviews. *JMIR mHealth and uHealth*, 6(1), e8873.

Mashhood, A., & Senapathi, M. (2021, March). Understanding the role of business analysts in digital transformation: A multivocal literature review. In 31st Australasian Conference on Information Systems (Vol. 34). Australasian Conferences on Information Systems (ACIS).

McKenna, K. Y., & Green, A. S. (2002). Virtual group dynamics. *Group Dynamics: Theory, Research, and Practice*, 6(1), 116.

Montali, L., Zulato, E., Frigerio, A., Frangi, E., & Camussi, E. (2021). Mirroring, monitoring, modelling, belonging, and distancing: Psychosocial processes in an online support group of breast cancer patients. *Journal of Community Psychology*, 50(2), 992–1007. https://doi.org/10.1002/jcop.22696

Moreno-Blanco, Diego, et al. (2021). Intelligent coaching assistant for the promotion of healthy habits in a multidomain mHealth-based intervention for brain health. *International journal of environmental research and public health*, 18(20), 10774.

Naz, H., Ilyas, N., & von Humboldt, S. (2022). Cyberpsychology and Older Adults. In Gu, D., & Dupre, M. (Eds.) *Encyclopedia of Gerontology and Population Aging* (pp. 1282–1286). Cham: Springer International Publishing.

Nguyen, M. H., Gruber, J., Marler, W., Hunsaker, A., Fuchs, J., & Hargittai, E. (2021). Staying connected while physically apart: Digital communication when face-to-face interactions are limited. *New Media & Society*, 24(9), 146144482098544. https://doi.org/10.1177/1461444820985442

Okdie, B. M., Guadagno, R. E., Bernieri, F. J., Geers, A. L., & Mclarney-Vesotski, A. R. (2011). Getting to know you: Face-to-face versus online interactions. *Computers in Human Behavior*, 27(1), 153–159.

Ricciardi, W., Pita Barros, P., Bourek, A., Brouwer, W., Kelsey, T., & Lehtonen, L. (2019). How to govern the DT of health services. *European Journal of Public Health*, 29(Suppl. 3), 7–12.

Riva, G. (2012). What is positive technology and its impact on CyberPsychology. *Studies in Health Technology and Informatics*, 181, 37–41. https://doi.org/10.3233/978-1-61499-121-2-37

Rossett, A., & Marino, G. (2005). If coaching is good, then e-coaching is. *T and D*, 59(11), 46.

Seixas, A. A., Olaye, I. M., Wall, S. P., & Dunn, P. (2021). Optimizing healthcare through digital health and wellness solutions to meet the needs of patients with chronic disease during the COVID-19 era. *Frontiers in Public Health*, 9, 667654.

Semwal, M., Whiting, P., Bajpai, R., Bajpai, S., Kyaw, B. M., & Tudor Car, L. (2019). Digital education for health professions on smoking cessation management: Systematic review by the Digital Health Education Collaboration. *Journal of Medical Internet Research*, 21(3), e13000.

Sequeira, L., Chu, C., Sprott, A., Srivastava, R., Strauss, J., & Strudwick, G. (2021). "This Is ME": Promoting person-centred care within the digital health environment. *Healthcare Quarterly*, 24(1), 69–75. https://doi.org/10.12927/hcq.2021.26462

Shutikova, M., & Beshenkov, S. (2020). Modern digital educational environment and media education – Platforms for transforming education system. *Media Education (Mediaobrazovanie)*, 60(4). https://doi.org/10.13187/me.2020.4.736

Singh, P., Bala, H., Dey, B. L., & Filieri, R. (2022). Enforced remote working: The impact of digital platform-induced stress and remote working experience on technology exhaustion and subjective wellbeing. *Journal of Business Research*, 151, 269–286.

Tahri Sqalli, M., & Al-Thani, D. (2020). Evolution of wearable devices in health coaching: Challenges and opportunities. *Frontiers in Digital Health*, 2, 545646.

Terblanche, N., Molyn, J., De Haan, E., & Nilsson, V. O. (2022). Coaching at scale: Investigating the efficacy of artificial intelligence coaching. *International Journal of Evidence Based Coaching & Mentoring*, 20(2), 20–36.

Valdagno, M., Goracci, A., Volo, S. di, & Fagiolini, A. (2014). Telepsychiatry: New perspectives and open issues. *CNS Spectrums*, 19(6), 479–481. https://doi.org/10.1017/S1092852913000916

Vial, G. (2021). Understanding digital transformation: A review and a research agenda. *Managing Digital Transformation*, 28, 13–66.

Weinberg, H., & Rolnic, A. (2020). *Theory and practice of online therapy: Internet-delivered interventions for individuals, groups, families, and organizations*. Routledge.

World Health Organisation (2016). *Monitoring and evaluating digital health interventions: A practical guide to conducting research and assessment*. Geneva. Licence: CC BY-NC-SA 3.0 IGO

World Health Organisation (2021). Global strategy on digital health 2020–2025. Geneva. Licence: CC BY-NC-SA 3.0 IGO

Walther, J. B. (2007). Selective self-presentation in computer-mediated communication: Hyperpersonal dimensions of technology, language, and cognition. *Computers in Human Behavior*, 23(5), 2538–2557.

van Nieuwerburgh, C., & Biswas-Diener, R. (2020). Positive psychology approaches to coaching. In Passmore, J. (Eds.), The Coaches' Handbook (pp. 314–321). Routledge: London.

Reid, D. J., & Reid, F. J. (2007). Text or talk? Social anxiety, loneliness, and divergent preferences for cell phone use. *CyberPsychology & Behavior*, 10(3), 424–435.

18

MOTIVATION; THE SELF, THE STICK, AND THE CARROT

Ciara Scott and Karen Morgan

> By annihilating the desires, you annihilate the mind. Every man without passions has within him no principle of action, nor motive to act.
>
> *– Claude Adrien Helvetius*

Defining motivation

The word motivation is derived from the Latin word motivus meaning "a moving cause." This reflects both the psychological and behavioural elements of motivation and the role that meaning, purpose, beliefs, and action play in determining it. Motivation is dynamic and subject to change over time in line with changes in our needs, beliefs, and values. Put simply, when we are motivated, we act. This action is designed to meet a need (e.g. hunger), bring about change (e.g. smoking behaviour) or move us closer to a goal or desired state (e.g. training for a sporting event). Specific motivations can be based on biological needs (e.g. food) or on learning (e.g. working towards a promotion at work). For healthcare professionals and coaches working with patients or clients, motivation is a key determinant of progress and success. Therefore, having a clear understanding of this complex construct and how to effectively assess and scaffold motivation is essential.

As with many other complex psychological constructs, there is no single or simple definition of motivation. The Oxford English dictionary describes it as "the reason why somebody does something or behaves in a particular way." The American Cambridge dictionary emphasises bidirectionality, defining motivation as "the willingness to do something, or something that causes such willingness." The fact that the thesaurus describes 46 synonyms including impetus, desire, drive, predetermination, incentive, encouragement, spur, and catalyst, speaks to the many faces of motivation. From a health psychology perspective, Morrison and Bennett (2021) define it as "memories, thoughts, experiences, needs and

DOI: 10.4324/9781003378426-21   282

preferences that act together to influence (drive) the type, strength and persistence of our actions".

In the early 1980s, Kelinginna compiled over one hundred definitions or statements about motivation dating as far back as 1884 and attempted to "resolve terminological confusion". The authors identified two categories which emphasised internal mechanisms, these were: phenomonogical (conscious or experiential processes) and physiological (internal physical processes). Three emphasised functional mechanisms: energising (energy arousal), directing and vector (energy arousal and direction), while two more were identified as restrictive (temporal-restrictive and process restrictive). Two categories emphasised the breadth of motivation (broad/balanced) or considered motivation the cause of all behaviour (all inclusive), (Kleinginna & Kleinginna, 1981). Despite efforts to identify, analyse, and categorise definitions of motivation, no consensus has been achieved to date.

Theories of motivation

Early theories

Theories of motivation have evolved over centuries and date back to the stoics and ancient philosophers. Aristotle hypothesised that "intellect in itself moves nothing" and that the faculty of desire (orektron) was responsible for movement or action (Hudson, 1981).

One of the early and most influential theories of motivation is drive reduction theory, proposed by Clark Hull in the 1940's. The theory is based on the concept of homeostasis and the idea that the body actively works to maintain a state of balance or equilibrium and within the range in which it functions well. Drives (which are unpleasant), e.g., thirst, produce a tension or state of arousal which impels action, resulting in a reward that reduces the drive. The concept of homeostasis is useful for understanding basic physiological drives; however, psychologists have recognised that we are also motivated by positive goals or incentives. For example, hunger is a drive which is satisfied by food, but we often use food as an incentive to eat past satisfaction, e.g. telling children to eat all their meal so the 'earn' a dessert as a reward. The incentive perspective also explains why success (e.g. creative, sporting, business) tends to create a greater desire or drive for success.

The Yerkes-Dodson law (named after the scientists that described it in the early 1900's) has been used to describe the phenomenon whereby we perform best when at the optimum level of arousal (intermediate). If we are under aroused we are sluggish or bored (in the 'comfort zone'), and if we are over aroused we find it difficult to focus and may be panicked. There is a 'goldilocks' or 'just right' zone of arousal at which we perform best. Essentially, increasing arousal levels helps focus motivation on a task, but only up to a certain point.

A century after the work of Yerkes and Dodson, the work of Carol Dweck (2008) on mindsets aligns developing a growth mindset with intentionally leaving our comfort zone, taking healthy risks to achieve positive outcomes. This work has further extended our understanding of drives, incentives, and human motivation.

Content and process theories of motivation

Currently, theories of motivation are often categorised as content theories or process theories. The former attempt to explain what motivation is, while the latter are concerned with how motivation occurs. Content theories include Herzberg's two-factor or motivation hygiene theory (Herzberg et al., 1957), McClelland's achievement motivation theory (1961) and Maslow's hierarchy of needs (1954). Process theories include Skinner's reinforcement theory (1958), Vroom's expectancy theory (1964) and Locke's goal setting theory (1968).

The field of positive psychology was developed to explore the understanding that happiness was not the absence of unhappiness (Seligman & Csikszentmihalyi, 2000). Similarly, Herzberg (1957) proposed that satisfaction at work was not the opposite of dissatisfaction. Whilst satisfaction was associated with intrinsic factors (motivators), he identified that dissatisfaction was associated with extrinsic factors, which he called hygiene factors. This differentiation between intrinsic motivation (something we innately do for flow or pleasure) and extrinsic motivation (something that is motivated by external forces, fears, or rewards), is common across theories of motivation.

McClelland's theory (1961) assumed that everyone has a dominant driving motivator; the motivation for achievement, for affiliation or for power and that these are developed through life experiences. He summarised that identifying drivers for motivation can be useful for setting goals, giving feedback, using incentives and rewards. Identifying individual drivers of motivation remains a central component of many behaviour change theories and interventions. Maslow (1954) theorised that motivation for survival is our primary need and people are not motivated towards higher needs (e.g. love, esteem) until their basic physiological and safety needs are fulfilled. Maslow also stated that whilst motivation to fulfil basic needs decreases as they are achieved (deficiency needs), meeting higher needs such as self-actualisation (growth needs) increases motivation. This theory is aligned with Fredrickson's broaden and build theory which posits that positive emotions enhance motivation, contributing to an upward spiral (Fredrickson, 2001). According to this theory, positive health behaviours can be practiced, developed, and shared and can positively impact psychological, cognitive, social, and physical resources. Resulting actions build enduring adaptive responses and personal resources such as optimism, resilience and social support and enhance health and flourishing. These responses can build social connection and positive spirals through groups and organisations (Fredrickson, 2001). Positive affective processes, i.e. positive emotions about exercise, such as enjoyment lead to sustainable health behaviours, more so than positive cognitive processes such as understanding the benefits (Van Cappellen et al., 2017).

The concept that we "learn from our mistakes" probably stems from Skinner's reinforcement theory. This theory proposed that people were more likely to repeat actions that had a positive outcome and less likely to repeat behaviour that had undesirable outcomes. He called this the "law of effect". Skinner's operant learning theory (Skinner, 1953) further identified that whilst positive reinforcement (reward) was strongly correlated with repeat behaviour, punishment only led to temporary changes in behaviour, even when the punishment was severe. This theory became known as "behaviourism." Vroom's expectancy theory of motivation (1964) also links the expected outcome to behaviour. Vroom assumed that behaviour was a conscious choice designed to maximise pleasure and minimise pain, hence people behaved in a way that maximised rewards.

Confucius has been quoted as saying, "When it is obvious that the goals cannot be reached, don't adjust the goals, adjust the action steps." Goal-setting is a core principle of coaching and positive psychology and authors have highlighted both that a growth mindset builds the motivation to achieve challenging goals (Dweck, 2009) and that failure to achieve goals and manage expectations can be disabling and demotivating (Fogg, 2019). Locke's goal setting theory rejected "behaviourism" and provided the theoretical framework for what is now more commonly known as SMART goals, first described by Doran in the 1980s (Doran, 1981). The theory holds that for goals to be successful they should have clarity (be specific), be open to evaluation of performance and success (measurable), be attainable (achievable) be realistic and reasonable (relevant) and be time-based or time sensitive (time bound). Learning goals (growth orientated) lead to higher performance than performance goals (outcome) and there are a number of moderators and mechanisms that support goal attainment. Locke also highlighted the strong correlation between motivation and goal setting (Locke, 1996). High self-efficacy and optimism can encourage people to have more confidence setting high reaching, long-term end goals. Whitmore (2010) outlines the benefits of using the SMART approach to develop smaller performance goals with incremental measures of success which can be celebrated, as success helps to maintain this motivation and confidence.

Motivation, health and behaviour change

Much of the work on motivation stems from studies of the workplace; however, motivation is also of much interest to health psychologists. Health psychology has evolved as a field of research and practice which tries to understand why individuals do or do not engage in certain health behaviours, as well as the factors that are associated with behaviour change (Prestwich et al., 2017). In 2014, Michie and colleagues compiled over 80 models and theories of behaviour change. Motivation or the factors which play a role in determining motivation are common components of many of these models and theories. Specific cognitive factors that feature include self-efficacy, autonomy, perceived control, mastery/competence and self-regulation (Michie et al., 2014).

Bandura defined self-efficacy as "personal beliefs that determine how well one can execute a plan of action" (Bandura, 1977). Whilst experiences of mastery and accomplishment support persistence and build self-efficacy, negative experiences and prolonged coping behaviours have the opposite effect.

Related to self-efficacy is the concept of perceived control which is a key feature of the theory of planned behaviour (TPB) another very popular theory from health psychology (Ajzen, 1991). According to TPB, behaviour is determined largely by intention which is in turn determined by attitudes, subjective norms and perceived behavioural control. Perceived behaviour control refers to the extent to which we feel able to perform a desired behaviour when faced with barriers (internal or external). Self-efficacy or belief in the ability to perform a behaviour, as well as external factors such as time, resources and the environment all impact perceived behavioural control. There is also some evidence to support the saying, "fake it 'till you make it." Self-belief can motivate actions that build positive emotions, resilience and confidence (Robertson, 2021).

Like self-determination theory (SDT), Bandura's social cognitive theory highlights the role of social and structural support in shaping positive health behaviours. Successful athletes recognise the importance of their training environment and fellow competitors. Motivating athletes to develop group meaning, belonging and social identity is often a key strategy in high performance sports (Slater et al., 2013). In the Irish longitudinal aging study (TILDA) social disengagement in later life was associated with more negative perceptions of ageing while engagement and cognitive stimulation was associated with more positive perceptions of ageing. Key components of ageing perceptions are beliefs about consequences and control (Robertson & Kenny, 2016). Other researchers have highlighted the association between autonomy and perception of control through the life course on positive health (Burke et al., 2022).

Bandura outlined the links between motivation, self-efficacy, confidence, and behaviour. Building confidence builds motivation (Bandura, 1997). People with high self-efficacy tend to be optimistic about the future and have higher levels of physical and psychological health (Seligman, 2006). Whilst self-efficacy defines the power of "I can" rather than "I will" and so is not directly attributable to behaviour, high self-efficacy can be associated with high functioning, high resilience, and reduced stress (Boniwell & Tunariu, 2019).

Motivation and positive psychology

Theories of positive psychology are also strongly correlated with theories of health behaviour. Positive psychology was developed to understand human flourishing and provides a lens for viewing humans as proactive, creative and self-determined, not passive individuals, dependent on external forces (Boniwell & Tunariu, 2019).

Like self-determination, positive psychology also aims to understand, test, develop and facilitate flourishing environments that support individuals and communities to thrive (Boniwell & Tunariu, 2019). Positive psychology provides a framework for broadening and building positive emotions, which in turn can broaden the scope for cognition and creativity and enhance resilience and coping in adversity (Fredrickson, 2001). Lastly, positive psychology also emphasises the bidirectional relationship between positive actions and positive emotions. Whilst positive emotions can enhance motivation, actions can also be a mechanism for developing motivation, meaning, purpose and positive emotions, building agency and progress (Seligman, 2006). Seligman describes agency as the mindset that we can accomplish goals now and in the future by drawing on our resources of efficacy, optimism, and imagination (Seligman, 2023). Both the concept of positive well-being (Ryff & Singer, 1998) and Seligman's PERMA model (Seligman, 2018) place meaning and purpose as central to eudaimonic positive health. Other theories have emphasised the role of hope and optimism for positive health behaviours and that like helplessness, optimism can be learnt by reframing our beliefs, as negative beliefs can have a detrimental effect on our emotions and subsequent behaviours (Boniwell & Tunariu, 2019).

Updated definitions of health also promote the dynamic nature of health as "the ability to adapt and self-manage" (Huber, 2011). Health and disease are not binary or mutually exclusive. Canguilhem theorised, "to be in good health means being able to fall sick and recover" (Canguilhem, 1991 Cited in Boyd, 2000). When health is viewed as an action rather than a status the role of motivation, autonomy, control, adaptability and resilience in being healthy become clear (Boyd, 2000). Positive emotions and eudaimonic happiness are associated with better positive habits such as sleep, exercise and positive relationships and are also associated with a reduction in negative habits such smoking and drinking alcohol excessively (Lianov et al., 2019). Ed Sheeran's song "Bad Habits" describes how good intentions can be overwhelmed by a downward spiral of one bad habit leading to another. There is evidence that the synergy between physical health, positive emotions and positive social connections collectively sustains an upward spiral effect (Kok et al., 2013). Intrinsic emotions can enhance motivation and positive behaviours, such as healthier dietary choices and improve physiological measures of health such as vagal tone and heart rate variability (Lianov, 2021).

Some models of behaviour deal specifically with health threats, e.g. protection motivation theory (Rogers, 1975, 1983). The theory holds that we assess the severity of an event, the probability that the event will occur if no protective behaviour is carried out and the availability and effectiveness of coping responses. The use of fear or threat to change attitudes and behaviour has been the subject of much research. The effectiveness of threat messages is closely linked with an individual's beliefs about their ability to act. Where people don't feel able to act, fear messages may just provoke worry.

These models represent the volume of research aimed at understanding the complexity of health behaviour over decades. They have common themes that help us understand how actions can be enabled or limited by beliefs, values, experiences, and support, which is valuable in understanding the complexity and bidirectional nature of how motivation works. Whilst many interventions place the onus on individuals to change, health has broad social, economic, commercial, political, and cultural determinants and an individual's attitudes, motivation, and behaviour can be enabled or limited by their support dyads and broader social norms (Duggan, 2019).

Bronfenbrenner (1979) developed a conceptual model for the layers of environmental factors that influenced a child's development. He described the microsystem as the immediate social and physical environment, broadening out through a mesosystem and ecosystem towards the broader social, environment, and cultural determinants of health, which he called the macrosystem. The model defines the links within and between these systems that set the context for growth.

Deci and Ryan's self-determination theory (SDT) (1985) outlined three core psychological needs: autonomy, relatedness (sense of belonging and connectedness) and competence, (sense of mastery over tasks). Autonomy is required for us to grow, learn, and reach our potential. SDT assumes that people are naturally orientated towards growth and strive to develop skills, independence, and connection with others, but rely on positive social environments to meet their basic psychological needs. For instance, babies naturally seek growth, learn to crawl, speak and demand attention to meet their needs, but there is also evidence that social and physical environments can threaten child development, causing both short-term adaptive responses and long-term effects on a child's capacity for learning, growth, forming relationships and their health and behaviour (Shonkoff et al., 2012). A meta-analysis that examined the impact of health interventions informed by SDT on health outcomes, measured small to medium changes in SDT constructs and health behaviours. Small positive changes in health outcomes were associated with autonomous motivation, but not controlled motivation or amotivation (Ntoumanis et al., 2021).

Health as a behaviour

Theories of positive psychology strongly correlate with theories of health behaviour. Theories of health behaviour identify the importance of motivation in health behaviours and the complex relationship with self-efficacy, actions, achievement, and positive emotions. Whilst we might assume that we need to feel motivated before we can do something these theories also suggest that positive emotions and actions build and sustain motivation. By contrast, Maier and Seligman (Maier & Seligman, 1976, 1967) described a "learned helplessness" effect. This effect occurs where individuals experience a negative uncontrolled situation and over time stop trying to change the situation (even if they have the ability to do so). This cycle is associated with all-or-nothing thinking. A lack of motivation is a common and important symptom of depression.

Developmental psychologists such as Erikson remind us of the importance of changes in health motivation across the lifespan. Adolescents, for example, are unlikely to be motivated by messages about long-term health. Agel (2016) concluded that the potential psychosocial determinants of oral health behaviour in adolescents were self-efficacy, intention, and social influences. For instance,

288

when making food choices in a secondary school environment (Browne et al., 2020), participants knew about the healthy eating policies and "what we should eat," but the social influence of sharing food and being part of a group swayed their food choices of discounted treats and snacks at local convenience stores. This example highlights the benefits of finding a tribe with shared values and that the gap between motivation, intention, and behaviour can be supported by positive social influences and supports.

Practice

Motivating others

Self-regulation refers to effortful control over one's thoughts, emotions, choices, impulses, and behaviours (Reed et al., 2020). There are three phases in self-regulation: goal awareness setting, goal pursuits and goal attainment, maintenance, or disengagement. Phase one may be supported by techniques such as motivational interviewing (MI). MI aims to evoke intrinsic motivation to change and is defined as:

> a collaborative, goal-oriented style of communication with particular attention to the language of change. It is designed to strengthen personal motivation for and commitment to a specific goal by eliciting and exploring the person's own reasons for change within an atmosphere of acceptance and compassion.
>
> *(Miller & Rollnick, 2013, p. 3)*

MI was originally developed for patients with addiction, but has been adapted and used for broader health behaviour change. It is patient-centred and can be used to explore ambivalence, resistance, or beliefs about health behaviour change. This process can be used to increase both patient and practitioner awareness of a patient's ambivalence or motivation before progressing to goal setting or what is called 'change talk'. MI recognises the importance of the patient's own motivation and readiness for change in successful behaviour change. If a patient is ambivalent, then just building rapport and awareness to reach a point where they are willing to contemplate change is most valuable.

In phase two, goal pursuit, feedback plays an important role in building confidence, self-efficacy, and maintaining awareness. Social support and learning from others also play a valuable role in broadening and building autonomy and competence. Bandura highlighted that people learn not just from their own experiences or from tuition, but are motivated by observing behaviours that others model and so learn vicariously from the positive and negative consequences of others' behaviour (Bandura, 1969). Goal ladders can be useful to build goal attainment. Consistent with the move towards a more patient-centred model of healthcare and shared decision-making, many practitioners are developing skills that support patients in being active participants in their own care. By definition, coaching conversations create a safe space for a non-directive, equal partnership where a client sets their own goals with support. The third phase of self-regulation involves goal attainment, maintenance, or disengagement. Attainment can mark the start of a new phase with the establishment of a new goal or if the goal has not been attained, the establishment of a new more attainable one.

The transtheoretical model (TTM) of behaviour change (Prochaska & DiClemente, 1982, 1992; Prochaska et al., 1994), one of the most common theories applied to understanding health behaviour (Michie et al., 2014), includes maintenance and relapse as one of its stages. The TTM describes the staged process by which individuals start to think about change, plan for change and start a new health behaviour. According to the theory there are five stages in the change cycle: pre-contemplation (not ready for the change), contemplation (thinking about the change), preparation (setting goals and preparing for action), action (taking action towards the new goal) and maintenance (maintaining a positive behaviour). The TTM outlines ten process of change that can prompt or support movement between stages. These include experiential processes such as consciousness raising and environmental revaluation, which are used more in the early stages of change and behavioural processes such as counterconditioning and reinforcement management which come into play in action and maintenance stages.

Authors have highlighted the importance of autonomy and independence, as well as the role the perception of support and control can play in subjective well-being and health behaviour (Burke et al., 2022). By example, one of the pillars of lifestyle medicine is exercise. We know physical activity is important for health, but clients may hold a belief that this activity is something they don't like or can't do. Coaching can bring awareness of what a client would be motivated by and what activity they may enjoy. Motivation to exercise may be very different for different people. Some may express how much they love the way they feel during exercise, some may say their motivation is how energised they feel afterwards (intrinsic motivation). For others, simply reframing this as movement may change their perception from something that is directed, such as a fitness class, to something that can be spontaneous like dancing. Some may be training towards a fitness goal, their incentive may be positive; for others it may be to reduce their health risk of osteoporosis or to lose weight (extrinsic motivation, fear or incentive). Some people love counting their steps or using data to measure their progress; for others it is the simple pleasure of nature, fresh air. Some people prefer time alone or activities that are creative such as gardening (Soga et al., 2017); for others joining a class or a team is motivating. Whilst collective effervescence was originally coined to describe the positive emotions and awe experienced from large religious gatherings, it has been more recently applied to the collective positive health benefits of group activities, teams and events (Gabriel et al., 2020). Understanding motivation is a key element in positive health and in supporting individuals to take positive steps towards better health. It is important also to bear in mind that goals that motivate us can be culturally based and reinforced. In collectivist cultures, the rights and responsibilities of the group take precedence over that of the individual. In individualistic cultures this is reversed.

Bandura's social cognitive theory has been expanded to describe "collective efficacy." Whilst this term was originally defined in educational settings, it has also been applied to the role of social and support networks in health behaviour and the management of chronic diseases (Vassilev et al., 2019). "The Frome Project" also demonstrated the health benefits of building compassion and positive emotions at a community level, with reduced levels of loneliness and depression and a reduction in hospital admissions (Abel, 2018). This project supports theories of group medicine and the benefits of collective motivation. In addition, Huta (2012) identified that hedonistic and eudaimonic motives for activities also positively impacted on close others, similar to the "positive ripple effect" described by Fredrickson (2001).

People may have very different motivations for participating in a particular health behaviour or not and it has been found that behaviours cluster in populations (Conry et al., 2011). The COM-B behaviour change wheel was developed to provide practitioners with a systematic approach to personalising health behaviour change interventions (Michie et al., 2011). It is a synthesis of 19 behaviour change frameworks, identified by systematic review. The COM-B model provides a simple framework for understanding behaviour, in which 'capability' (physical and psychological), 'opportunity' (physical and social) and 'motivation' (automatic and reflective) are conceptualised as three essential conditions for behaviour (Michie et al., 2011). When using the wheel, a client identifies the broader social, physical, psychological and support elements that they will benefit from in planning and actioning positive health changes. At stage one (understand the behaviour) the client is encouraged to identify what needs to change and select a target behaviour. Stage two (identify intervention options) focuses on designing and evaluating interventions using the APEASE criteria for the goals they have set (acceptability, practicality, effectiveness, affordability, safety, and equity). In stage three (identify content and implementation options) specific behaviour change techniques are identified (again, considering APEASE criteria). This tool provides a practical toolkit for behaviour change.

Conclusion

It seems that there has never been more interest in understanding the complex construct that is motivation. The pandemic highlighted the importance of both adaptability and self-management: we observed the habits of people and groups and we questioned the motives of scientists, healthcare workers and governments. We have learned that complex public health challenges require multiple *f*its levels of intervention and "cannot be solved by simply focussing on individual responsibility and behavioural interventions" (Thomas & Daube, 2023). This chapter has outlined some of the models and theories that enhance our understanding of the complexity of motivation and its role in health behaviour. Multiple stakeholders in healthcare provision benefit from understanding and applying behavioural science in strategies to enhance positive health.

Takeaways

General

- Motivation is strongly associated with action and with values, beliefs, competence, self-efficacy, experience, and social support.
- Sustainable behaviour change is easiest when it taps into intrinsic motivation or autonomic motivation rather than relying on control.
- Language that patients and clients perceive to be supportive of autonomy is more effective in supporting behaviour change than language that can be perceived as controlling.

Practical

- Focus on getting started. Agency and progress build motivation.
- It can be difficult to motivate others; listen to understand their motivation, values, and beliefs and what has worked well for them before, so that they can set achievable goals. Is the motivation driven by intrinsic motivation (the self) a positive reward (the carrot) or by fear and compliance (the stick)?
- Positive and health psychology provide frameworks and a "toolbox" for emphasising the positive effects of health and building agency. Use tools to maintain and sustain motivation over time.
- It is helpful to look at alignment between values and external influences on motivation. Feedback that supports autonomy can improve self-regulation.
- People can learn from what motivates them and makes them feel successful in one area of their life and apply this to other goals. If someone feels "demotivated" find out what inspires and energises them as practicing positive habits rebuilds agency.

Wicked questions

1 Which comes first motivation or action?
2 What happens when motivations clash or compete?
3 What can people learn from being in flow in the past that can help them to understand what motivates them?

References

Abel, J. (2018). Compassionate Frome. *BMJ*, 363, k4299.

Agel, M. (2016). Psychosocial determinants of oral health behaviour in adolescents. *Evidence-Based Dentistry*, 17(3), 72.

Ajzen, I. (1991). The theory of planned behaviour. *Organisational Behaviour and Human Decision Processes*, 50, 179–211.

Bandura, A. (1969). Social-learning theory of identificatory processes. In D. A. Goslin (Ed.), *Handbook of socialization theory and research* (pp. 213–262). Rand McNally & Company.

Bandura, A. (1977). Self-efficacy: Toward a unifying theory of behavioral change. *Psychological Review*, 84(2), 191–215.

Bandura, A. (1997). *Self-efficacy: The exercise of control.* W H Freeman/Times Books/ Henry Holt & Co.

Boniwell, I., & Tunariu, A. D. (2019). *Positive psychology: Theory, research and applications.* McGraw-Hill Education.

Boyd, K. M. (2000). Disease, illness, sickness, health, healing and wholeness: Exploring some elusive concepts. *Medical Humanities*, 26, 9–17.

Bronfenbrenner, U. (1979). *The ecology of human development: Experiments by nature and design.* Harvard University Press.

Browne, S., Barron, C., Staines, A., & Sweeney, M. (2020). 'We know what we should eat but we don't...': A qualitative study in Irish secondary schools. *Health Promotion International*, 35(5), 984–993.

Burke, T. J., Young, V. J., & Duggan, A. (2022). Recognizing the blurred boundary between health-related support and control in close relationships. *Personal Relationships*, 29(4), 644–673.

Canguilhem, G. (1991). *The normal and the pathological.* Zone Books.

Conry, M.C., Morgan, K., Curry, P. et al. (2011). The clustering of health behaviours in Ireland and their relationship with mental health, self-rated health and quality of life. *BMC Public Health*, 11, 692. https://doi.org/10.1186/1471-2458-11-692

Deci, E. L., & Ryan, R. M. (1985). *Intrinsic motivation and self-determination in human behavior.* Springer Science & Business Media.

Doran, G. T. (1981). There's a SMART way to write management's goals and objectives. *Journal of Management Review*, 70, 35–36.

Duggan, A. P. (2019). *Health and illness in close relationships.* Cambridge University Press.

Dweck, C. (2008). *Mindset: The new psychology of success* (1st ed.). Random House.

Dweck, C. (2009). Mindsets: Developing talent through a growth mindset. *Olympic Coach*, 21, 4–7.

Fogg, B. J. (2019). *Tiny habits: The small changes that change everything.* Eamon Dolan Books.

Fredrickson, B. L. (2001). The role of positive emotions in positive psychology: The broaden-and-build theory of positive emotions. *American Psychologist*, 56(3), 218.

Gabriel, S., Naidu, E., Paravati, E., Morrison, C. D., & Gainey, K. (2020). Creating the sacred from the profane: Collective effervescence and everyday activities. *The Journal of Positive Psychology*, 15(1), 129–154.

Herzberg, F., Mausner, B., Peterson, R. O., & Capwell, D. F. (1957). *Job attitudes. Review of research and opinion.* Psychological Service of Pittsburgh.

Huber, M., Knottnerus, J. A., Green, L., van der Horst, H., Jadad, A. R., Kromhout, D., Leonard, B., Lorig, K., Loureiro, M. I., van der Meer, J. W., Schnabel, P., Smith, R., van Weel, C., & Smid, H. (2011). How should we define health?. *BMJ (Clinical research ed.)*, 343, d4163. https://doi.org/10.1136/bmj.d4163

Hudson, S. D. (1981). Reason and motivation in Aristotle. *Canadian Journal of Philosophy*, 11(1), 111–135.

Huta, V., Pelletier, L. G., Baxter, D., & Thompson, A. (2012). How eudaimonic and hedonic motives relate to the well-being of close others. *The Journal of Positive Psychology*, 7(5), 399–404.

Kleinginna, P. R., & Kleinginna, A. M. (1981). A categorized list of motivation definitions, with a suggestion for a consensual definition. *Motivation and Emotion*, 5, 263–291. https://doi.org/10.1007/BF00993889

Kok, B. E., Coffey, K. A., Cohn, M. A., Catalino, L. I., Vacharkulksemsuk, T., Algoe, S. B., Brantley, M., & Fredrickson, B. L. (2013). How positive emotions build physical health: perceived positive social connections account for the upward spiral between positive emotions and vagal tone. *Psychological Science*, 24(7), 1123–1132. https://doi.org/10.1177/0956797612470827

Lianov L. (2021). A powerful antidote to physician burnout: Intensive Healthy Lifestyle and Positive Psychology Approaches. *American Journal of Lifestyle Medicine*, 15(5), 563–566. https://doi.org/10.1177/15598276211006626

Lianov, L. S., Fredrickson, B. L., Barron, C., Krishnaswami, J., & Wallace, A. (2019). Positive Psychology in Lifestyle Medicine and Health Care: Strategies for Implementation. *American journal of lifestyle medicine*, 13(5), 480–486. https://doi.org/10.1177/1559827619838992

Locke, E. A. (1968). Toward a theory of task motivation and incentives. *Organizational Behavior and Human Performance*, 3(2), 157–189.

Locke, E. A. (1996). Motivation through conscious goal setting. *Applied & Preventive Psychology*, 52(2), 117–124.

Maier, S. F., & Seligman, M. E. (1976). Learned helplessness: Theory and evidence. *Journal of Experimental Psychology: General*, 105(1), 3.

Maslow, A. H. (1954). *Motivation and personality*. Harper & Row Publishers.

McClelland, D. C. (1961). The achieving society. University of Illinois at Urbana-Champaign's Academy for Entrepreneurial Leadership Historical Research Reference in Entrepreneurship.

Michie, S., van Stralen, M. M., & West, R. (2011). The behaviour change wheel: A new method for characterising and designing behaviour change interventions. *Implementation Science*, 6(42). https://pubmed.ncbi.nlm.nih.gov/21513547/

Michie, S., West, R., Campbell, R., Brown, J., & Gainforth, H. (2014). *ABC of behaviour change theories*. Silverback Publishing.

Miller, W. R., & Rollnick, S. (2013). *Motivational interviewing: Helping people to change* (3rd ed.). Guilford Press.

Morrison, V., & Bennett, P. (2021). *Health psychology* (5th ed.). Pearson.

Ntoumanis, N., Ng, J. Y. Y., Prestwich, A., Quested, E., Hancox, J. E., Thøgersen-Ntoumani, C., Deci, E. L., Ryan, R. M., Lonsdale, C., & Williams, G. C. (2021). A meta-analysis of self-determination theory-informed intervention studies in the health domain: Effects on motivation, health behavior, physical, and psychological health. *Health Psychology Review*, 15(2), 214–244.

Prestwich, A., Conner, M., & Kenworthy, J. (2017). Health behavior change: Theories, methods and interventions (1st ed.). Taylor and Francis.

Prochaska, J. O., & DiClemente, C. C. (1982). Transtheoretical therapy: Toward a more integrative model of change. *Psychotherapy: Theory, Research and Practice*, 19(3), 276–288.

Prochaska, J. O., & DiClemente, C. C., & Norcross, J. C. (1992). In search of how people change: Applications to addictive behaviour. *American Psychologist*, 47, 1102–1114.

Prochaska, J. O., Redding, C. A., Harlow, L. L., & Rossi, J. S., & Velicer, W. F. (1994). The transtheoretical model of change and HIV prevention: A review. *Journal of Consulting and Clinical Psychology*, 21, 471–486.

Reed, R. G., Combs, H. L., & Segerstrom, S. C. (2020). The structure of self-regulation and its psychological and physical health correlates in older adults. *Collabra. Psychology*, 6(1), 23. https://doi.org/10.1525/collabra.297

Robertson, I. (2021). *How confidence works: The new science of self-belief*. Random House.

Robertson, D. A., & Kenny, R. A. (2016). "I'm too old for that"—The association between negative perceptions of aging and disengagement in later life. *Personality and Individual Differences*, 100, 114–119.

Rogers, R. W. (1975). A protection motivation theory of fear appeals and attitude change. *Journal of Psychology*, 91, 93–114.

Rogers, R. W. (1983). Cognitive and physiological processes in fear appeals and attitude change: A revised theory of protection motivation. In C. J. & P. R. (Eds.), *Social Psychophysiology* (pp. 153–177). Guilford Press.

Ryff, C. D., & Singer, B. (1998). The contours of positive human health. *Psychological Inquiry*, 9(1), 1–28.

Seligman, M. (2018). PERMA and the building blocks of well-being. *The Journal of Positive Psychology*, 13(4), 333–335.

Seligman, M. E. (2006). *Learned optimism: How to change your mind and your life.* Vintage.

Seligman, M. (2023). Psychological history and predicting the future. *Possibility Studies & Society*, 1(1–2), 206–210. https://doi.org/10.1177/27538699221128224

Seligman, M. E., & Csikszentmihalyi, M. (2000). Positive psychology: An introduction. *American Psychological Association*, 55(1), 5–14.

Seligman, M. E., & Maier, S. F. (1967). Failure to escape traumatic shock. *Journal of Experimental Psychology*, 74, 1–9.

Shonkoff, J. P., Richter, L., van der Gaag, J., & Bhutta, Z. A. (2012). An integrated scientific framework for child survival and early childhood development. *Pediatrics*, 129(2), e460–e472.

Skinner, B. F. (1953). *Science and human behaviour.* Free Press.

Skinner, B. F. (1958). Reinforcement today. *American Psychologist*, 13(3), 94–99.

Slater, M. J., Evans, A. L., & Barker, J. B. (2013). Using social identities to motivate athletes towards peak performance at the London 2012 Olympic Games: Reflecting for Rio 2016. *Reflective Practice: International and Multidisciplinary Perspectives*, 14(5), 672–679. doi: 10.1080/14623943.2013.835725

Soga, M., Gaston, K. J., & Yamaura, Y. (2017). Gardening is beneficial for health: A meta-analysis. *Preventive Medicine Reports*, 5, 92–99.

Thomas, S. & Daube, M. (February 2023). New times, new challenges for health promotion, Health Promotion International, 38(1), daad012. https://doi.org/10.1093/heapro/daad012

Van Cappellen, P., Rice, E. L., Catalino, L. I., & Fredrickson, B. L. (2017). Positive affective processes underlie positive health behaviour change. *Psychology & Health*, 33(1), 77–97.

Vassilev, I., Rogers, A., Kennedy, A., Oatley, C., & James, E. (2019). Identifying the processes of change and engagement from using a social network intervention for people with long-term conditions. A qualitative study. *Health Expect*, 22, 173–182.

Vroom, V. H. (1964). *Work and motivation.* Wiley.

Whitmore, J. (2010). *Coaching for performance: The principles and practice of coaching and leadership* (25th ed.). Nicholas Brealey Publishing.

19

POSITIVE PSYCHOLOGY FOR HEALTH EQUITY

Qadira M. Ali, Alyssa M. Vela and David Bowman

Positive psychology through a health equity lens

Positive Psychology: A Natural Partner in the Movement Toward Health Equity

As understanding of the multitude of factors contributing to racial and ethnic health disparities deepens, the call for health equity demands an increasingly multidisciplinary, broad-based approach. According to the Robert Wood Johnson Foundation (RWJF), "health equity means that everyone has a fair and just opportunity to be as healthy as possible" (RWJF, 2017). Achieving health equity requires focused, ongoing societal efforts to address avoidable inequities, historical and contemporary injustices, and the elimination of health and health care disparities (Braveman & Gruskin, 2003; Kelly, 2022). Positive psychology offers an underutilized approach in the health equity space (Sanders et al., 2021).

Racism - in its structural and interpersonal forms - functions as one of the most pernicious contributors to racial and ethnic physical and mental health disparities. Dr. Camara Jones, esteemed physician-researcher and racism expert, has described racism as "a system of structuring opportunity and assigning value based on the social interpretation of how one looks (which is what we call 'race'), that unfairly disadvantages some individuals and communities, unfairly advantages other individuals and communities, and saps the strength of the whole society through the waste of human resources" (Jones, 2000; APHA, n.d.). It is well-documented that racial minority groups, notably Black, Hispanic, and Indigenous individuals, experience discrimination and adverse physical and mental health outcomes at higher rates than white (typically majority group) individuals (Sanders et al., 2021). The biopsychosocial model of racism positions it as a significant stressor associated with psychological and physiological stress responses linked to numerous negative physical and mental health effects (Clark et al., 1999).

DOI: 10.4324/9781003378426-22   296

Microaggressions represent another contributor to psychological harm among racially diverse populations. Sue et al. (2007) defined microaggressions as "everyday verbal and nonverbal slights, snubs, or insults, whether intentional or unintentional, which communicate hostile, derogatory, or negative messages ... based solely upon marginalized group membership." Exposure to microaggressions has been associated with numerous detrimental psychological health effects, including eroded self-esteem, depressive symptoms, and psychological distress (Blume et al., 2012; Mercer et al., 2011; Nadal et al., 2014).

Among the proposed mechanisms for these differential outcomes, allostatic load and cumulative toxic stress function as triggers of chronic inflammation, which is considered the maladaptive progenitor of the most common chronic diseases in the Western world. This concept of unbridled chronic stress extending from exposure to racism highlights a promising intervention point for positive psychology within racially diverse populations (Guidi et al., 2021). The life course perspective offers a sobering reflection that children who begin to experience racism early in life accumulate high toxic stress exposure over time, thereby increasing their risk of potential adverse health effects (Jones & Neblett, 2017).

Positive psychology interventions (PPIs) may provide beneficial, healthful coping strategies for historically oppressed groups most affected by racial discrimination and health disparities. Overall, various PPIs have been associated with improved health outcomes, including lower rates of hypertension, anxiety, depression, cardiovascular disease, stroke, and inflammation (Kim et al., 2016). Even life expectancy benefits have been demonstrated in the context of PPIs focused on optimism (Lee et al., 2019). Given that historically marginalized communities of color typically experience worse outcomes of the aforementioned conditions and others, the potential utility of adding PPIs to the standard of care for medically vulnerable populations is clear.

Just as significantly, positive psychology may function as an approach to address prejudicial attitudes and discriminatory behavior among perpetrators (Sanders et al., 2021). The work of getting to the root of discrimination on an individual level complements the usual application of PPIs in helping minoritized groups build resilience against unfair treatment. Contrary to the focus of the past two decades of PPIs within racially minoritized groups, the burden of navigating discrimination should not be borne alone by marginalized community members, who may experience "racial battle fatigue" (Jones & Neblett, 2017; Sanders et al., 2021). Positive psychology must explore the drivers of, and psychological effects on, individuals who engage in discrimination. In a methodical process, clinicians may help to guide perpetrators of discrimination to a place more likely to be aligned with core values, like love, empathy, and compassion – all of which reside at the very heart of positive psychology (Drustrup, 2021).

Moreover, the field of positive psychology would miss an opportunity to promote one of its six core virtues – justice – by not proactively addressing how its clinicians may be leaders in health equity promotion. In more ways than one, the convergence of positive psychology and health equity promises to achieve more than solely helping historically oppressed groups cope better with challenging circumstances. This interplay promises to help disrupt one of the most hazardous social ills present today: racism.

Special considerations when applying a health equity lens to positive psychology

The field of positive psychology has been critiqued over the past two decades for its often lacking acknowledgement of the social determinants of health (SDOH), or those contextual factors that highly influence an individual's state of mental and physical health (Sanders, et al., 2021; van Zyl & Rothmann, 2022). According to the World Health Organization, social determinants are "the conditions in which people are born, grow, live, work and age. These circumstances are shaped by the distribution of money, power and resources at global, national and local levels" (WHO, 2012). Social determinants include social and economic conditions (e.g. education, income/employment, racism/discrimination, community safety, adverse childhood experiences), physical environment (e.g. pollution, transportation, food access), and health care access and quality (Kelly, 2022; WHO, 2012). It has been estimated that SDOH cumulatively account for more than 70–80% of health outcomes with the remaining 20–30% resulting from individual-level health behaviors, like nutrition, exercise, and smoking status (Hood et al., 2016). While the heart of many PPIs rests in affirming an individual's ability to thrive despite myriad life adversities, inadequate assessment, affirmation and addressing of the uniquely challenging circumstances experienced disproportionately by many communities of color falls short of health equity-driven practice.

Applying a health equity lens to PPIs additionally warrants an intersectional framework approach in order to fully capture the various sources of psychological stressors and strengths within diverse populations (Stevens-Watkins et al., 2014). Intersectionality acknowledges that an individual has multiple, intersecting social identities (e.g. race, gender, sexual orientation, socioeconomic status) that may interact to potentiate an individual's experience of oppression or privilege (Bowleg, 2012; Moradi & Subich, 2003). An intersectional framework helps to explain why some members of historically oppressed populations experience even higher levels of psychological distress in the course of daily life, given their multiple intersecting and oppressed identities. Using this more nuanced lens, clinicians may learn to approach diverse populations with deeper cultural humility, which is an approach characterized by a self-reflective, compassionate willingness to learn about others in a manner that aims to acknowledge and fix power imbalances (Yeager & Bauer-Wu, 2013). Multiple levels of oppression must be examined simultaneously to garner a full and complete picture of the context in which individuals live (Moradi & Subich, 2003).

While many communities of color shoulder a heavy burden as it relates to adverse SDOH, individuals from racially and ethnically diverse groups may simultaneously possess noteworthy culturally propagated protective factors that increase stress tolerance and foster well-being (Banks & Kohn-Wood, 2007; Jones & Neblett, 2017). For example, a strong sense of Black racial identity has been repeatedly associated with reduced negative mental health effects of racial discrimination exposure (Sellers et al., 2003). Spirituality and religiosity – values entrenched in many communities of color – may boost positive emotions like hope, optimism, and gratitude, all of which bolster individuals against adversity (McIntosh et al., 2021). Connecting with nature embeds a sense of groundedness found throughout diverse communities the world over. However, in the United States a "nature gap" exists along racial lines wherein predominantly Black areas may be three times as likely to be nature deprived (lacking in natural green spaces) as compared to majority white ones, yet another historical by-product of systemic racism (Rowland-Shea et al., 2020).

Since its establishment as a field, positive psychology has most often been studied in white, well-educated, Western samples (Ryff, 2022). This general population's experiences largely informed a presumed universal notion of well-being that is rife with potential for being culturally biased (van Zyl & Rothmann, 2022). As the application of positive psychology expands and diversifies through clinical encounters, research and training clinicians, the present moment necessitates adopting an attitude of cultural humility as all previously established tenets of PPIs may not resonate in more diverse populations (Ryff, 2022).

Resilience: a resource and a risk in combating inequities

Discrimination does not discriminate

As described in the previous section, people who experience discrimination, including those of minoritized race ethnicity, gender identity, and/or sexual orientation, often experience worse mental and physical health outcomes. Immigrants, people with disabilities and people with obesity are also at risk of worse mental health and suboptimal well-being due to stereotypes, prejudice, and discrimination. Among people with diverse sexual orientations and gender identities, forms of marginalization predict a host of negative outcomes, including lower life satisfaction and purpose, and worse psychological distress as suggested by a higher rate of suicide attempts (Sanders et al., 2021). While the following sections largely focus on the African American population, the underlying theme that marginalized groups experience worse health outcomes is broadly applicable across diverse minoritized populations.

In the sections that follow, notable themes relevant to the intersection of positive health, race, and resilience factors will be explored. The guiding query for what follows is: "In what ways has this historically marginalized racial group cultivated resilience despite entrenched racism?"

Positivity and optimism in African-Americans

African Americans demonstrate many of the same health benefits of optimism, emotional and social support as their white counterparts. Some data suggest that optimism and positivity portend improved psychological health, lower mortality, and improved cardiovascular health in African Americans (Lee et al., 2022;

Sims et al., 2019; Steinhardt et al., 2015). However, clinicians may unintentionally contribute to feelings of negativity toward patients who are not successful by labeling them "non-compliant." The health care team, in their attempts to support their patients to make meaningful lifestyle changes, must be aware of how their own attitudes and perspectives may influence positive (or negative) emotions in their patients. (Steinhardt et al., 2015). As such, screening patients for psychosocial stressors may help clinicians to develop more culturally sensitive lifestyle management plans. Interventions to support positive psychological well-being (such as positive emotions, active coping, and social support) are warranted to address modifiable barriers (Brewer et al., 2018).

The impact of social inequalities vs. lifestyle habits on health

In the traditional medical model, health is influenced by personal health behaviors, genetics, and access to health care. However, the Bay Area Regional Health Inequities Initiative (2020) developed a conceptual framework connecting social inequalities and health. The framework notes that the factors related to direct medical care account for less than 30% of health outcomes; the other 70% of health outcomes are accounted for by the social, political, and economic environment. The rules and practices that sociopolitical and environmental systems enact and promote determine who has (and who does not have) access to resources and opportunities. The health of racial and ethnic minorities therefore is not solely a direct result of their behaviors and actions. Rather, the environments in which individuals live and the policies surrounding them play a significant role in shaping opportunities to influence what choices they can make (Kelly, 2022).

For example, food insecurity – or the state of being without reliable access to a sufficient quantity of affordable, nutritious food to live an active, healthy life – is known to disproportionately affect Black and Hispanic individuals (Walker et al., 2021). This economic condition may heighten chronic stress levels and constrain opportunities for healthful food choices – all of which increase risk for chronic disease (Myers, 2020). Accordingly, lifestyle medicine interventions should integrate validated screening for food insecurity, or consider nutrition security screening as a more nuanced method to assess consistent access to health-promoting foods (Mozaffarian, 2023).

Resilience, spirituality and mental health stigma

Within the African American community, spirituality may manifest through interconnectedness (with God and others). Faith operates as a mechanism through which to reframe adversities as conquerable struggles that can lead to personal empowerment. Spiritual practices (e.g. prayer, singing hymns) strengthen the relationship with God by encouraging people to be emotionally, physically, and spiritually engulfed in the experience of worship. Thus, spirituality has been found to be a meaningful coping mechanism among many communities of color, including African Americans and Latinos. (Drolet & Lucas,

2020; Herren et al., 2019). There is evidence that frequent spiritual experiences are associated with improved inflammatory responses and less severe depressive symptomatology, which are associated with better neurocognitive performance in those who are exposed to physiological and psychological stress (Herren et al., 2019). Aspects of spirituality in the African American community have developed to directly oppose racism and oppression and offer unique means for combatting the harmful effects of racism (Drolet & Lucas, 2020). Many African Americans and others in the African diaspora seek guidance and mental wellness from their faith as opposed to seeking medical attention, in part due to stigma surrounding mental illness (Codjoe et al., 2021). Given the impact of stigma on deterring some members of this population from seeking mental health treatment, spirituality may be an alternative, culturally relevant intervention to address depression and improve resilience - when broached with cultural humility (Herren et al., 2019).

Resilience and race

Belonging to a minoritized racial group is a risk factor for negative outcomes such as poor physical health, unemployment, and discrimination (Steinhardt et al., 2015). As such, African Americans experience more adversity than white individuals, and subsequently, more opportunities for resilience. Resilience denotes a greater ability to bounce back from adversity. Resilience also emerged as a common theme among African American respondents in the face of unemployment, incarceration, and discrimination. Older African Americans' experiences of surviving and enduring racism are central to their responses to life threatening illnesses. Strength and perseverance acquired in response to racism may explain the higher level of resilience (Steinhardt et al., 2015).

Resilience and John Henryism

The Social Stress Paradigm postulates that socially disadvantaged groups will experience poor physical and mental health due to increased exposure to stressors, yet fewer financial resources and coping resources. However, these expectations are not always reflected in African Americans' health patterns. One of the culturally relevant coping approaches is John Henryism, which may buffer the adverse impact of stress on health. The John Henryism construct derives from both folk legend, "John Henry," a Black steel driver, and a real-life 1940s-era sharecropper, John Henry Martin (James, 1994; Robinson & Tobin, 2021). John Henry utilized all his resources to successfully beat out a machine for railroad construction, but he died right afterwards from physical and mental exhaustion. John Henry Martin similarly suffered health deterioration while trying to achieve financial security during the Jim Crow era. John Henryism may have emerged as a coping strategy during the racially fraught Jim Crow and segregation eras to overcome the effects of systemic racism – through glorifying hard work and perseverance.

301

While John Henryism is a culturally relevant form of coping (and is not limited to African Americans), this construct may be both a physical and mental health risk and resource (Robinson & Tobin, 2021). John Henryism is considered a persistent high-energy, active coping style to overcome adversity (James, 1994). Someone with high John Henryism would actively face adversity with vigor and determination; on the other hand, someone with low John Henryism would tend to feel more discouraged and easily overcome by life's struggles (Robinson & Tobin, 2021). John Henryism may contribute to physical health problems, while simultaneously promoting positive mental health. High levels of John Henryism may be psychologically protective because it cultivates a greater sense of mental fortitude and perseverance through difficult times. Robinson and Tobin further discussed that while this high effort coping approach may be physiologically strenuous, it could potentially promote healthy behaviors, such as a healthy diet and exercise (2021). On the contrary, in the environmental affordances model, some psychologically protective coping strategies, such as substance use and consumption of unhealthy foods, may be key contributing factors to poor physical health among Black Americans. This suggests that Black Americans may engage in a wide range of coping strategies that are distinct to this population and may be health-promoting and health-challenging at the same time (Robinson & Tobin, 2021).

The superwoman schema: resilience and Black women

In an article by Allen et al., African American women have been described as balancing traditionally hard traits of self-reliance, independence, hard work, achievement, assertiveness, and strength with traditionally soft roles of nurturer and caregiver (2019). Sojourner Truth in the mid-19th century became a symbol of strength and resilience among African American women. In her speech, "Ain't I a Woman?," she describes her need to develop a toughness that enabled her to "work [the fields]...as much as a man....and bear the lash [endure the pain/whippings of slavery] as well!" She was simultaneously responsible for motherhood and caretaking without the conveniences of white womanhood, such as being "helped into carriages" and "lifted over ditches." Thus, African American women are often treated like their male counterparts, while simultaneously being prohibited from expressions of weakness or vulnerability for the sake of survival (Allen et al., 2019).

This image of the strong Black woman has persisted throughout generations and is described, even today, as an asset that allows African American women to manage their lives in a race- and gender-conscious society. Among African American women, being strong has been described as (1) feeling an obligation to present an image of strength, even when one didn't feel strong, (2) feeling an obligation to suppress emotions, (3) resistance to being vulnerable or dependent on others, (4) determination to succeed despite limited resources, and (5) obligation to help others (Allen et al., 2019). The "superwoman schema" may be a double-edged sword for African American women, providing them with the fortitude and determination to withstand and support others in the context of race and gender specific stressors. However, it may simultaneously increase the risk for stress-related adverse health outcomes due to activation of the hypothalamic–pituitary–adrenal (HPA) axis, chronic inflammation, and abdominal obesity, which increases risk for cardiometabolic diseases (Allen et al., 2019).

In the study by Allen et al. (2019), feeling an obligation to present an image of strength and an obligation to suppress emotions was protective among those reporting high levels of racial discrimination. On the contrary, having an intense motivation to succeed and feeling an obligation to help others exacerbated the health risk associated with racial discrimination. Future studies on positive psychology in African American women should consider the unique experience that they face while dealing with the burdens and blessings of the superwoman schema.

The previously discussed positive psychology factors may be useful culturally specific assets to consider as public health efforts continue to evolve around eliminating health disparities – rather than focusing primarily on racial or cultural risk factors (Hurtado-de-Mendoza et al., 2022).

Positive psychology applications and adaptations for diverse populations and cultures

Applications of positive psychology have been studied with, and for, an extensive range of challenges, groups, formats, and identities. A rich body of literature explores the opportunities to apply positive psychology principles and theory to interventions that address barriers to psychological well-being, while emphasizing a strengths-based approach to care (Carr et al., 2019; Hendriks et al., 2020). Interventions, a selection of which will be discussed in this chapter, have been developed, implemented, and studied in individual and group formats, considered at broader community and population levels, applied to various types of health care (e.g. federally qualified health care centers - FQHCs) and community settings (e.g. churches). The potential impact of PPIs is far reaching. Yet, attention to the psychosocial context in which interventions are recommended and applied is also essential, with strengths-based approaches, contextualized alongside SDOH and well-studied barriers to psychological well-being (e.g. racism). PPIs that are delivered with awareness, and appreciation for such context, or that are tailored to culture, communities, and/or settings, can be especially impactful (Carey et al., 2019; Sanders et al., 2021).

PPIs have the opportunity to support health equity at individual and community levels in a variety of ways. Refer to Table 19.1 for specific examples. Some of the most well-studied interventions include: mindfulness practices, meditation, gratitude practices, and other mind–body interventions. While the full scope of PPIs is beyond the scope of this chapter, several of these types of interventions have been studied in application for historically underrepresented peoples, groups, communities and settings, the results of which are relevant to reducing health disparities and promoting health equity. Specifically, PPIs can

Table 19.1 Select positive psychology interventions (PPIs) among diverse and under-represented samples

Study	Population and intervention	Area(s) of impact	PPI outcome(s)
Basurrah, A. A., Di Blasi, Z., Lambert, L., Murphy, M., Warren, M. A., Setti, A.,... & Shrestha, T. (2022). The effects of positive psychology interventions in Arab countries: A systematic review. *Applied Psychology: Health and Well-Being*.	Systematic review of 44 RCTs and quasi-experimental studies of PPIs in ten Arab countries.	PPI area of focus: mindfulness, positive thinking, strengths, hope, optimism, self-compassion, positive traits, multiple areas.	– PPIs appear effective for improvement of well-being – Effectively address mental health (e.g. anxiety, stress, depression) – 91% of studies noted cultural adaptation, without providing details
Burnett-Zeigler, I., Hong, S., Waldron, E. M., Maletich, C., Yang, A., & Moskowitz, J. (2019). A mindfulness-based intervention for low-income African American women with depressive symptoms delivered by an experienced instructor versus a novice instructor. *The Journal of Alternative and Complementary Medicine, 25*(7), 699–708.	Feasibility and efficacy of adapted MBSR for 31 African American women at an urban FQHC; eight-week group-based mindfulness intervention	Depressive symptoms	– Decrease in depressive symptoms at 8 weeks and 16 weeks – Increase in self-acceptance and growth
Hendriks, T., Schotanus-Dijkstra, M., Hassankhan, A., Sardjo, W., Graafsma, T., Bohlmeijer, E., & de Jong, J. (2020). Resilience and well-being in the Caribbean: Findings from a randomized controlled trial of a culturally adapted multi-component positive psychology intervention. *The Journal of Positive Psychology, 15*(2), 238–253.	Culturally-adapted multi-component PPI RCT, six-sessions for multi-ethnic employees	Resilience	– Large effect on resilience, mental well-being, negative affect – Moderate effect on depression, positive affect – Small effect on anxiety – No effect on stress, financial distress, psychological flexibility

(Continued)

Table 19.1 (Continued)

Study	Population and intervention	Area(s) of impact	PPI outcome(s)
Hernandez, R., Cheung, E., Carnethon, M., Penedo, F. J., Moskowitz, J. T., Martinez, L., & Schueller, S. M. (2018). Feasibility of a culturally adapted positive psychological intervention for Hispanics/Latinos with elevated risk for cardiovascular disease. *Translational behavioral medicine, 8*(6), 887–897.	8 weekly 90-minute sessions, culturally-tailored PPI, in Spanish, by LCSW	Emotional well-being, cardiovascular health,	– Engagement in happiness-inducing behaviors – Emotional vitality – Subjective happiness
Ho, Mui, M., Wan, A., Ng, Y., Stewart, S. M., Yew, C., Lam, T. H., & Chan, S. S. (2016). Happy Family Kitchen II: a cluster randomized controlled trial of a community-based positive psychology family intervention for subjective happiness and health-related quality of life in Hong Kong. *Trials, 17*(1), 367–367. https://doi.org/10.1186/s13063-016-1508-9	Community-based family-level intervention offered in 31 schools and social service units to align with collectivist culture	Family intervention program emphasized: joy, gratitude, flow, savoring, and listening for potential impact on happiness and QOL	– Improvement in subjective happiness – No change in mental or physical QOL
Waldron, E. M., Miller, E. S., Wee, V., Statton, A., Moskowitz, J. T., & Burnett-Zeigler, I. (2022). Stress, coping and the acceptability of mindfulness skills among pregnant and parenting women living with HIV in the United States: A focus group study. *Health & Social Care in the Community.*	Focus groups of pregnant and parenting women living with HIV, engaged in community-enhanced case management program to adapt a mindfulness intervention.	Mindfulness skills for coping with stressors.	– Stressors, coping skills, access, acceptability of care, and motivation/trust in care engagement were all relevant to PPI adaptation. – Openness to mindfulness skills for stress – Preference for group PPIs

(*Continued*)

Table 19.1 (Continued)

Study	Population and intervention	Area(s) of impact	PPI outcome(s)
Waters, L. (2020). Using positive psychology interventions to strengthen family happiness: A family systems app	RCT of 2 PPIs, 300 families in 6 countries, systems approach with environmental context considerations	Individual change, relational/ family change	Increase in happiness for intervention group, positive practices can change system elements and result in family-level outcomes

Note: RCT= randomized controlled trial, MBSR = mindfulness-based stress reduction (an evidence-based intervention), FQHC= federally qualified health center, LCSW = licensed clinical social worker, QOL = quality of life.

be employed as strengths-based approaches that prioritize cognitive, behavioral, and psychosocial strengths. For example, Sanders et al. (2021) argue that PPIs have some overlap with interventions targeting reduction in prejudice, offering the opportunity to support coping with oppression, as well as potentially reducing oppression itself by effecting oppressors (i.e. historically majority groups).

PPIs have demonstrated efficacy in settings, and for populations and conditions, in which historically marginalized groups are disproportionately affected by structural and systemic bias and racism. For example, a review of PPIs in the workplace revealed their utility to support employee well-being and performance, as well as a trend toward a positive impact of PPIs on stress, burnout, anxiety, and depression (Meyers et al., 2013). Given the commonality of bias and discrimination in the workplace, team or system-level PPIs could benefit those most affected by such treatment, both directly and indirectly. Historically marginalized individuals are also disproportionately impacted by many of the leading causes of death, disability, and quality of life adjusted years lived, such as cancer, cardiovascular disease, and mental illness. Specifically, behavioral interventions, including PPIs, can be leveraged to support quality of life and reduce cardiovascular health disparities, given the higher rates of cardiovascular conditions experienced by Black, Latinx, and Asian Americans (Chirinos et al., 2022).

PPIs can influence well-being in a variety of ways - from helping individuals with minoritized identities cope with the effects of discrimination to influencing members of majority groups to support a reduction in prejudice, and ultimately oppression (Sanders et al., 2021). For example, research on the elements and impact of PPI has found that loving-kindness meditation is associated with enhanced well-being, intergroup attitudes, and reduced bias and prejudice. Positive psychology frameworks have also been utilized to develop and apply intervention that foster healthy social identity development by attending to the influences of cultural context, environment, and intersectionality on identity and engagement in PPIs. This intersectional lens is especially important for individuals with multiple, intersection, marginalized aspects of identity, such as race, gender, and ability/disability (Carey et al., 2019). Positive psychology approaches to care and PPIs utilized in clinical practice, can also intentionally acknowledge and address discrimination in order to foster a strengths-based approach to care to offset the effects of discrimination, restore cultural dignity, and promote strengths and resilience within the context of discrimination and cultural stressors (Klibert & Allen, 2019). As an example, narrative therapy, a multi-story approach to clinical care that helps a patient draw meaning from experiences that align with their identity, has been studied as an effective approach to supporting individuals to cope with social barriers to well-being, including discrimination (Klibert & Allen, 2019).

In contrast, given the history of positive psychology research and some limitations in diversity of study samples and settings, many evidence-based PPIs have required, or will require, adaptation in approach, technique, and other delivery, to allow for consideration of the unique lived experiences and practices of historically marginalized populations. Cultural adaptation, community-engaged interventions, and application to diverse implementation settings, are all approaches that have supported the reach and benefit from PPIs. For example, attention to, and intentional incorporation of spiritual and religious practices, may bolster the interest and uptake of PPIs for some groups and communities. In fact, many of the central tenets of PPIs and spiritual practices are the same, such as hope, gratitude, and compassion (Falb & Pargament, 2014).

Select positive psychology interventions

Table 19.1 outlines several examples of PPIs in application to historically marginalized groups at the individual level (Burnett-Zeigler et al., 2019; Hernandez et al., 2018; Waldron et al., 2022), systems or community level (Hendriks et al., 2020; Ho et al., 2016; Waters, 2020), or population level (Basurrah et al., 2022). Many of these PPIs explore the need for, or include a cultural adaptation framework to optimize PPIs. Cultural adaptation allows for cultural tailoring and study of interventions that have been well studied in majority western populations, or to specifically target the communities, families, or groups they are being offered to. The present science also indicates the need for additional research in cultural adaptation of PPIs to meet the needs of diverse participants and to consider the setting and environmental context in which interventions are offered. For example, the PPIs discussed in Table 19.1 occurred in community health care settings, an FQHC, and in schools. The results of these select studies, and other references in this chapter, indicate the potential global impact and benefit from PPIs, the utility across languages and cultures, and potential utility in both clinical and non-clinical populations. For example, a 2019 meta-analysis assessed the efficacy of PPIs to enhance well-being among adults and children in 41 countries. Results of the entire study sample of over 72,000 individuals indicated positive effects of PPIs on depression, anxiety, quality of life, stress, strengths, and overall well-being. Interestingly, the effect of PPIs on quality of life was stronger for children and adolescents than for adults, while the effect of PPIs on well-being and depression was stronger for older adults than for those in earlier life stages. Additionally, the country or origin and engagement did moderate the effect of PPIs on well-being, strengths, QOL, anxiety, and depression, with greater effects identified in non-western countries (Carr et al., 2020).

A practical approach to integrating health equity into the field of positive psychology

Promoting holistic well-being of all individuals and communities demands that the positive psychology field grapples with pressing societal factors that subvert health attainment, including racism and discrimination. Opportunities for effective, antiracism-oriented intervention exist on every level of society - from the macro level (i.e. politics, education, health care) to the micro level (i.e. clinic visits, workplace and community-based interpersonal interactions). Clinicians ought to proactively consider how positive psychology may be a tool to advance health equity and to mold a more just society (Bartoli & Pyati, 2009).

White clinicians of positive psychology must reckon with their own internal blocks to antiracist action prior to helping clients do the same. The same process described by Drustrup (2021) as a model for addressing racism within a therapeutic setting should be completed by both clinician and client. This model for all-white dyads in a therapeutic alliance to engage with topics of race and racism involves five steps - beginning with racial literacy and ending with proactively seeking to engage in social spaces outside of traditionally white ones (Drustrup, 2021). In order for the clinician to operate from a place of authentic antiracism, she must engage in a lifelong process of racial reckoning. This journey need not be perfect, but it must be embarked upon earnestly and with a genuine desire to be a change agent for a more just society (Drustrup, 2021).

Positive psychology-oriented research presents key opportunities to investigate questions relevant to more diverse populations, query the influence of SDOH like racism on well-being, and to expand understanding of culturally specific resources of importance to psychosocial well-being. For example, including measures of microaggressions, prejudice and discrimination (e.g. the Daily Life Experiences Scale) would help to examine linkages between these experiences and elements of positive psychology. Research in this field has historically left unaddressed the role of race and ethnicity, socioeconomic status and culture on optimal well-being; these gaps are essential to fill as a stepping stone toward better understanding how positive psychology may be a meaningful contributor to health equity work (van Zyl & Rothmann, 2022).

Research on the impact of engaging in discriminatory behavior on an individual's well-being is scant. This area of inquiry is wide open for further investigation into the well-being consequences of perpetrating prejudice. How does prejudice impact an individual's ability to thrive holistically? How might positive psychology help to buffer against potential harmful effects of engaging in discrimination? These questions and others warrant further exploration as the field of positive psychology seeks to expand its application to furthering antiracism work and health equity (Sanders et al., 2021).

In closing,

> we call on positive psychologists to embrace the opportunity to expand the relevance of our scholarship to the dire problem of marginalization, not only in attempts to promote coping among those who are marginalized, but to understand the ways that positive characteristics and experiences might help reduce inequality.
>
> *(Sanders et al., 2021)*

Takeaways

- Positive psychology may contribute toward health equity in several ways, including by reducing the psychological and physical toll of chronic discrimination on minoritized racial groups and by offering approaches to reduce prejudice among perpetrators of discrimination.
- Resilience in the face of inequities may function as both a health risk and resource for African Americans and other minoritized groups, by simultaneously improving mood and negatively affecting physical health due to chronic stress associated with overcoming adversities.
- PPIs have demonstrated evidence to support and improve well-being for diverse peoples and groups and in diverse settings, such as community settings, federally qualified health centers, and for families.
- PPIs can, and do, benefit from cultural adaptation to uniquely support specific identities, communities, and settings.

Wicked questions

1 What value may researchers studying human strengths, happiness, and fulfillment offer to the problems of prejudice and discrimination?
2 How may the field of Positive Psychology espouse and advocate for an antiracist approach in scholarship, education and training, and clinical care?
3 What PPIs have been effectively used in diverse populations to address health disparities?
4 What resources and attributes may be cultivated by racial-ethnic minorities in order to enhance their resilience to psychological distress?
5 How can positive psychology be leveraged to reduce inequality in our society?

References

Allen, A. M., Wang, Y., Chae, D. H., Price, M. M., Powell, W., Steed, T. C., Rose Black, A., Dhabhar, F. S., Marquez-Magaña, L., & Woods-Giscombe, C. L. (2019). Racial discrimination, the superwoman schema, and allostatic load: Exploring an integrative stress-coping model among African American women. *Annals of the New York Academy of Sciences*, 1457(1), 104–127.

American Public Health Association. (n.d.) Racism and health. Retrieved February 2, 2023, from https://www.apha.org/topics-and-issues/health-equity/racism-and-health.

Banks, K. H., & Kohn-Wood, L. P. (2007). The influence of racial identity profiles on the relationship between racial discrimination and depressive symptoms. *Journal of Black Psychology*, 33(3), 331–354.

Bartoli, E., & Pyati, A. (2009). Addressing clients' racism and racial prejudice in individual psychotherapy: Therapeutic considerations. *Psychotherapy (Chic)*. 46(2), 145–57.

Basurrah, A. A., Di Blasi, Z., Lambert, L., Murphy, M., Warren, M. A., Setti, A.,... & Shrestha, T. (2022). The effects of positive psychology interventions in Arab countries: A systematic review. *Applied Psychology: Health and Well-Being*. 15(2), 803–821. https://doi.org/10.1111/aphw.12391

Bay Area Regional Health Inequities. (2020). *A public health framework for reducing health inequities.* https://www.barhii.org/barhii-framework

Blume, A. W., Lovato, L. V., Thyken, B. N., & Denny, N. (2012). The relationship of microaggressions with alcohol use and anxiety among ethnic minority college students in a historically White institution. *Cultural Diversity and Ethnic Minority Psychology*, 18(1), 45–54. https://doi.org/10.1037/a0025457

Bowleg, L. (2012). The problem with the phrase women and minorities: Intersectionality-an important theoretical framework for public health. *American Journal of Public Health*, 102(7), 1267–1273. https://doi.org/10.2105/AJPH.2012.300750

Braveman, P., & Gruskin, S. (2003). Defining equity in health. *Journal of Epidemiology and Community Health*, 57(4), 254–258.

Brewer, L. C., Redmond, N., Slusser, J. P., Scott, C. G., Chamberlain, A. M., Djousse, L., Patten, C. A., Roger, V. L., & Sims, M. (2018). Stress and achievement of cardiovascular health metrics: The American Heart Association Life's simple 7 in blacks of the Jackson Heart Study. *Journal of the American Heart Association*, 7(11), e008855. https://doi.org/10.1161/JAHA.118.008855

Burnett-Zeigler, I., Hong, S., Waldron, E. M., Maletich, C., Yang, A., & Moskowitz, J. (2019). A mindfulness-based intervention for low-income African American women with depressive symptoms delivered by an experienced instructor versus a novice instructor. *The Journal of Alternative and Complementary Medicine*, 25(7), 699–708.

Carey, C. D., Pitt, J. S., Sánchez, J., Robertson, S., & Mpofu, E. (2019). Exploring positive psychological interventions as race, gender and disability intersect. In L.E. Van Zyl & S. Rothman (Eds.), *Theoretical Approaches to Multi-Cultural Positive Psychological Interventions* (pp. 261–280). Springer Cham. https://doi.org/10.1007/978-3-030-20583-6

Carr, A., Cullen, K., Keeney, C., Canning, C., Mooney, O., Chinseallaigh, E., & O'Dowd, A. (2021). Effectiveness of positive psychology interventions: A systematic review and meta-analysis. *The Journal of Positive Psychology*, 16(6), 749–769.

Chirinos, D. A., Vargas, E., Kamsickas, L., & Carnethon, M. (2022). The role of behavioral science in addressing cardiovascular health disparities: A narrative review of efforts, challenges, and future directions. *Health Psychology*, 41(10), 740.

Clark, R., Anderson, N. B., Clark, V. R., & Williams, D. R. (1999). Racism as a stressor for African Americans: A biopsychosocial model. *American Psychologist*, 54(10), 805.

Codjoe, L., Barber, S., Ahuja, S., Thornicroft, G., Henderson, C., Lempp, H., & N'Danga-Koroma, J. (2021). Evidence for interventions to promote mental health and reduce stigma in Black faith communities: Systematic review. *Social Psychiatry and Psychiatric Epidemiology*, 56(6), 895–911. https://doi.org/10.1007/s00127-021-02068-y.

Drolet, C. E., & Lucas, T. (2020). Perceived racism, affectivity, and C-reactive protein in healthy African Americans: Do religiosity and racial identity provide complementary protection?. *Journal of Behavioral Medicine*, 43(6), 932–942. https://doi.org/10.1007/s10865-020-00146-1

Drustrup D. (2021). Talking with white clients about race. *Journal of Health Service Psychology*, 47(2), 63–72.

Falb, M. D., & Pargament, K. I. (2014). Religion, spirituality, and positive psychology: Strengthening well-being. In J. Teramoto Pedrotti & L.M. Edwards (Eds.), *Perspectives on the Intersection of Multiculturalism and Positive Psychology* (pp. 143–157). Springer Science + Business Media. https://psycnet.apa.org/doi/10.1007/978-94-017-8654-6_10

Guidi, J., Lucente, M., Sonino, N., Fava, G. A. (2021). Allostatic load and its impact on health: A systematic review. Psychotherapy and Psychosomatics, 90(1), 11–27.

Hendriks, T., Schotanus-Dijkstra, M., Hassankhan, A., Sardjo, W., Graafsma, T., Bohlmeijer, E., & de Jong, J. (2020). Resilience and well-being in the Caribbean: Findings from a randomized controlled trial of a culturally adapted multi-component positive psychology intervention. *The Journal of Positive Psychology*, 15(2), 238–253.

Hendriks, T., Schotanus-Dijkstra, M., Hassankhan, A., De Jong, J., & Bohlmeijer, E. (2020). The efficacy of multi-component positive psychology interventions: A systematic review and meta-analysis of randomized controlled trials. *Journal of Happiness Studies*, 21, 357–390.

Hernandez, R., Cheung, E., Carnethon, M., Penedo, F. J., Moskowitz, J. T., Martinez, L., & Schueller, S. M. (2018). Feasibility of a culturally adapted positive psychological intervention for Hispanics/Latinos with elevated risk for cardiovascular disease. *Translational behavioral medicine*, 8(6), 887–897.

Herren, O. M., Burris, S. E., Levy, S. A., Kirk, K., Banks, K. S., Jones, V. L., Beard, B., Mwendwa, D. T., Callender, C. O., & Campbell, A. L. (2019). Influence of spirituality on depression-induced inflammation and executive functioning in a community sample of African Americans. *Ethnicity & Disease*, 29(2), 267–276. https://doi.org/10.18865/ed.29.2.267

Ho, Mui, M., Wan, A., Ng, Y., Stewart, S. M., Yew, C., Lam, T. H., & Chan, S. S. (2016). Happy Family Kitchen II: a cluster randomized controlled trial of a community-based positive psychology family intervention for subjective happiness and health-related quality of life in Hong Kong. *Trials*, 17(1), 367–367. https://doi.org/10.1186/s13063-016-1508-9

Hood, C. M., Gennuso, K. P., Swain, G. R., & Catlin, B. B. (2016). County health rankings: Relationships between determinant factors and health outcomes. *American Journal of Preventive Medicine* 50(2), 129–135. https://doi.org/10.1016/j.amepre.2015.08.024

Hurtado-de-Mendoza, A., Gonzales, F., Song, M., Holmes, E. J., Graves, K. D., Retnam, R., Gómez-Trillos, S., Lopez, K., Edmonds, M. C., & Sheppard, V. B. (2022, December). Association between aspects of social support and health-related quality of life domains among African American and White breast cancer survivors. *Journal of Cancer Survivorship*, 16(6), 1379–1389. https://doi.org/10.1007/s11764-021-01119-2. Epub 2021 Oct 16. PMID: 34655040.

James S. A. (1994). John Henryism and the health of African-Americans. *Culture, Medicine and Psychiatry*, 18(2), 163–182. https://doi.org/10.1007/BF01379448

Jones C. P. (2000). Levels of racism: A theoretic framework and a gardener's tale. *American Journal of Public Health*, 90(8), 1212–1215. https://doi.org/10.2105/ajph.90.8.1212.

Jones, S. C. T., & Neblett, E. W. (2017). Future directions in research on racism-related stress and racial-ethnic protective factors for Black youth. *Journal of Clinical Child & Adolescent Psychology*, 46(5), 754–766.

Kelly, Jennifer F. (2022). Building a more equitable society: Psychology's role in achieving health equity. *American Psychologist*, 77(5); 633–645.

Kim, E. S., Hagan, K. A., Grodstein, F., DeMeo, D. L., De Vivo, I., & Kubzansky, L. D. (2016). Optimism and cause-specific mortality: A prospective cohort study. *American Journal of Epidemiology*, 185(1), 21–29.

Klibert, J., & Allen, B. (2019). Taking a strengths-based approach to address discrimination experiences in a clinical context. In L.E. Van Zyl & S. Rothman (Eds.),

Theoretical Approaches to Multi-Cultural Positive Psychological Interventions (pp. 21–50). Springer, Cham. https://doi.org/10.1007/978-3-030-20583-6_2

Lee, H. H., Kubzansky, L. D., Okuzono, S. S., Trudel-Fitzgerald, C., James, P., Koga, H. K., Kim, E. S., Glover, L. M., Sims, M., & Grodstein, F. (2022). Optimism and risk of mortality among African-Americans: The Jackson heart study. *Preventive Medicine*, 154, 106899. https://doi.org/10.1016/j.ypmed.2021.106899

Lee, L. O., James, P., Zevon, E. S., Kim, E. S., Trudel-Fitzgerald, C., Spiro, A. 3rd, Grodstein, F., Kubzansky, L. D. (2019, September 10). Optimism is associated with exceptional longevity in 2 epidemiologic cohorts of men and women. *Proceedings of the National Academy of Sciences of the United States of America*,116(37), 18357–18362.

McIntosh, R., Ironson, G., & Krause, N. (2021). Keeping hope alive: Racial-ethnic disparities in distress tolerance are mitigated by religious/spiritual hope among Black Americans. *Journal of Psychosomatic Research*, 144, 110403.

Mercer, S. H., Zeigler-Hill, V., Wallace, M., & Hayes, D. M. (2011). Development and initial validation of the inventory of microaggressions against black individuals. *Journal of Counseling Psychology*, 58(4), 457–469. https://doi.org/10.1037/a0024937

Meyers, M. C., van Woerkom, M., & Bakker, A. B. (2013). The added value of the positive: A literature review of positive psychology interventions in organizations. *European Journal of Work and Organizational Psychology*, 22(5), 618–632.

Moradi, B., & Subich, L. M. (2003). A concomitant examination of the relations of perceived racist and the sexist events to psychological distress for African American women. *The Counseling Psychologist*, 31(4), 451–469. https://doi.org/10.1177/0011000003031004007

Mozaffarian, D. (2023, March 30). Measuring and addressing nutrition security to achieve health and health equity. Health policy brief. *Health Affairs*. https://doi.org/10.1377/hpb20230216.926558

Myers, C. A. (2020). Food insecurity and psychological distress: A review of the recent literature. *Current Nutrition Reports*, 9, 107–118. https://doi.org/10.1007/s13668-020-00309-1

Nadal, K. L., Griffin, K. E., Wong, Y., Hamit, S., & Rasmus, M. (2014). The impact of racial microaggressions on mental health: Counseling implications for clients of color. *Journal of Counseling & Development*, 92(1), 57–66. https://doi.org/10.1002/j.1556-6676.2014.00130.x

Robert Wood Johnson Foundation. (2017). *What is health equity? A definition and discussion guide*. Available at: https://www.rwjf.org/en/insights/our-research/2017/05/what-is-health-equity-.html#:~:text=In%20a%20report%20designed%20to,be%20as%20healthy%20as%20possible. Accessed on March 1, 2023.

Robinson, M. N., & Thomas Tobin, C. S. (2021). Is John Henryism a health risk or resource?: Exploring the role of culturally relevant coping for physical and mental health among black Americans. *Journal of Health and Social Behavior*, 62(2), 136–151. https://doi.org/10.1177/00221465211009142

Rowland-Shea, J., Doshi, S., Edberg, S., Fanger, R. (2020, July 21). The nature gap: Confronting racial and economic disparities in the destruction and protection of nature in America. Report by Center for American Progress. Available at: https://www.americanprogress.org/article/the-nature-gap/. Accessed on March 15, 2023.

Ryff, C. D. (2022). Positive psychology: Looking back and looking forward. *Frontiers in Psychology*, 13, 840062.

Sanders, C. A., Rose, H., Booker, J. A., & King, L. A. (2021). Claiming the role of positive psychology in the fight against prejudice. *The Journal of Positive Psychology*, 18(1), 61–74.

Sellers, R. M., Caldwell, C. H., Schmeelk-Cone, K. H., & Zimmerman, M. A. (2003). Racial identity, racial discrimination, perceived stress, and psychological distress among African American young adults. *Journal of Health and Social behavior*, 44(3), 302–317.

Sims, M., Glover, L. M., Norwood, A. F., Jordan, C., Min, Y. I., Brewer, L. C., & Kubzansky, L. D. (2019). Optimism and cardiovascular health among African Americans in the Jackson Heart Study. *Preventive Medicine*, 129, 105826. https://doi.org/10.1016/j.ypmed.2019.105826

Steinhardt, M. A., Dubois, S. K., Brown, S. A., Harrison, L., Jr, Dolphin, K. E., Park, W., & Lehrer, H. M. (2015). Positivity and indicators of health among African Americans with diabetes. *American Journal of Health Behavior*, 39(1), 43–50. https://doi.org/10.5993/AJHB.39.1.5

Stevens-Watkins, D., Perry, B., Pullen, E., Jewell, J., & Oser, C. B. (2014). Examining the associations of racism, sexism, and stressful life events on psychological distress among African-American women. *Cultural Diversity & Ethnic Minority Psychology*, 20(4), 561–569. https://doi.org/10.1037/a0036700

Sue, D. W., Capodilupo, C. M., Torino, G. C., Bucceri, J. M., Holder, A. M., Nadal, K. L., & Esquilin, M. (2007). Racial microaggressions in everyday life: Implications for clinical practice. *The American Psychologist*, 62(4), 271–286. https://doi.org/10.1037/0003-066X.62.4.271

van Zyl, L. E., & Rothmann, S. (2022). Grand challenges for positive psychology: Future perspectives and opportunities. *Frontiers in Psychology*, 13, 833057.

Waldron, E. M., Miller, E. S., Wee, V., Statton, A., Moskowitz, J. T., & Burnett-Zeigler, I. (2022). Stress, coping and the acceptability of mindfulness skills among pregnant and parenting women living with HIV in the United States: A focus group study. *Health & Social Care in the Community*. 30(6), e6255–e6266. https://doi.org/10.1111/hsc.14063

Walker, R. J., Garacci, E., Dawson, A. Z., Williams, J. S., Ozieh, M., & Egede, L. E. (2021). Trends in food insecurity in the United States from 2011–2017: Disparities by age, sex, race/ethnicity, and income. *Population Health Management*, 24(4), 496–501.

Waters, L. (2020). Using positive psychology interventions to strengthen family happiness: A family systems approach. *The Journal of Positive Psychology*. 15(5), 645–652. https://doi.org/10.1080/17439760.2020.1789704

World Health Organization (WHO). (2012). What are the social determinants of health? Available at: http://www.who.int/social_determinants/sdh_definition/en/. Accessed on February 1, 2023.

Yeager, K. A., & Bauer-Wu, S. (2013). Cultural humility: Essential foundation for clinical researchers. *Applied Nursing Research*, 26(4), 251–256.

20

APPLYING POSITIVE PSYCHOLOGY AND THE PILLARS OF LIFESTYLE MEDICINE

Liana Lianov

The role of positive psychology in healthcare and self-care

The implementation of positive psychology approaches in healthcare has the potential to address multiple goals. Among these are boosting positive provider–patient and healthcare team interactions, managing stress, strengthening mood disorder treatment, promoting emotional well-being, and facilitating healthy behaviors. Using these approaches in self-care helps with stress management, emotional well-being and sustaining healthy habits. This chapter will examine the role of positive psychology in health behavior change and the pillars of lifestyle medicine – a predominantly plant-based eating pattern, physical activity, adequate and high-quality sleep, avoiding risky substance use, managing stress, and social connection. The chapter concludes with practical approaches for applying positive psychology in clinical settings.

Positive affect and health behavior change

The root of lifestyle medicine and other healthcare specialties is health behavior change. Yet, the struggle to make these changes greatly challenges self-care, as well as the care provided by health professionals. We can look to positive psychology for helpful solutions. Research demonstrates that positive affective processes can drive positive behavior change. The upward spiral theory of lifestyle change explains how positive affect can promote long-term adherence to healthy behaviors, namely by triggering nonconscious motivation for those behaviors. When positive emotions are associated with target behaviors, individuals pay greater attention to those behaviors and make decisions to engage in them repeatedly. Moreover, based on the broaden-and-build-theory, these positive emotions build resources which reinforce the positive experience and

DOI: 10.4324/9781003378426-23   314

further increase nonconscious motivation (Fredrickson, 2004; Van Cappellen et al., 2018).

In addition to this dynamic that promotes healthy behaviors, positive emotions are also shown to directly influence physical health. One trial investigated these mechanisms of action. Participants were randomly assigned to an intervention group of loving-kindness meditation or to a waiting-list control group. The intervention group participants increased positive emotions more than those in the control group. Increased positive emotions produced increase in vagal tone – a proxy for physical health – and were mediated by social interactions. The researchers concluded that positive emotions, social connections, and physical health influence one another in a self-sustaining upward-spiral dynamic (Kok et al., 2013; Van Cappellen et al., 2018).

Health coaches were the early adopters in healthcare who harnessed the power of positive psychology for behavior change. They lead the way for positive psychology advances in medicine. Not only does the association of positive affect with desired behaviors lead to greater behavioral achievement and sustainability, but also positive activities - activities that produce positive affect, improving emotional well-being and increasing happiness levels can be prescribed. Happier people – those with high positive affect and life satisfaction and low negative affect – tend to exercise, not smoke, use seat belts, eat healthy food and avoid risky alcohol use. Moreover, happier people do well across other life domains, including work performance, social relationships and resilience in the face of adversity (Kansky & Diener, 2017).

In summary, the theoretical and empirical literature suggests that positive affect and positive psychology constructs play a key role in health behavior change that is foundational to improved health outcomes. Hence, coaching with positive psychology techniques and prescribing interventions to increase positive affect may represent essential tools in medicine and these activities can easily be incorporated into self-care.

Positive psychology in each lifestyle medicine pillar

Positive emotions boost healthy behaviors and vice versa; hence, positive psychology can play a key role in the lifestyle medicine pillars. Let's take a look at the empirical evidence for these reinforcing, reciprocal links and how positive psychology constructs can be harnessed for addressing each pillar.

Eating patterns

Eating healthy food such as vegetables and fruits is associated with positive affect, happiness or vitality (Fararouei et al., 2013; Mujcic & Oswald, 2016). Optimism, in particular, has been found as a powerful construct associated with the consumption of healthier food (Ait-Hadad et al., 2020; Boehm et al., 2018; Hingle et al., 2014; Kelloniemi et al., 2005), healthy body weight and less snacking (Ait-Hadad et al., 2020; Hingle et al., 2014; Pänkäläinen et al., 2018).

When examining longitudinal food diaries of 12,385 randomly sampled Australian adults and making adjustments for changing incomes and personal circumstances, researchers found that increased fruit and vegetable consumption was predictive of increased happiness, life satisfaction and well-being within a 24-month period. An increase of 0.24 life-satisfaction points was gained for an increase of eight portions a day; this effect equals the psychological gain of moving from unemployment to employment. Motivation to eat healthy food can be enhanced by well-being improvements, which occur more immediately than physical health effects (Mujcic & Oswald, 2016).

Research on quantities of plants-based foods needed to see a meaningful effect on emotional and mental well-being is scant. One survey found meaningful changes in affect in students consuming at least 7–8 servings of fruit or vegetables per day. These effects predicted positive affect the next day, suggesting that healthy foods were driving affective experiences (Blanchflower, Oswald & Stewart-Brown, 2013; White, Horwath &Conner, 2013).

Moreover, it appears that feeling more positively can help individuals eat more healthfully (Ait-Hadad et al., 2020; Hingle et al., 2014; Pänkäläinen et al., 2018; Whatnall et al., 2019). In the upward spiral theory, participants are more likely to maintain healthy habits when they perceive positive emotions during the activity (Van Cappellen et al., 2018). A cautionary note is needed here, as some studies have found that positive emotions are associated with increased caloric intake during socializing or celebrations (Bongers et al., 2013; Cardi et al., 2015; Evers et al., 2013, 2018).

Semi-structured interviews of adults with metabolic syndrome exploring the relationship of eating and positive psychology constructs, such as gratitude, identified five themes: eating healthfully leads to positive psychology constructs, positive psychology constructs lead to eating healthfully, eating healthfully prevents negative emotions, healthy behaviors are associated with a healthy diet, and an upward healthy eating spiral (Carrillo et al. 2022).

Also, positive thoughts and feelings may help build additional resources, such as learning to cook healthy recipes, to support eating healthfully (Fredrickson, 2004). Greater feelings of self-efficacy and perceived control, ongoing self-monitoring, active coping strategies, enhanced social interactions, and increased self-regulation and motivation are possible mechanisms for achieving and maintaining a healthy diet (Carrillo et al., 2022; Huffman et al., 2021). Therefore, helping people cultivate positive emotions may help them improve their adherence to a healthy diet.

During coaching, emphasizing the role of enjoyment versus health benefits of foods can successfully leverage the mood and food consumption relationship. Mood influences the choice between healthy versus indulgent foods through its impact on the weights people put on long-term health benefits versus short-term mood management benefits when making dietary choices. Studies show that a positive mood increases the salience of long-term goals such as health, leading to greater preference for healthy foods (Gardner et al., 2014; Mujcic &

Oswald, 2016). Motivation to eat healthy food can also be enhanced by emotional well-being improvements, which occur more immediately than physical health effects (Mujcic & Oswald, 2016). Conversely, a negative mood increases the salience of immediate, concrete goals such as mood management, leading to greater preference for indulgent foods (Gardner et al., 2014; Mujcic & Oswald, 2016).

Future studies should focus on bolstering specific positive psychological constructs to help individuals improve their dietary patterns and boost self-perceptions of healthy habits. Studies should also examine ways to enhance participants' positive experiences when engaging in healthy eating behaviors.

Physical activity

The second major pillar of a healthy lifestyle and in lifestyle medicine is physical activity. A mountain of evidence has been building about the impact of physical activity on mood and mental health for both populations with and without mental illness. In fact, physical activity is shown to be an effective depression treatment.

The most robust and convincing evidence of the key role of physical activity on emotional and mental well-being is its capacity to prevent and treat depression (Babyak et al., 2000; Blumenthal et al., 2007; Cooney et al., 2013; Ernst et al., 2006; Mammen & Faulkner, 2013; McKercher et al., 2014; Rimer et al., 2012). Physical activity is also observed to increase positive moods and emotional well-being.

Commonly cited among healthy, nonpsychiatric patients is the runner's high - a euphoric state resulting from long-distance running (Boecker et al., 2008). Mood improvements in healthy adults have been noted with as little as 10 minutes of exercise and with other forms of exercise besides running. For example, improvements in the Profile of Mood States Inventory have been observed after just 10 minutes of cycling (Hansen et al., 2001). A self-report survey of 11,637 individuals in 15 European countries, adjusting for sex, age, country, general health, relationship status, employment and education, showed that increasing physical activity volume was associated with higher levels of happiness in a dose-response relationship (Richards et al., 2015).

Both exercise and daily movement can contribute to mood improvement. Self-reports of happiness and physical activity from over 10,000 participants, as well as passive data from users' phone accelerometers, revealed that those who were more physically active – through both exercise and nonexercised activities – were happier. Further, individuals are happier in the moments when they are more physically active (Lathia et al., 2017).

As with healthy eating, when we promote physical activity, we need to keep in mind its powerful reciprocal link with positive affect. A systematic review of 24 studies demonstrated that affective responses during and after exercise had a reliable correlation with affective judgments about future physical activity (Rhodes & Kates, 2015).

Interviews of study participants who have undergone metabolic/bariatric surgery revealed specific contexts that increased positive emotions during physical activity, such as doing an enjoyable type of exercise, and social interactions, mindfulness during exercise, and a sense of mastery performing the exercise, whereas negative affect lowered engagement. Hence, interventions that lead to positive affect and address factors that lead to negative affect have the potential to effectively increase physical activity after metabolic/bariatric surgery (Feig et al., 2022).

These studies provide just a few examples of the mounting literature that physical activity and positive mood appear to be strongly linked, and lifestyle medicine practitioners can take advantage of this link to facilitate this important lifestyle behavior for prevention and treatment of lifestyle related disease.

Sleep

Clinical evidence suggests that sleep and emotion interact. As with the other pillars of lifestyle medicine, sleep has a reciprocal, reinforcing relationship with mood. When one is anxious, sad or stressed, one might not be able to get to sleep or might awaken early. In turn, poor quality and inadequate sleep is associated with increases sadness, anger, and irritability. Hence, sleep hygiene is an essential element of emotional well-being.

Most experts would agree that for the average healthy adult requires between seven and seven and a half hours with a range of seven to nine hours for deriving physiologic and emotional benefits of sleep. Evaluations of more than a thousand scientific articles have led to the consensus by the American Academy of Sleep Medicine and Sleep Research Society jointly" (Watson et al., 2015; Worley, 2018).

Inadequate sleep can take a toll on psychological well-being, significantly affecting our emotional interpretation of events and increasing stress levels. One explanation is that sleep deprivation effects emotional memory nudging a tendency to focus on and remember negative experiences. Those who were sleep-deprived responded to low stressors in a similar way as those without sleep deprivation tend to respond to high stressors (Worley, 2018).

When healthy young adults had their sleep restricted 33% below habitual sleep duration, to an average under five hours per night for seven consecutive nights, they demonstrated mental exhaustion and mood disturbances, which returned to normal after two nights of habitual sleep duration (Dinges et al., 1997).

Hence, sleep deprivation is associated with impaired emotion regulation and generation. Sleeping one and a half to two hours less than usual can lead to individuals becoming more impulsive and experiencing less positive affect (Saksvik-Lehouillier et al., 2020). Moreover, insomnia can be a risk factor for development of anxiety disorders (Neckelmann et al., 2007) and depression (Riemann & Voderholzer, 2003). On the other hand, habitual duration sleep enhances mood and affect states and positive emotion expression (Lollies et al., 2022; Yoo et al., 2007).

In addition to managing negative emotions that can interfere with sleep, positive psychological states may act as protective factors, buffering the impact of psychological distress. Hence, both positive affect and eudaimonic well-being are shown to be associated with good sleep. The relationships are bidirectional, with disturbed sleep engendering lower positive affect and reduced psychological well-being, and positive psychological states promoting better sleep (Steptoe et al., 2008). However, empirical data on the association between positive affect and sleep in clinical populations is limited and more high-quality research is needed (Ong et al., 2017).

Substance use

A healthy lifestyle includes avoidance of risky substance use to avoid physical and mental sequalae. Substance use, such as alcohol, has been linked with mental health consequences. For example, a self-report survey of 7,937 German participants found associations between moderate alcohol consumption (i.e., not increased or no alcohol consumption), nonsmoking, higher frequency of physical and mental activity, a body mass index within the range of normal to overweight (i.e. not underweight or obese) and better mental health (Velten et al., 2014). Moreover, as a central nervous system depressant, it is no surprise that alcohol use is associated with depression. Alcohol use disorder co-occurs with depression disorders more frequently than what would be expected by chance (McHugh & Weiss, 2019).

Although lifestyle medicine practitioners are not addiction specialists, they can offer brief interventions to individuals with mild to moderate substance use problems. Often individuals turn to substance use to escape unpleasant or negative life experiences or memories of traumatic events. Boosting positive experiences can help counter this process. It is important for some individuals to seek the help of a trauma informed psychologist, psychiatrist or therapist if they continue to suffer from previous traumatic events or have diagnoses requiring the expertise of a trained mental health professional.

Having the capacity to envision a positive future with life purpose, good work, pleasant experiences, and positive social relationships can serve as the keystone for turning to productive habits and away from substance use. Mild to moderate substance use disorder can be treated as a behavioral disorder and behavior change strategies can be implemented as with other behavior change challenges using motivational interviewing, cognitive behavioral and positive psychology techniques.

Reframing the use of alcohol or other drug use as a lifestyle behavior that can be changed has the potential to free up the individual to view decreases in substance use, or avoidance altogether, as attainable. A driver for empowering change is the positive psychology goal of a pleasant, engaged and meaningful life. Early small steps of change include reframing one's mindset to seek what is going well in one's life and practicing gratitude. Additional positive psychology approaches, including leveraging character strengths and positive affect, which have been implemented in recovery for alcohol use, smoking and other drug addictions (Krentzman, 2013).

Positive psychology aligns with known factors that support recovery from substance use disorder and can be incorporated into systems of care. Many individuals do not seek traditional therapy due to societal stigma and other barriers; hence positive psychology approaches can be self-initiated and conducted online increasing access to recovery care. PPIs in clinical settings and self-care, as well as in online, digital and community programs may offer an effective framework for addiction treatment and prevention strategies. (Crookes, 2018; Krentzman, 2013).

Stress management

Positive psychology approaches can serve as important interventions for managing stress by increasing positive emotions that can buffer against physiologically harmful stress and can be prescribed to address this pillar of a healthy lifestyle. Studies show that multiple-component positive affect interventions both increase positive affect and decrease negative affect and are useful in addressing health-related and other types of stress (Moskowitz et al., 2012).

Positive psychology skills to increase positive affect can be taught and can lead to improved positive affect and indirectly decrease stress. Moskowitz and colleagues studied an aggregated array of research-informed positive psychology skills to help individuals cope with life stressors, targeting individuals with serious illnesses, such as HIV and metastatic breast cancer, affective disorders and other major stressors, including drug addiction and caregiving. Key skills in most interventions included noticing, savoring or planning positive experiences, improving relationships, and pursuing meaningful or personal development goals. The authors concluded that it is possible to teach positive affect interventions while avoiding unconditional cheerfulness or dismissing negative affect that can help bring attention to needed self-care (Saslow et al., 2014).

A systematic review of 50 randomized controlled trials published between 1998 and August 2018 found evidence for the efficacy of multi-component positive psychology interventions (MPPIs) in improving subjective well-being, depression, psychological well-being, anxiety and stress. However, the limited number of studies on anxiety and stress precluded definitive conclusions and further studies were recommended for diverse populations (Hendriks et al., 2020). Hence, research has uncovered that stress plays a role in unhealthy behaviors which underlie the conditions treated by lifestyle medicine. Research also suggests that PPIs have the potential to help counter the stress reactions related to adverse experiences and medical conditions. However, much more research is needed to sort out which PPIs are effective in diverse populations and circumstances.

Social connection

Multiple robust cohort studies have confirmed that social isolation has been associated with greater morbidity, including increased depression, and mortality.

Empirical evidence of the inverse is also strong. Social connection is associated with healthy body mass index, control of blood sugars, improved cancer survival, decreased cardiovascular mortality, decreased depressive symptoms, mitigated posttraumatic stress disorder symptoms, improved overall mental health and physical health, and greater happiness and longevity (Martino et al., 2017).

In a meta-analytic review social isolation, loneliness, and living alone corresponded to a 29%, 26% and 32% increased likelihood of mortality, respectively, with no differences between measures of objective and subjective social isolation. Results remained consistent across gender, length of follow-up, and world region (Holt-Lunstad et al., 2015). The inverse association of social connection with health and longevity was indicated in another meta-analytic review of 148 studies (308,849 participants) in which participants with stronger social relationships had a 50% increased likelihood of survival, with consistency across age, sex, initial health status, cause of death and follow-up period (Holt-Lunstad et al., 2010).

One of the best-known and longest cohort studies of factors contributing to well-being is the Harvard Adult Development Study. Over more than eight decades of follow-up and still ongoing, the study has collected data on a variety of potential well-being contributors from self-report, health records and direct assessments. Hence, they were able to control for a wide spectrum of cofounders and isolate that the single most important factor in health, well-being, happiness and longevity is social connection (Valliant, 2002).

A key mechanism of action for these social connection well-being effects that researchers have posited is increases in vagal tone. In an "upward spiral," autonomic flexibility – represented by vagal tone – facilitates social and emotional opportunities, which lead to higher connection. Studies have shown that those with initially higher vagal tone levels increased their connectedness and positive emotions more rapidly than others on follow-up. Also, increases in connectedness and positive emotions predicted increases in vagal tone, independent of the initial level. Hence, social connection and psychosocial well-being reciprocally and prospectively predict one another (Kok & Fredrickson, 2010; Kok & Fredrickson, 2016).

Activities that promote these links between good relationships and health have been identified as positive interpersonal processes, such as having fun together, sharing laughs, doing kind things for one another and expressing gratitude (Algoe, 2019). Interactions with acquaintances or even strangers have been shown to contribute to well-being in addition to strong ties with family and friends. In a study by Sandstrom and Dunn (2014), on the days students interacted with more classmates than usual, they reported greater happiness and feelings of belonging. In subsequent studies of daily interactions, the researchers also found that weak ties are related to poor emotional well-being.

In recognition of these striking empirical findings, a proactive healthy lifestyle needs to intentionally increase positive social interactions. Lifestyle medicine and other practitioners can counsel on increasing social connections, prescribe greater connections, and assess the quantity and quality of social interactions to help patients improve their health and promote longevity and health and well-being (Martino et al., 2016).

Health and medical applications

The theoretical underpinnings of mechanisms of action and empirical findings to date on the role of positive psychology in health and specifically the life-style medicine pillars deserves attention by health practitioners for application in healthcare, as well as self-care. Although further research is needed to delineate effective practices and impact in healthcare settings and for diverse populations, a proactive and comprehensive healthy lifestyle approach should implement these positive psychology mindsets and activities. This approach appears to be especially relevant for lifestyle medicine due to the link with the six pillars of the field.

Moreover, conditions commonly treated in lifestyle medicine, especially cardiovascular disease, have shown up prominently in the positive psychology literature. With some of the most robust studies showing the link between positive psychology constructs and cardiovascular disease, PPIs and mindfulness programs should be included in health maintenance and cardiovascular disease treatment plans (Kubzansky et al., 2018).

In addition to the role of positive emotions in the six pillars and its powerful force to drive health behavior change – the key to successful lifestyle treatment, positive activities, such as expressing gratitude and practicing generosity, may serve as independent protective health factors. Positive activities promote well-being by boosting positive emotions, positive thoughts, positive behaviors and need satisfaction (Lyubomirsky & Layous, 2013), as well as having physiological effects (Kok et al., 2013). Intentional positive activities can lead to these effects and be taught in self-care, health education programs, and can instill in youth positive patterns of emotions, thoughts and behaviors that may serve them over their lifetimes. Certain positive activities might be particularly well suited to certain individuals and to specific risk factors. This research is evolving. In the meantime, a practical approach is self-selection of activities, such as gratitude practice, acts of kindness, mindfulness and savoring, by individuals based on their culture, interests, personality, and more (Layous et al., 2013).

Positive psychology constructs can be incorporated in most elements of a clinical practice including assessment, interactions during clinical encounters, health coaching, health maintenance and treatment prescriptions, and referrals to behavioral health, community and digital resources. Medical practices routinely screen for and monitor negative emotions, depression, anxiety and stress. They can include brief positive psychology assessments, such as the satisfaction with life scale. They can also assess and monitor frequency of positive activities, starting the dialogue with patients about their readiness to engage in the activities. For the interested patients, activities can be prescribed as with any other lifestyle interventions.

Lifestyle medicine and most effective clinical practices rely on the broader health team. Hence, after the primary provider makes the recommendation or prescription, the nurses, health coaches, and others can work with the patients to develop specific action plans. The clinical encounter itself and interactions between patients, providers and health team members can serve as role models for positive interactions that boost the parasympathetic nervous system and broaden and build problem solving. The patients will have a positive experience and recall positive emotions that can nudge their adherence to the treatment recommendations. Last, but not least, growing credible resources, community programs and apps can support patients with these treatment and self-care plans (Lianov, 2019).

Conclusion

In this chapter, the empirical evidence for the link of positive psychology to each of the six pillars of lifestyle medicine, as well as health behavior changes were covered. In addition, recommendations were made for applications in self-care and healthcare. Future research will further develop the evidence and best practices for positive psychology in medicine.

The overarching conclusion is that the application of positive psychology to physical health and in lifestyle medicine and healthcare is promising. A short-term goal is to harness the field's research-informed approaches, activities and interventions based on the individual's interests, while the work to build the evidence base within healthcare continues (Park et al., 2016; Pressman et al., 2019). Medical practitioners and positive psychologists can advance the integration of positive psychology into medicine and healthcare by collaborating on translational research, disseminating research-informed educational and training programs and developing practical clinical applications.

Takeaways

General

- Not surprisingly, this chapter which reviews the role of positive psychology in lifestyle medicine and beyond, reinforces key take-aways in Chapter 2 which describes lifestyle medicine breakthroughs, including the application of positive psychology approaches.
- Positive affect has a reinforcing, reciprocal link with healthy behaviors, which are essential to the successful implementation of lifestyle medicine.
- Positive psychology constructs can be integrated into health coaching techniques for more effective behavior change, as well as increasing nonconscious motivation for healthy behaviors.
- PPIs, not only have a role in behavior change, but also represent an independent pillar of lifestyle medicine, by serving as additional protective factors for physical health.
- Practical positive psychology approaches can be implemented into lifestyle medicine practice, as well as healthcare more broadly.
- The combination of the best of lifestyle medicine and positive psychology science can lead to positive health, a state of well-being, beyond what can be achieved by solely addressing traditional risk factors.

Practical

- Healthy lifestyles, including healthy eating, physical activity, sleep, avoiding or managing risky substance use, managing stress, and promoting social connection can be reinforced with positive emotions, mindsets and experiences associated with the desired behaviors. Health behavior change counselling can be enhanced with positive psychology approaches. These approaches can be interwoven with traditional counselling techniques, such as motivational interviewing, including positive visioning and linking the behaviors with PERMA elements.
- Activities that boost positive affect – referred to as positive activities or PPIs – lead to physiologic benefits and can be prescribed as part of health maintenance and treatment plans.
- Positive psychology approaches can be incorporated into major elements of healthcare, including emotional well-being assessments, positive clinical encounters, coaching with positive psychology techniques, and PPI prescriptions.

Wicked questions

1 How can PPIs be incorporated into healthy lifestyles and the clinical flow of medical practice to ensure high levels of use and engagement?
2 What specific elements of self-care and healthcare can harness the power of positive psychology most effectively and efficiently and serve as role models for implementation?
3 In what ways can early adopters of positive psychology in medicine and other stakeholders serve as champions for transforming healthcare that emphasizes positive health?
4 What translational research questions, when answered, will garner greatest interest and credibility to the role of positive psychology in healthcare?

References

Ait-Hadad, W., Bénard, M., Shankland, R., Kesse-Guyot, E., Robert, M., Touvier, M., Hercberg, S., Buscail, C., & Péneau, S. (2020). Optimism is associated with diet quality, food group consumption and snacking behavior in a general population. *Nutr. J.*, 19(1):6.

Algoe, S.B. (2019). Positive interpersonal processes. *Curr. Dir. Psychol. Sci.*, 28(2):183–188.

Babyak, M., Blumenthal, J.A., Herman, S., Khatri, P., Doraiswamy, M., Moore, K., Craighead, W.E., Baldewicz, T.T., & Krishnan, K.R. (2000). Exercise treatment for major depression: Maintenance of therapeutic benefit at 10 months. *Psychosom. Med.*, 62:633–638.

Blanchflower, D., Oswald, A., & Stewart-Brown, S. (2013). Is psychological wellbeing linked to the consumption of fruit and vegetables? *Soc. Indic. Res.*, 114:785–801.

Blumenthal, J.A., Babyak, M.A., Doraiswamy, P.M., Watkins, L., Hoffman, B.M., Barbour, K.A., Herman, S., Craighead, E., Brosse, A.L., Waugh, R., Hinderliter, A., & Sherwood, A. (2007). Exercise and pharmacotherapy in the treatment of major depressive disorder. *Psychosom. Med.*, 69(7):587–596.

Boecker, H., Sprenger, T., Spilker, M.E., Henriksen, G., Koppenhoefer, M., Wagner, K.J., Valet, M., Berthele, A., & Tolle, T.R. (2008). The runner's high: Opioidergic mechanisms in the human brain. *Cereb. Cortex.*, 18(11):2523–2531.

Boehm, J.K., Chen, Y., Koga, H., Mathur, M.B., Vie, L.L., & Kubzansky, L.D. (2018). Is optimism associated with healthier cardiovascular-related behavior? Meta-analyses of 3 health behaviors. *Circ. Res.*, 122(8):1119–1134.

Bongers, P., Jansen, A., Houben, K., & Roefs, A. (2013). Happy eating: The single target implicit association test predicts overeating after positive emotions. *Eat Behav.*, 4(3):348–355.

Cardi, V., Leppanen, J., & Treasure, J. (2015). The effects of negative and positive mood induction on eating behaviour: A meta-analysis of laboratory studies in the healthy population and eating and weight disorders. Neurosci. Biobehav. Rev., 57:299–309.

Carrillo, A., Feig, E.H., Harnedy, L.E., Huffman, J.C., Park, E.R., Thorndike, A.N., Kim, S., & Millstein, R.A. (2022). The role of positive psychological constructs in diet and eating behavior among people with metabolic syndrome: A qualitative study. Health Psychol. Open., 9(1): 20551029211055264.

Cooney, G.M., Dwan, K., Greig, C.A., Lawlor, D.A., Rimer, J., Waugh, F.R., McMurdo, M., & Mead, G.E. (2013). Exercise for depression, *Cochrane Database Syst. Rev.*, 9: CD004366..

Crookes, A.E. (2018). Perspectives: Positive psychology and the field of addiction - A proposal for a culturally relevant framework. *Middle East J. Posit. Psychol.*, 4(1), 29–49.

Dinges, D.F., Pack, F., Williams, K., Gillen, K.A., Powell, J.W., Ott, G.E., Aptowicz, C., & Pack, A.I. (1997). Cumulative sleepiness, mood disturbance, and psychomotor vigilance performance decrements during a week of sleep restricted to 4–5 hours per night. *Sleep.*, 20(4):267–277.

Ernst, C., Olson, A.K., Pinel, J.P., Lam, R.W., & Christie, B.R. (2006). Antidepressant effects of exercise: Evidence for an adult-neurogenesis hypothesis? *J. Psychiat. Neurosci.*, 31(2):83–92.

Evers, C., Denise, M.A., de RidderJessie, T.D., & de Witt Huberts, C. (2013). Good mood food. Positive emotion as a neglected trigger for food intake. *Appetite* 68(1):1–7.

Evers, C., Dingemans A., Junghans A.F., & Boevé. (2018). Feeling bad or feeling dood, does emotion affect your consumption of food? A meta-analysis of the experimental evidence. *Neuroscience & Behavioral Reviews.* 92:195-208.

Fararouei, M., Brown, I.J., Akbartabar, T.M., Haghighi, R.E., & Jafari, J. (2013). Happiness and health behavior in Iranian adolescent girls. *J. Adolesc.*, 36(6):1187–1192.

Feig, E.H., Harnedy, L.E., Golden, J., Thorndike, A.N., Huffman, J.C., & Psaros, C.A. (2022). Qualitative examination of emotional experiences during physical activity post-metabolic/bariatric surgery. *Obes. Surg.*, 32(3):660–670.

Fredrickson, B.L. (2004). The broaden-and-build theory of positive emotions. *Philos. Trans. R Soc. Lond B Biol. Sci.*, 359(1449):1367–1378.

Gardner, M.P., Wansink, B., Kim, J., & Park, S.B. (2014). Better moods for better eating? How mood influences food choice. *J. Consum. Psychol.*, 24(3):320–335.

Hansen, C.J., Stevens, L.C., & Coast, R. (2001). Exercise duration and mood state: How much is enough to feel better? *Health Psychol.*, 20(4):267–275.

Hendriks, T., Schotanus-Dijkstra, M., Hassankhan, A., de Jong, J., & Bohlmeijer, E. (2020). The efficacy of multi-component positive psychology interventions: A systematic review and meta-analysis of randomized controlled trials. *J. Happiness Stud.*, 21(1):357–390.

Hingle, M.D., Wertheim, B.C., Tindle, H.A., Tinker, L., Seguin, R.A., Rosal, M.C., & Thomson, C.A. (2014). Optimism and diet quality in the women's health initiative. *J. Acad. Nutr. Diet.*, 114(7):1036–1045.

Holt-Lunstad, J., Smith, T.B., Baker, M., Harris, T., & Stephenson, D. (2015). Loneliness and social isolation as risk factors for mortality: A meta-analytic review. *Perspect. Psychol. Sci.*, 10(2):227–237.

Holt-Lunstad, J., Smith, T.B., & Layton, J.B. (2010). Social relationships and mortality risk: A meta-analytic review. *PLOS Medicine*, 7(7):e1000316..

Huffman, J. C., Millstein, R. A., Mastromauro, C.A., Moore, S.V., Celano, C.M., Bedova, C. A.,Suarez, L., Boehm, J.K., & Januzzi, J.L (2916). Patients with an acute coronary syndrome: Treatment development and proof-of-concept trial. *J Happiness Stud.*, 17(5):1985–2006.

Huffman, J.C., Golden, J., Massey, C.N., Feig, E.H., Chung, W.J., Millstein, R.A., Brown, L., Gianangelo, T., Healy, B.C., Wexler, D.J., Park, E.R., & Celano, C.M., (2021). A positive psychology-motivational interviewing program to promote physical activity in type 2 diabetes: The BEHOLD-16 randomized trial. *Gen. Hosp. Psychiatry*, 68:65–73.

Kansky, J., & Diener, E. (2017). Benefits of well-being: Health, social relationships, work and resilience. *J. Posit. Psychol. Well-being*, 1(2):129–169.

Kelloniemi, H., Ek, E., & Laitinen, J. (2005). Optimism, dietary habits, body mass index and smoking among young Finnish adults. *Appetite*, 45(2):169–176.

Kok, B.E., Coffeey, K.A., Cohn, M.A., Catalino, L.I., Vacharkulksemsuk, T., Algoe, S.B., Brantley, M., & Fredrickson, B.L. (2013). How positive emotions build physical health: Perceived positive social connections account for the upward spiral between positive emotions and vagal tone. *Psychol. Sci.*, 24:1123–1132.

Kok, B.E., & Fredrickson, B.L. (2010). Upward spirals of the heart: Autonomic flexibility, as indexed by vagal tone, reciprocally and prospectively predicts positive emotions and social connectedness. *Biol. Psychol.*, 85:432–436.

Kok, B.E., & Fredrickson, B.L. (2016). Corrigendum to "Upward spirals of the heart: Autonomic flexibility, as indexed by vagal tone, reciprocally and prospectively predicts positive emotions and social connectedness" [*Biol. Psychol.*, 85(3) (2010) 432–436]. *Biol. Psychol.*, 117:240.

Krentzman, A.R. (2013). Review of the application of positive psychology to substance use, addiction, and recovery research. *Psychol. Addict. Behav.*, 27(1), 151–165.

Kubzansky, L.D., Huffman, J.C., Boehm, J.K., Hernandez, R., Kim, E.S., Koga, H.K., Feig, E.H., Lloyd-Jones, D.M., Seligman, M.E.P., & Labarthe, D.R. (2018). Positive psychological well-being and cardiovascular disease. JACC health promotion series. *J. Am. Coll. Cardiol.*, 72(12), 1382–1396.

Lathia, N., Sandstrom, G.M., Mascolo, C., & Rentfrow, P.J. (2017). Happier people live more active lives: Using smartphones to link happiness and physical activity. *PloS One.*, 12(1):e0160589.

Layous, K., Chancellor, J., & Lyubomirsky, S. (2013). Positive activities as protective factors against mental health conditions. *J. Abnorm. Psychol.*, 123:2–12.

Lianov, L. (Ed.). (2019). *Roots of Positive Change, Optimizing Healthcare with Positive Psychology*. Chesterfield, MO: American College of Lifetsyle Medicine.

Lollies, F., Schnatschmidt, M., Bihlmeier, I., Genuneit, J., In-Albnon, T., Holtmann, M., Legenbauer, T., & Schlarb, A.A., (2022). Associations of sleep and emotion regulation processes in childhood and adolescence - A systematic review, report of methodological challenges and future directions. *Sleep Sci.*, 15(4):490–514.

Lyubomirsky, S., & Layous, K. (2013). How do simple positive activities increase well-being? *Curr. Dir. Psychol. Sci.*, 22(1):57–62.

Mammen, G., & Faulkner, G. (2013). Physical activity and the prevention of depression: A systematic review of prospective studies. *Am. J. Prev. Med.*, 45(5):649–657.

Martino, J., Pegg, J., & Frates, E.P. (2017). The connection prescription: Using the power of social interactions and the deep desire for connectedness to empower health and wellness. *Am. J. Lifestyle Med.*, 11(6):466–475.

McHugh, R.K., & Weiss, R.D. (2019). Alcohol use disorder and depressive disorders. *Alcohol Res.*, 40(1):arcr.v40.1.01.

McKercher, C., Sanderson, K., Schmidt, M.D., Otahal, P., Patton, G.C., Dwyer, T., & Venn, A.J. (2014). Physical activity patterns and risk of depression in young adulthood: A 20-year cohort study since childhood. *Soc. Psychiatry Psychiatr. Epidemiol.*, 49(11):1823–1834.

Moskowitz, J.T., Hult, J.R., Duncan, L.G., Cohn, M.A., Maurer, S., Bussolari, C., & Acree, M. (2012). A positive affect intervention for people experiencing health-related stress: Development and non-randomized pilot test. *J. Health Psychol.*, 17(5):676–692.

Mujcic, R., & Oswald, A.J. (2016). Evolution of well-being and happiness after increases in consumption of fruit and vegetables. *Am. J. Public Health.*, 106(8):1504–1510.

Neckelmann, D., Mykletun, A., & Dahl, A.A. (2007). Chronic insomnia as a risk factor for developing anxiety and depression. *Sleep*, 30(7):873–880.

Ong, A.D., Kim, S., Young, S., & Steptoe, A. (2017). Positive affect and sleep: A systematic review. *Sleep Med. Rev.*, 35:21–32.

Pänkäläinen, M., Fogelholm, M., Valve, R., Kampman, O., Kauppi, M., Lappalainen, E., & Hintikka, J. (2018). Pessimism, diet, and the ability to improve dietary habits: A three-year follow-up study among middle-aged and older Finnish men and women. *Nutr. J.*, 17(1):92.

Park, N., Peterson, C., Szvarca, D., Vander Molen, R.J., Kim E.S. & Collon K. (2016). Positive Psychology and physical health. *Am. J. Lifestyle Med.*, 10(3):200–206.

Pressman, S., Jenkins, B.N., & Moskowitz, S.D. (2019). Positive affect and health: What do we know and where next should we go? *Ann. Rev. Psychol.*, 70:627–650.

Rhodes, R.E., & Kates, K.A. (2015). Can the affective response to exercise predict future motives and physical activity behavior? A systematic review of published evidence. *Ann. Behav. Med.*, 49(5):715–731.

Richards, J., Jiang, X., Kelly, P., Chau, J., Bauman, A., & Ding, D. (2015). Don't worry, be happy: Cross-sectional associations between physical activity and happiness in 15 European countries. *BMC Public Health*, 15:53.

Riemann, D., & Voderholzer, U. (2003). Primary insomnia: A risk factor to develop depression? *J. Affect. Disorders.*, 76(1–3):255–259.

Rimer, J., Dwan, K., Lawlor, D.A., Greig, C.A., McMurdo, M., Morely, W., & Mead, G.E. (2012). Exercise for depression. *Cochrane Db Syst. Rev.*, 11(7):CD004366.

Saksvik-Lehouillier, I., Saksvik, S.B., Dahlberg, J., Tanum, T.K., Ringen, H., Karlsen, H.R., Smedbøl, T., Sørengaard, T.A., Mailen Stople, M., Kallestad, H., & Olsen, A. (2020). Mild to moderate partial sleep deprivation is associated with increased impulsivity and decreased affect in young adults. *Sleep*, 43(10):zsaa078.

Sandstrom, G.M., & Dunn, E.W. (2014). Social interactions and well-being: The surprising power of weak ties. *Pers. Soc. Psychol. B.*, 40:910–922.

Saslow, L.R., Cohn, M., & Moskowitz, J.T. (2014). Positive affect interventions to reduce stress: Harnessing the benefit while avoiding the pollyanna. In J. Gruber & J.T. Moskowitz (Eds.). *Positive emotion: Integrating the light sides and dark sides*, p. 515–532. Oxford University Press.

Steptoe, A., O'Donnell, K., Marmot, M., & Wardle, J. (2008). Positive affect, psychological well-being, and good sleep. *J. Psychosom. Res.*, 64(4):409–415.

Valliant, G.E. (2002). *Aging well: Surprising guideposts to a happier life from the landmark Harvard study of adult development.* Boston, MA: Little, Brown.

Van Cappellen, P., Rice, E.L., Catalino, L.I., & Fredrickson, B.L. (2018). Positive affective processes underlie positive health behaviour change. *Psychol. Health.*, 33(1):77–97.

Velten, J., Lavalle, K.L., Scholten, S., Meyer, A.H., Zhang, K.C., Schneider, S., & Margraf, J. (2014). Lifestyle choices and mental health: A representative population survey. *BMC Psychol.*, 2:58.

Watson, N.F., Badr, M.S., Belenky, G., Bliwise, D.L., Buxton, O.M., Buysse, D., Dinges, D.F., Gangwisch, J., Gardner, M.A., Kushida, C., Malhotra, R.K., Martin, J.L., Patel, S.R., Quan, S.F., & Tasali, E. (2015). Recommended amount of sleep for a healthy adult: A joint consensus statement of the American Academy of Sleep Medicine and Sleep Research Society. *Sleep*, 38(6):843–844.

Whatnall, M.C., Patterson, A.J., Siew, Y.Y., Kay-Lambkin, F., & Hutchesson, M.J. (2019). Are psychological distress and resilience associated with dietary intake among Australian University students? *Int. J. Environ. Res. Public Health*,16(21):4099.

White, B.A., Horwath, C.C., & Conner, T.S. (2013). Many apples a day keep the blues away—Daily experiences of negative and positive affect and food consumption in young adults. *Brit. J. Health Psychl.*, 8(4):782–798.

Worley, S.L. (2018). The extraordinary importance of sleep. The detrimental effects of inadequate sleep on health and public safety drive an explosion of sleep research. *Pharmacy and Therapeutics*, 43(12): 758–763.

Yoo, S.S., Gujar, N., Hu, P., Jolesz, F.A., & Walker, M.P. (2007). The human emotional brain without sleep—A prefrontal amygdala disconnect. *Curr. Biol.*, 17(20):877–878.

INDEX

Note: **Bold** page numbers refer to tables and *Italic* page numbers refer to figures.

For Product Safety Concerns and Information please contact our EU
representative GPSR@taylorandfrancis.com
Taylor & Francis Verlag GmbH, Kaufingerstraße 24, 80331 München, Germany